FRENCH MEDICAL CULTURE
IN THE NINETEENTH CENTURY

THE WELLCOME INSTITUTE SERIES
IN THE HISTORY OF MEDICINE

Already Published

Doctors, Politics and Society: Historical Essays
Edited by Dorothy Porter and Roy Porter

Doctors, and Ethics:
The Earlier Historical Setting of Professional Ethics
Edited by Andrew Wear, Johanna Geyer-Kordesch and Roger French

Forthcoming Titles

The History of Health and the Modern State
Edited by Dorothy Porter

The History of Medical Education in Britain
Edited by V. Nutton and Roy Porter

Medicine in the Enlightenment
Edited by Roy Porter

Academic inquiries regarding the series should be addressed to
the editors W. F. Bynum and Roy Porter at the
Wellcome Institute for the History of Medicine,
183 Euston Road, London NW1 2BE, UK

FRENCH MEDICAL CULTURE
IN THE NINETEENTH CENTURY

Edited by
Ann La Berge and Mordechai Feingold

Amsterdam – Atlanta GA 1994

First published in 1994
by Editions Rodopi B. V., Amsterdam – Atlanta, G A 1994.

© 1994 A. La Berge and M. Feingold

Design and Typesetting by Christine Lavery, the Wellcome Trust
Printed and bound in the Netherlands by Editions Rodopi B. V.,
Amsterdam – Atlanta, G A 1994.

British Library Cataloguing in Publication Data
A catalogue record for this book is available from the British Library
ISBN 90-5183-561-2 (BOUND)

CIP-Gegevens Koninklijke Bibliotheek, Den Haag

French
French Medical Culture in the Nineteenth Century / ed. by
Ann La Berge and Mordechai Feingold.
Amsterdam – Atlanta G A 1994: Rodopi. – Ill.
(Clio Medica 25 / The Wellcome Institute Series
in the History of Medicine)
Met index, lit. opg.
ISBN 90-5183-561-2 (BOUND)
Trefw.: geneeskunde; Frankrïjk,
geschiedenis; 19e eeuw.

© Editions Rodopi B. V. Amsterdam – Atlanta GA 1994
Printed in the Netherlands

Contents

Acknowledgements

We would like to thank the College of Arts and Sciences and the Center for the Study of Science in Society at Virginia Polytechnic Institute and State University for generously funding the conference at Blacksburg that gave rise to this book.

We would also like to thank Bill Bynum of the Wellcome Institute for helping us prepare the text for publication, Sally Bragg of the Wellcome Institute for expediting our task and Dr Kim Cross and her colleague Christine Lavery at The Wellcome Trust for their technical skill and expertise in getting this work to press.

Notes on Contributors

Laurence Brockliss was born in 1950 and educated at Cambridge University. For ten years he taught history at the University of Hull, until he moved to Oxford in 1984 and became a Fellow and Tutor in Modern History at Magdalen College. For twenty years he has worked on the history of education, science and medicine in early-modern France and has published widely in the field. From 1985 to 1992 he was also editor of the annual publication *History of Universities*. His most important work to date is *French Higher Education in the Seventeenth and Eighteenth Centuries: A Cultural History* (Oxford: Oxford University Press, 1987). At present he is completing a social and cultural history of French medicine in the early-modern period, which he is writing with Professor Colin Jones of Exeter University. The essay in this present collection reflects his interest in using hitherto unknown archival material to recover the reality of medical practice. His address is Magdalen College, Oxford OX1 4AU, UK.

Jacalyn Duffin is the Hannah Professor of the History of Medicine at Queen's University, Kingston, Canada. A historian and practising hematologist, her research interests include concepts of disease, especially in nineteenth-century French and Canadian medicine. Her computer-assisted analysis of a Canadian practice, *Langstaff: A Nineteenth-Century Medical Life*, was published by the University of Toronto Press in 1993. She is now working on an intellectual biography of René Laennec. Her address is History of Medicine, Old Medical Building, Queen's University, Kingston, Ontario K7L 3N6, Canada.

Mordechai Feingold is Associate Professor of Science and Technology Studies at Virginia Polytechnic Institute and State University. A historian of science, he is currently working on a history of the Royal Society and the diffusion of Newtonianism. His address is Center for the Study of Science in Society, Price House, Virginia Polytechnic Institute and State University, Blacksburg, Virginia 24061, USA.

Toby Gelfand is Hannah Professor of the History of Medicine at the University of Ottawa, where he holds a joint appointment in the medical faculty and the department of history. His current research deals with Charcot's Salpêtrière school. He is collaborating on a new biography of Charcot, and is co-editor of *Freud and the History of Psychoanalysis* (Analytic Press, 1992). He has taught at the universities of Minnesota and Princeton. His publications focusing on the history of French medicine include *Professionalizing Modern Medicine: Paris Surgeons and Medical Science and Institutions in the Eighteenth Century* (Greenwood Press, 1980). His address is Faculty of Medicine, University of Ottawa, 451 Smyth, Ottawa, Ontario, Canada K1H 8M5.

Jan Goldstein is professor of modern European history at the University of Chicago and author of *Console and Classify: The French Psychiatric Profession in the Nineteenth Century* (New York: Cambridge University Press, 1987, 1990), which received the Herbert Baxter Adams Prize of the American Historical Association. She is editor of, and a contributor to, a collection of essays, *Foucault and the Writing of History*, to be published by Blackwell's. She is currently working on a book that examines competing theories of psychology and the politics of selfhood in France during the half-century following the Revolution. Her address is Department of History, 1126 East 59th St., University of Chicago, Chicago, IL 60637, USA.

Caroline Hannaway is currently Historical Consultant to the National Institutes of Health History Office, Bethesda, Maryland. She is editing books on the Paris Clinical School of the nineteenth century (with Ann La Berge) and on the history of tropical and colonial medicine. Her address for correspondence is 316 Suffolk Rd., Baltimore, MD 21218, USA.

Joy Harvey is an Associate Editor on the Darwin Project at Cambridge University. She has taught History of Science and Science and Society, most recently at Virginia Polytechnic Institute and State University. Her publications have focused on French Darwinism, nineteenth-century anthropology and medicine, and women in science and medicine. She is currently finishing a book on Clémence Royer, Darwin's French translator and is preparing a series of essays on Dr Mary Putnam Jacobi. Her address is Darwin Letters Project, Manuscript Room, Cambridge University Library, Cambridge CB3 9DR, UK.

Martha L. Hildreth is Associate Professor of History at the University of Nevada, Reno and adjunct professor at the University of Nevada School of Medicine. She is the author of a wide range of articles on the history of medicine and public health in late nineteenth and early twentieth-century France. Most recently she has written on the topic of influenza etiology, prevention and therapy. She is the author of a book, *Doctors, Bureaucrats and Public Health in France, 1888–1902* (New York: Garland, 1987) and is currently working on the incorporation of germ theory and heredity into medical thought and practice in the early twentieth century. Her address is: Department of History, University of Nevada, Reno, NV 89557, USA.

Ann La Berge is Assistant Professor of Humanities and Science and Technology Studies at Virginia Polytechnic Institute and State University. She is the author of *Mission and Method: The Early Nineteenth-Century French Public Health Movement* (New York: Cambridge University Press, 1992) and has written on *puériculture* and the medicalization of child care in France. She is currently editing (with Caroline Hannaway) a work on the Paris Clinical School of the nineteenth century and is working on the history of medical microscopy and medical statistics in nineteenth-century France. Her address is Center for the Study of Science in Society, Price House, Virginia Tech, Blacksburg, VA 24061, USA.

Anne Marie Moulin is director of research at the National Centre for Scientific Research (CNRS) in Paris and associate professor at the Medical School of Geneva. She was trained both as a philosopher and a physician. As a parasitologist she worked in Central Africa and in the Arab world. Her main work is on the history of immunology, *Le dèrnier langage de la médecine. L'immunologie de Pasteur au SIDA* (Paris: Presses universitaires de France, 1991). She has co-edited a volume *Science and Empires* for the Boston Studies in Philosophy of Science (Boston: Kluwer, 1991). She is currently writing a book on the history of the Pasteur Institute and has recently contributed a paper called 'Death and Resurrection of Immunology at the Pasteur Institute (1917–1940)' for the book *Immunology: Pasteur's Inheritance*, (ed.) Wiley Eastern, P. A. Cazenave, and P. Talwer (New Delhi, 1991). Her address is Inserm U 158, Hôpital des Enfants-Malades, Pavillon Archambault, 149, rue de Sèvres, Paris 75015, France.

Matthew Ramsey is Associate Professor of History at Vanderbilt University. He is the author of articles on the social history of medicine in the eighteenth and nineteenth centuries and of *Professional and Popular Medicine in France, 1770–1830: The Social World of Medical Practice* (New York: Cambridge University Press, 1988). He is now completing a companion volume on the development of professional monopoly in French medicine. His address is Department of History, Vanderbilt University, Nashville, TN 37235, USA.

George Weisz is Professor of the History of Medicine at McGill University. He received his Ph.D. in History from the State University of New York at Stony Brook and his Doctorat de 3e Cycle in Sociology from the University of Paris. His books include: *The Organization of Science and Technology in France, 1803–1914,* (ed.) with Robert Fox (New York: Cambridge University Press, 1980); *The Emergence of Modern Universities in France, 1863–1914* (Princeton: Princeton University Press, 1983); *Social Science Perspectives on Medical Ethics* (Dordrecht and Boston: Kluwer, 1990); and the forthcoming *The Medical Mandarins: The French Academy of Medicine in the Nineteenth and Twentieth Centuries*. His address is Department of Social Studies of Medicine, 3655 Drummond St., Montreal, Quebec, H3G 1Y6, Canada.

Preface

This volume – a collaborative effort of established scholars in French history and the history of medicine – brings together the dominant themes of French medical culture in all its disparate strands viewed from several perspectives: inside the medical community itself; within the broader context of French society and culture; and the outsider's view. While a couple of recent collections have addressed particular aspects of French medical culture, such as the relationship of the professions – including medicine – to the French state and the Pasteurian revolution, no volume has attempted a multifaceted coverage.[1] Useful collections have also been published for sixteenth-, seventeenth-, and eighteenth-century medicine, but none of them has a French focus.[2] So far no collection has restricted itself to French medicine, addressing the principal themes of the French medical experience.

This collection serves an important professional role by defining a developing sub-specialty at the intersection of French cultural and intellectual history, the history of medicine and science, and the social history of medicine. Although it is becoming increasingly popular – and often most appropriate – to bridge national boundaries and look at topics like medicine from an international and comparative perspective, it is clear that there was something distinctive about the nineteenth-century French medical experience which influenced and reflected sociopolitical developments within French society. Not only was France the birthplace of modern scientific medicine, but France was different from other European countries demographically, politically, and socioeconomically. Indigenous problems and practices such as depopulation and wet nursing – just to cite two well-known examples – were sociomedical and required medical expertise for their investigation and solution. For these reasons the present volume, by exploring the singularity of the French model, will also serve as the basis for a future integrative and comparative approach.

The eleven essays in this volume illustrate the richness, complexity, and diversity of French medical culture in the nineteenth century, a period that witnessed the 'medicalization' of French society. Medical themes permeated contemporary culture and politics, and medical discourse infused many levels of French society from the bastions of science – the medical faculties and research institutions – to novels, the theatre, and the daily lives of citizens as patients.

We have not tried to impose uniformity of spelling and punctuation. Consequently, the reader will find British spelling and punctuation styles in some articles, American in others. We assume a cosmopolitan readership and trust that our readers will be familiar with both and not be troubled by these minor differences.

Notes

1. Gerald L. Geison, (ed.), *Professions and the French State, 1700–1900* (Philadelphia: University of Pennsylvania Press, 1984). This volume includes articles on French medicine by Toby Gelfand, Jan Goldstein, and Matthew Ramsey. On the Pasteurian revolution, see Claire Salomon-Bayet, (ed.), *Pasteur et la révolution pastorienne* (Paris: Payot, 1986).

2. For example, see Andrew Wear, R. K. French, and I. M. Lonie, (eds), *The Medical Renaissance of the Sixteenth Century* (New York: Cambridge University Press, 1985); Roger French and Andrew Wear, (eds), *The Medical Revolution of the Seventeenth Century* (New York: Cambridge University Press, 1989); Andrew Cunningham and Roger French, (eds), *The Medical Enlightenment of the Eighteenth Century* (New York: Cambridge University Press, 1990).

Introduction

Ann La Berge and Mordechai Feingold

Medical themes and medical discourse permeated nineteenth-century French society, culture, and politics – from the conception of the city as a pathogenic organism in the first half of the century to the predilection to advance medical explanations for France's decline following its defeat in the Franco-Prussian War. Medical ideas coloured popular perceptions, shaped public policies and informed literature, theatre, and art. One visible manifestation of this 'medicalization' of French society was the transforming of many physicians into political agents and arbiters of national values.[1]

After 1830, physicians and other social observers increasingly referred to Paris as a diseased city whose 'dangerous classes' were seen as a threat to social order and political stability.[2] Such observers believed that the lower classes, carriers of civic contamination, had to be 'civilized', which came increasingly to mean medicalized or hygienized. The aim of such cleansing measures was the 'embourgeoisement', of the lower classes, to 'make them like us'. The mode of implementation was public health and private hygiene. Consequently, hygienism, or the ideology of public health, emerged as the secular religion of the Third Republic. Legislators, social critics, reformers, and physicians all offered medical reasons to rationalize the defeat in the Franco-Prussian War, to account for French depopulation, and to explain the perceived moral and physical degeneracy of the French people. This widespread tendency to view France as fundamentally disease-ridden prompted the new Republic to look to physicians to solve those socio-medical afflictions believed to be at the root of military, economic, and moral weakness. Consequently, alcoholism, tuberculosis, venereal disease, and high infant mortality – were all cited as causes of degeneracy and depopulation – dominated public discourse and stood high on the national agenda of matters on which action was needed.[3]

Such thoroughgoing medicalization can be partly attributed to the prestige that Paris medicine enjoyed in the first half of the century. The capital was an international centre for medical study and a major exporter of clinical and public health ideas and practices. Numerous centralized hospitals served as training centres for medical students and physicians at all levels, who passed from hospital to hospital as they studied patients and diseases in the Paris free clinics. Students returning to England, Scotland, and the United States took with them their experiences in the dissection rooms and clinics of Paris as well as the exposure to (and some training in) such new technologies as medical statistics and microscopy.[4] For example, John Hughes Bennett, having studied microscopy with Alfred Donné in Paris, returned to Edinburgh to become an eminent teacher and champion of medical microscopy. In the domain of public health, the French influence on Britain's William Farr and Edwin Chadwick in vital statistics has recently been demonstrated. (French influence on Britain, however, was not one-way, for French physicians borrowed much from British colleagues as well.)[5] By 1900 the establishment of Pasteur Institutes in some of the French colonies and in the United States ensured the rapid dissemination of the ideas and practices of the Pasteurians. And in the domain of psychiatry and pediatrics Paris initiated the spread of innovative views and techniques.

French medical culture reflected dominant themes of contemporary society and politics. The dialectic which ran throughout the century between liberalism and socialism – both legacies of the French Revolution – appeared in medical terms as tension between liberal medicine (private practice) and social, bureaucratic medicine. It was evident in the unease between the right to public health on the one hand and private property on the other. French medical culture also reflected the old strain between Paris and the provinces, between the efforts of the Parisian government to impose centralization and bureaucracy on the provinces and regional efforts to preserve cultural diversity in local customs and institutions. Both patients and medical practitioners in the provinces sensed a fundamental tension between their individual rights and the capital's bid for cultural and political dominance. Attempts to promote public health reform show the extent of the conflict between Paris and the provinces, the 'princes of medicine' – the élite of Parisian public health – made hygienism the cornerstone of their programme. In the name of national security and social order, they sought to impose their views and practices on the country at large. The provinces resisted. To them such a policy was yet another attempt by power-hungry Parisian physicians to control the provinces by the imposition of centralized order, which, they believed, would intrude into the domain of the family and private life and deprive physicians and families of individual liberties.[6]

A pervasive ideology of science also characterized French society. In medicine this appeared as an attempt by some physicians to transform medicine into medical science by incorporating the accessory sciences such as medical chemistry and microscopy and developing a medicine grounded in the laboratory as well as the clinic. The dichotomy between a scientific/laboratory approach and a clinical orientation existed in French medicine until after the Second World War. Likewise, physicians sought to apply scientific principles and practices to public health to transform public hygiene into a scientific discipline. Scientific hygiene emerged in full-blown form after 1875 as hygienism. The dominance of scientism was exemplified late in the century by attempts of intellectuals to develop a biomedical discourse on topics such as race as well.

Medical discourse infused all areas of French society from the bastions of science – the academies and research institutions – to newspapers, novels and the theatre, to the daily lives of citizens as patients. Learned medical discourse was initiated and carried out in the Academy of Medicine, the most prestigious and influential institution of the French medical establishment. The Academy provided the most important forum for the discussion of medical and public health issues. The discussions themselves illustrate the function of scientific debate and the role rhetoric played in framing it.[7]

Lengthy debates in the Academy of Medicine, such as that of 1837 over the introduction of statistics into medicine and of 1854–5 over the utility of the microscope for pathology and clinical medicine turned academic medicine into a spectacle. Writing in 1855, Paul Broca called these debates 'great scientific tournaments'.[8] Within the Academy issues were raised and debated but rarely resolved. Indeed, resolution was not the main purpose of academic debate. Far more important was the viability of a forum to exchange information and discuss ideas. Equally crucial was the medium the Academy offered for the dissemination of ideas discussed internally by the medical elite to the scientific community at large. When Paul Broca chronicled for the *Moniteur des hôpitaux* the debate on the microscope, he maintained that to expect a pragmatic result from an academic debate would be to misunderstand its function. The purpose of such debates was not to change the opinions of the participants, but rather to articulate the state of knowledge at any given time on key issues. Moreover, such debates publicized the results of scientific research and allowed the public to form an opinion on issues hitherto confined to a small circle of investigators.

3

Academic debates, Broca held, also functioned as archives, marking the successive stages of scientific progress for future historians.[9]

In addition to serving as a forum for the élite of French medicine, the Academy also functioned as the public health advisory board to the national government. Permanent commissions were established to gather information as well as to advise on and manage epidemics, vaccination, mineral water and secret remedies. Matthew Ramsey shows how the mandarins of French medicine confronted popular culture over the issue of secret remedies. The crusade to control secret remedies had originated in the Royal Society of Medicine in the 1780s and, once the Society was resuscitated as the Academy in 1820, the institution took up the problem again. Members of the Academy claimed that in the name of public health the state had the right and the duty to pronounce on the efficacy, novelty, and safety of such remedies. For their part, the people maintained their right to choose their own therapies. The ensuing debate underscores the dialectic between the claims of public health *vis-à-vis* that of private property and individual rights.[10]

The problem of secret remedies is explored by Ramsey's discussion of a purgative known as the remedy Leroy (which had been recognized as dangerous following several deaths) and of the widely used anti-syphilitic, the *rob Laffecteur*. Widespread use of the remedy Leroy illustrated the popular demand for strong medicine – interventionist remedies that produced visible results, such as purging and puking. In 1823 the Academy, citing well-documented dangers to public health, recommended suppression of the remedy Leroy. This recommendation was endorsed by the Minister of the Interior in a circular sent to prefects asking them to ban its prescription except by pharmacists. Notwithstanding this effort, the remedy Leroy continued to generate a large volume of sales. The masses, accustomed to self-medication and disinterested in the public health programme of the national government, resisted medical and state intrusion. Nor did further attempts to ban the remedy lessen demand. Like many proprietary formulae, the Leroy – like opium in nineteenth-century England – was a 'people's remedy', firmly entrenched in popular culture. As with opium, it was not until superior alternative therapies became available that the efforts to eradicate drugs deeply rooted in popular culture succeeded.[11]

In the end, then, although the secret remedy commission analyzed many remedies – some 60 were investigated between 1825 and 1834 – the Academy failed in its efforts to ban dangerous remedies. The Academy itself had no regulatory power, functioning merely as an advisory agency. National public health policy was in the domain of the Minister of the Interior (a responsibility transferred after 1830 to the Minister of Commerce). Throughout the Restoration and the July Monarchy regulation was in the hands of a non-interventionist regime. In this, as in other areas of public health, the national government preferred to leave regulation of remedies in the hands of local authorities.[12]

The problem of secret remedies should be considered within the broader framework of the public health movement and the professionalization of medicine. The public health movement was statist and regulatory. The academic medical establishment promoted public health, even though its implementation was at odds with the liberal concern for property rights. Within this context the regulation of remedies was a desirable goal. Similarly, the move toward the professionalization of medicine made the need to regulate the dispensation of remedies desirable. First, since professionalization required the implementation of a new code of ethics – including standards of expertise and open communication – secret remedies were, by definition, antithetical to such reform. Second, the oversupply of physicians in Paris and some areas of France resulted in a professional strategy that sought to restrict practice to licensed physicians and eliminate charlatanism. In this way the glut of doctors could be eased, and members of the medical profession could corner the large market of popular and domestic medicine. Thus self-interest joined with the enlightened humanitarian ideology of public health in an effort to eradicate secret remedies and those practitioners that dispensed them.[13]

Ultimately the campaign against secret remedies could not have been successful before alternative and 'safe' therapies were made available. Popular culture triumphed as long as the 'people' willingly kept the managers of proprietary remedies in business by purchasing their products while thwarting the efforts of academic medicine to assume control. The crusade against secret medicine and popular resistance to it also illuminates the larger issue of the overall relations between physicians and patients.

Traditionally, historians of medicine have devoted much of their attention to famous physicians. More recently they have delved into the lives and practices of lesser-known practitioners, such as provincial physicians, midwives, and folk healers.[14] Until recently history of medicine was written primarily from the practitioner's point of view. Only in the last two decades have medical historians begun applying the methods of social and cultural historians to patients.[15] Taking the patient's perspective as their focus, these studies have enriched our understanding of the evolution of the doctor–patient relationship. The two case studies by Laurence Brockliss and Jacalyn Duffin illustrate this new scholarship. Both scholars utilize exceptionally rich – but not necessarily unique – case records that not only make their respective analyses important, but indicate the potential of further such investigations. Brockliss's study is based on the correspondence of the early eighteenth-century Parisian physician, Etienne-François Geoffroy. Duffin uses the extensive manuscript case records and personal papers of the nineteenth-century physician-researcher, René Théophile Hyacinthe Laennec. Both essays help us view the evolution of the physician–patient relationship from the eighteenth to the nineteenth century within the broader framework of rapidly changing Parisian medicine.

In the early eighteenth century, physicians like Geoffroy evaluated the patient by observation and the patient's narrative. As the century progressed, the surgical-anatomical approach to disease began to change the focus of some physicians, who introduced physical examination of patients into their practices. By the early nineteenth century new diagnostic tools such as the thermometer, stethoscope, and microscope became available. With the emergence of the Paris clinics, where patients served as laboratory animals, the research physician's focus began to shift from patient to disease.[16]

Geoffroy practised medicine among élite Parisians in the 1720s, but also catered to provincial patients with whom he carried on consultations by letter, a common form of medical practice in the eighteenth-century, and one still used a century later by fashionable physicians like Laennec. Consultation by letter offered a unique doctor–patient interaction which could succeed because patients and practitioners understood the same medical discourse. Consultation typically involved an intermediary, a referral from another physician, a relative, or a friend – and although letters were often written by individuals other than the patient, they nonetheless convey the patient's perspective and illuminate the dynamics of the doctor–patient relationship.

Geoffroy was the typical Hippocratic physician in terms of the therapies he prescribed and how he tailored them to individual patients. In his practice both physician and patient exercised considerable power. Geoffroy prescribed, but the client was free to follow or ignore advice. Patients did what they wished and were often noncompliant. At the same time Geoffroy represented a new breed of physician. As Brockliss demonstrates, he was among the first generation of French physicians to wield 'practitioner power', through which Parisian physicians came not only to command respect, but to elevate their status and power. This was a significant new development in French medicine. Hitherto, upper class patients treated their physicians as lackeys. Geoffroy's generation was the first to benefit from a shift in the power structure of physician–patient relations, a shift made possible by the rise of the professional classes that accompanied the emergent absolutist and bureaucratic sovereign state.

The medical practice of Laennec one hundred years later was quite different. Like Geoffroy, Laennec was a member of elite Parisian medical culture and treated many notable patients, such as Mme de Stael, Mme Récamier, René Chateaubriand, Lamennais, Cardinal Fesch, Victor Cousin and the Duchesse de Berry. Many of Laennec's private patients – both clergymen and aristocrats – selected him for religious and political reasons. Laennec was a devout Catholic and royalist, belonging to that group Duffin labels physician–royalists. In addition, Laennec also treated and studied a large number of patients in public hospitals, invariably members of the working classes.

A notable feature of Duffin's study is her emphasis on the intricate connection between Laennec's hospital patients and his research on the stethoscope. Since Laennec needed a large number of cases in order to correlate the sounds he heard using his instrument with the lesions he observed after patients' deaths, he relied on public hospital patients. Ironically, the tension between research and practice determined the difference between Laennec's relationship with his public and private patients. With the former, the success of his research was contingent upon his patients dying. The large body of archival material unearthed by Duffin clearly reveals the sharp contrast between the individual care provided by Laennec to his private patients – reminiscent of eighteenth-century practices – and the calculated research-oriented nature of his hospital work, where his patients were primarily the object of scientific investigation.

Although Laennec and his private patients still shared the common bond of elite medical culture, where both physician and client shared power, hospital patients were not necessarily stripped of all power. A tacit contractual relationship existed between the patients on the one hand and physicians and institutions on the other. Patients relinquished their power in return for medical care. Ultimately, their willingness to enter the Paris hospitals was critical to the success of the clinical enterprise and to the improvement of diagnostic techniques.

George Weisz's paper moves us to the physician's perspective as he examines the development of medical specialization in Paris by looking at physicians' self-perceptions of their knowledge, expertise and practices. Weisz seeks to identify specialties by looking at the way nineteenth-century physicians defined themselves rather than by superimposing categories based on our twentieth-century differentiations. If we employ the latter approach, as many medical historians such as Erwin Ackerknecht have done, then, argues Weisz, we shall see a greater continuity than actually existed and, even worse, we shall miss the unique fluid character of nineteenth-century medicine. Likewise, an attempt to define specialties by looking at professional associations and journals, would render the specialties more organized than they really were, and again, would result in a failure to fully appreciate the chaotic nature of medical specialization. Using as a principal source medical guidebooks, such as Henri Meding's 1852 *Paris Médical*, and, later in the century, the *Annuaire Roubaud* and the *Guide Rosenwald*, Weisz identifies three stages of specialty development. From 1800 to about 1860, few physicians considered themselves specialists. Specialization carried negative connotations, being linked with charlatanism and patent remedies. In the early nineteenth century only obstetrics – with its institutional foundations (La Maternité), its faculty chairs, its own special patient population, and the object of state attention – had any legitimacy as a specialty. Specialized hospitals, such as the Enfants-Malades and St Louis (skin diseases) and a variety of public and private institutions for the mentally ill, antedated physicians' self-definition of themselves as specialists.[17]

Public health emerged as a medical specialty during the 1820s, with the first specialized journal, the *Annales d'hygiène publique et de médécine légale* (1829 –), chairs at the three medical faculties, and its own institution, the Paris health council. But by the end of the century, public health was no longer recognized as a *medical* specialty, since by then specialties had become associated with clinical hospital and private practice. By comparison, before 1860, mental illness had institutions and a journal, the *Annales médico-psychologiques* (1843 –) but no curricular basis in the medical faculties.[18]

Until the 1860s, developing specialties were typically taught in public and private courses which were offered outside – but complemented – the regular medical curriculum. Such was the case with accessory sciences like microscopy, for example. In the second phase of medical specialization from the 1860s to the 1880s, new subjects were introduced into the formal medical curriculum so that by the 1880s seven chairs in clinical specialties had been established at the Paris Faculty of Medicine. Weisz argues that this curriculum reform was not, however, in response to physicians' needs and demands, but rather an attempt to counter the perceived decline of French science and medicine.[19]

Only after the 1880s, Weisz's third phase, did institutional and educational developments determine and foster specialization of practice among the Parisian medical élite. Thus, intellectual, academic and institutional specialization preceded the specialization of practice. This institutional support distinguished the medical élite from other physicians, who, in the absence of regulation, could call themselves specialists with or without specialized training and institutional affiliations.

While the study of such physicians as Geoffroy and Laennec and the development of medical specialization illustrate the nature of Parisian medical culture, the capital was not typical of France. Throughout the eighteenth and nineteenth centuries, Paris medicine embodied certain distinctive traits, such as an emphasis on research and specialization, that distinguished it from provincial medicine. Outside of Paris most professional medical care was provided by what Martha Hildreth calls the average general practitioner, or the family practitioner. Both the family practitioner and the physician–scientist emerged as contrasting icons in nineteenth-century French culture. The former came to represent humane, patient-centered medicine, and the latter, a Pasteurian hero who personified the contributions of science to medicine and society.

Hildreth analyses French 'social theatre', the large number of nineteenth-century plays that utilized medical science and practice as key themes and physicians as principal characters. The plays reveal a culture that idolized 'scientism' and its practitioners. Yet this adulation of the new scientific medicine was offset by the threat that the new order posed to the more traditional and personal medical care exemplified by the provincial family practitioner. Hildreth emphasizes that family medicine as practised by an idealized family physician was perceived as the cultural alternative to the laboratory and scientific medicine represented by Paris. Her essay, like that of Brockliss, emphasizes the patient's point of view, illustrating how patients – as much as physicians – were consequential actors in medical culture. Hildreth's interpretation challenges the standard account of the doctor–patient relationship, which argues for the decreasing importance and power of patients that accompanied the rise of scientific technological medicine.[20]

After 1880 physicians shifted their attention from social and environmental factors to micro-organisms and heredity in their attempts to account for disease. Hildreth uses this context to analyse the division between the approach of the family practitioner, who located the site of hereditary disease in the family and the scientist–hero who looked for disease in the laboratory. This contrast was an oversimplification, but it defined what physicians and the French people in general saw as two distinct approaches to medicine and disease. In the 'social theatre' the two types of physician were pitted against each other.

After 1870, when scientific laboratory medicine legitimated physicians' diagnostic and preventive expertise, a new form of medical discourse, focusing on degeneracy and decline, pervaded French society. Hildreth identified 25 plays with medical themes performed between 1900 and 1910. Such themes include the tragedy of inherited disease and its power to disrupt families; the power of physicians and medicine; and the contrast between scientific/laboratory and patient-oriented medicine, highlighting both the power of the laboratory to cure disease and the fear of human experimentation in the service of the new medicine. Both Hildreth and Anne Marie Móulin find widespread awareness within popular culture of both trends, with the people and the patients taking an active part in the larger medical discourse. But whereas Moulin concludes that the Pasteurians and the Pasteur Institute enjoyed wide popular support, Hildreth emphasizes a contrary trend – that of the provincial family practitioners who, by manipulating idealized images, were elevated to the level of popular heroes. Correspondingly, Parisian bureaucratic, scientific medicine and the various public health institutions were depicted as major threats to private practice.

The interaction between medical and literary discourse appeared in novels as well as plays. Balzac, Sue, Flaubert, Zola and, later, Proust appropriated medical themes and metaphors and adopted the physician as a key literary figure. Diseases such as tuberculosis and syphilis and mental illnesses such as hysteria became fashionable literary and dramatic themes. As with plays, novels not only reflected the influence of medical ideas, but also transmitted medical themes to popular and bourgeois audiences. This allowed a wider segment of society to participate in medical discourse.

Jan Goldstein examines the relationship between literary and medical discourse by looking at the uses each made of male hysteria. Hysteria was a gendered disease, traditionally associated with women. Citing examples from correspondence between Gustave Flaubert and George Sand, Goldstein shows how Flaubert, by considering himself a hysterical woman, opened the way for a subversion of gender stereotypes (a first step in easing the differences between genders). In contrast, for the psychiatrists, who operated within the norms of medical culture, gendered diseases continued to reinforce traditional stereotypes.

Flaubert's many references to hysteria illustrate how medical discourse interacted with literary discourse. The interaction was one-sided: novelists and playwrights were knowledgeable about and influenced by medical discourse, while physicians were rarely influenced by literary culture. Yet, Goldstein points out striking similarities noted by physicians between their psychiatric case histories and fictional stories. Certainly in the work of Pierre Janet and Sigmund Freud scientific and medical writing integrated reportage and literary narrative.

The uses of hysteria varied from literary to medical discourse. Goldstein suggests that when male physicians applied the term 'hysteria' to female patients, they used the disease categorization for their own empowerment, with resulting patient repression. By contrast, within literary culture, a male's diagnosis of himself as afflicted with a gendered disease could be liberating. Just as for women hysteria had traditionally been associated with a malfunction of the procreative organs, so now for men it came to explain writer's block or a general stifling of the creative impulse. Consequently, within literary culture hysteria symbolized a move toward androgyny – a disintegration of gender barriers and stereotypes, and the creation of a gender-free common ground.

An awareness of the role of gender within medical culture necessitates further consideration of the patient–physician relationship. For, in addition to differentiating physicians and patients according to class and geographical region, a further distinction based on gender is needed. After all, the naming of a disease empowered the physician, investing him with diagnostic and therapeutic expertise. But in cases of gendered diseases, labelling a disease further contributed to the disempowerment of a female patient. Since such a disease was associated with an 'inferior' sex, it assumed a second-class status – the 'other' – in relation to the male norm. Consequently, if a man was diagnosed as suffering from a disease typically associated with females, such as hysteria, then he, like the disease, was stigmatized. Thus, in contrast with literary culture, the governing paradigms of physicians and the constraints of their social milieu dictated that the only males who could be afflicted with such a culturally undesirable disease were members of the lower class.

Ultimately then, although literary and medical culture interacted, they preserved their separate identities. Literary culture was more tolerant of gender differences and more accepting of the positive feminine contribution to literary endeavours, whereas physicians clung to rigid gender stereotypes. A good example from medical culture is Charcot, who in the 1870s and 1880s made hysteria a fashionable and common disease. Although about one-fourth of his hysterical patients were male, this did not contribute to Charcot's degendering the disease. Instead, Charcot attempted to fulfill the Enlightenment vision of deriving natural laws of disease from empirical evidence, arguing that the laws governing hysteria were universal. His interest was not in gender redefinition but in claiming that the diagnostic entity of hysteria was one and the same, irrespective of time, place, race or gender.

Just as hysteria was associated by most physicians with gender, so was pathology associated with race. Toby Gelfand's paper allows us to consider the role of race in medical culture and how French society found in biomedical discourse explanations and justifications for racist theories. Gelfand focuses on the career and writings of Jules Soury in order to examine the connection between medical epistemology and the constitution of racial beliefs about Jews and to address the broader question of the confluence of pathology and race in late nineteenth-century France. And his paper illustrates how literary and medical culture were fused in the work and thought of Soury.

Soury was a prolific writer, who began his career as a specialist in the history of religions and then became an expert in the physiology of the central nervous system. Soury moved from a historical to a biomedical analysis of Jews in an attempt to show that racial differences were grounded in physiology. The Dreyfus Affair acted as a catalyst to bring his latent anti-Semitism to the fore. There emerged in Soury's thought a synthesis of science and racial anti-Semitism based on the notion that there were physical, organic differences between Jews and Aryans which could be found by histological and biochemical analyses of nerve tissues. Thus, with Soury, anti-Semitism gained a scientific, material, organic basis. That biomedical science could buttress anti-Semitism and that race could be linked with pathology was also suggested by the clinical studies of Charcot, who noted the prevalence of various nervous diseases among Jews.

The introduction of the concept of race in the nineteenth-century sciences of anthropology and ethnography provided the context for biomedical examination of racial differences and the biomedical discourse on Jews: Jewish vitality, Jewish natural immunities, and a variety of pathological conditions all came up for consideration. Charcot, for example, observed Jewish neuropathologies. In line with the increasing emphasis on inherited diseases, noted by Hildreth, the assumption of inherited pathological tendencies among Jews became a common theme in the medical literature of the late nineteenth century.

Soury followed a long medical tradition of physicians trying to find a physical, organic basis for disease – the tradition of pathological anatomy – as well as the older Hippocratic tradition of associating diseases with race, nationality, sex, age and life condition. But this kind of accepted medical thinking took on a new virulence in late nineteenth-century France when racism against Jews came to a head with the Dreyfus Affair.

If literary and medical culture did not merge in the case of Goldstein's investigation of differing concepts of hysteria, they coalesced in the work and thought of Soury, who bridged the gap between the humanities and the sciences. His work epitomized the influence of medical discourse on the thought of Third Republic France and showed how a concept of race could be constructed on a scientific basis and biological anti-Semitism based on the physiology of the nervous system. Soury's anti-Semitism flowed directly from his scientific ideology, according to which racial differences that had formerly been discussed primarily within the context of history and religion could now be located in the anatomy and physiology of the nervous system and illustrated by differing pathologies.

Hildreth and Goldstein contend that plays and novels were crucial in transmitting medical ideas to a popular audience. And as Gelfand shows, Soury conveyed his biomedically-based anti-Semitism to the reading public as well. The medical community, too, needed stable channels through which to transmit and diffuse medical ideas. Historians differ in their evaluations of the manner in which new techniques such as microscopy or a paradigm such as Pasteurian germ theory were disseminated. Some argue that ideological pre-conditioning was necessary prior to the successful diffusion of these new ideas, while others stress social and institutional factors in accounting for the acceptance of, or resistance to, innovation. In any case, it is clear that a myriad of political, social, economic and institutional constraints combined to obstruct the development of research laboratories within the medical community and hamper the coveted synthesis of teaching, research and practice of laboratory and hospital medicine.

Caroline Hannaway's paper on eighteenth-century medical research provides a preview of educational and research methods and problems that would characterize and bedevil French medicine throughout the nineteenth century. One of the principal concerns was the absence of institutional support, especially for laboratory facilities. The continuity of this problem for well over one hundred years is striking. But so was the persistence of Vicq d'Azyr's medical vision, a latter-day incarnation of which would be the interdisciplinary Pasteurian approach.

Félix Vicq d'Azyr, the epitome of Enlightenment medicine, was a comparative anatomist and key figure in articulating the goals of the late eighteenth-century Royal Society of Medicine, the man whose vision of medicine was destined to presage nineteenth-century French medical culture. His plan for a national medical programme was institutionalized in the Royal Society of Medicine, which later became the model for the Academy of Medicine. The nineteenth-century Academy, however, was not an exact replica of Vicq d'Azyr's design, for he had envisaged a far more truly national programme in which a large network of physicians would correspond with the Society on a regular basis. The nineteenth-century Academy emulated Vicq d'Azyr's model only in so far as it established epidemic and vaccine commissions that gathered information from correspondents throughout the nation. But as the institution became entrenched during the Restoration and July Monarchy, a Parisian élite medical culture emerged in line with the general French political and cultural model, which thwarted the implementation of a truly national cooperative effort. Hannaway aims to discuss Vicq d'Azyr's views on comparative anatomy and veterinary medicine as part of his broad programme for medicine and public health in order to delineate his significant contribution to medical education.

In the eighteenth as in the nineteenth century, many educational opportunities for medical students were located outside the Faculty of Medicine. Public and private courses on a variety of medical and scientific topics, often taught by professors from the Faculty or one of the other scientific institutions, such as the Jardin du Roi or the

Collège Royale, were plentiful and complemented faculty offerings. These courses were at the 'cutting edge' of medical training, typically covering material not incorporated into the official medical curriculum. Thus, before a chair in pathological anatomy was established at the Faculty in 1835, that subject could be studied only outside the formal curriculum. The same was true of microscopy and later, bacteriology. Private courses were usually taught in rented rooms. In just such a venue, Vicq d'Azyr taught his anatomy courses in the 1770s and Hermann Lebert, his microscopy classes in the 1840s. Half a century later microscopy and bacteriology were taught in a similar manner as practical courses at the Pasteur Institute.

Lack of adequate institutional support for laboratory facilities plagued French medicine from the 1770s into the twentieth century. One possible explanation for such neglect may be the pervasiveness of the clinical mentality – which sought to maintain a large number of Parisian hospitals to serve as clinical laboratories at the expense of scientific, experimental, laboratory medicine. But while such an interpretation appears to be convincing, Hannaway's essay suggests that the lack of research facilities was a more deep-seated institutional problem, ante-dating the great era of French clinical medicine.

Public and private courses provided the institutional setting in which medical microscopy was introduced into Paris medicine in the 1830s and 1840s. Like the stethoscope earlier and Pasteurian science later, the introduction of medical microscopy provides an instructive case study for the appraisal of the acceptance and diffusion of new medical technologies and scientific theories. A careful study of microscopy also enables us to analyse the tension that existed between medical research and medical practice. In the first two decades of the century microscopy was practised in France mainly by chemists, botanists and embryologists. Within a couple of years of the introduction of the new compound, achromatic microscope in the late 1820s, however, Alfred Donné became the first French physician to take a serious interest in medical microscopy, focusing initially on the analysis of body fluids. In 1837 Donné offered the first series of lectures on medical microscopy in Paris, a public course he taught in one of the amphitheatres of the Faculty of Medicine. By the 1840s there were four microscopy teachers, and research was expanded to include the solid parts of the body, with particular attention given to the differentiation of malignant and benign tumours. The microscope also made possible the identification of a variety of plant and animal parasites that caused common skin diseases, such as thrush. The use of the instrument spread rapidly among a small group of research-minded Parisian physicians. But while these few physicians readily accepted certain specific uses of the microscope – to analyse blood or to identify skin parasites, for example – more general application of the instrument to medical practice, to preventive and therapeutic medicine, seemed to hold little promise.

The microscope met with greater resistance among Parisian physicians than did the stethoscope. Both instruments were similar in that they were difficult to use and required considerable skill and training. But while the stethoscope offered diagnostic accuracy for the leading nineteenth-century disease – tuberculosis – as well as for a variety of lung and heart problems, the diagnostic benefits of the microscope were far less obvious. Dermatological diseases caused by parasites were less spectacular and were usually not fatal, thereby offering only limited opportunities for pathological anatomy. Only if physicians had been able to use the microsocpe with assurance to distinguish malignant from benign tumours or to diagnose tuberculosis in its early stages by an analysis of sputum or blood, might the instrument have assumed a central place within the Paris school. But some of the most experienced surgeons like Alfred-Armand Velpeau claimed that the microscope provided no more certain knowledge than naked-eye observation. Concurrently, practitioners did not see that the microscope offered any obvious advantages for patients. Nor did the instrument fit into prevailing theories of disease causation, which were primarily environmental and social. For practitioners and public health reformers, the germ theory never really displaced the stronghold which environmental and social etiologies held in French medicine and society. The germ theory was at best incorporated into the existing etiological framework which was redefined but not overturned. Even when micro-organisms were identified as breeding particular diseases, still, the predisposing causes were sought within the social and environmental domain. Bacteriology strengthened the public health position by providing further justification for public health reform. But as Anne Marie Moulin's paper makes clear, it is not at all certain when, or whether, it is possible to speak of a 'Pasteurian revolution' within the context of French medical culture and French society at large.

While it was recognized that the microscope increased research opportunities, most physicians still doubted the utility of both the instrument and the germ theory in medical practice. However, for many élite Paris physicians the dichotomy between research and practice was artificial. Most of them were engaged in both – medical research reinforcing their private practice – as Duffin's study of Laennec makes clear. But outside this elite group, and especially outside Paris, most medical practitioners were not research-oriented; for them the advantages of instrument and theory were far less obvious. It was only in the 1890s, with the advent of diphtheria serotherapy, that an increasing number of common practitioners began to see the merits of utilizing the microscope in their medical practices.[21]

Anne Marie Moulin tackles the twin issues of the Pasteurian revolution and the pasteurization of France by carefully evaluating the manner in which Pasteur's views were transmitted and adopted by French physicians and by the culture at large. French society, she argues, was more easily 'pasteurized' than were French physicians, a conclusion challenging Hildreth's inference from her study of social theatre. The two points of view need not be at odds. Whereas Moulin fixes her attention on elite Parisian physicians – who were, with few exceptions, receptive to Pasteurian ideas and who attempted to incorporate them into their research and practices – she did not study the large group of ordinary provincial physicians who comprised the sample examined by Hildreth and who resisted pasteurization until the 1890s. 1894 proved to be a turning point, because for the first time it was possible to identify the germ of diphtheria, to offer a diagnosis, and to treat (and cure) the disease through the administration of a serum. Only at this juncture, when an immediate practical application was made visible, did pasteurism begin to attract ordinary physicians.

Moulin's study challenges the received view in the history of medicine which contends that Pasteur's germ theory brought about an immediate revolution in medical theory and practice. She argues instead for a synthesis rather than a revolution, suggesting that the great achievement of Pasteurism was the fusion of contagionist and infectionist theory. In such a way, the prevailing social and environmental notions of disease causation could easily be made to accommodate the germ theory. Dirt and bad smells were redefined as *'tas de microbes'*, and the rationale for public health reform could be sustained without resort to the germ theory. Moulin labels this approach 'restricted Pasteurism', but the overall impression is one of continuity rather than revolution.

The Pasteurian programme was sponsored by the Parisian medical élite and community leaders, when Pasteur himself asserted that he was attempting not to infringe on the physicians' domain but only to expand their realm of theory and practice. Various groups of physicians were able to incorporate germ theory into their theories of disease causation. Pathologists integrated germ theory into pathology, identifying micro-organisms as one of four major causes of disease. Surgeons, for their part, began to practise first antisepsis, and later asepsis, though the major influence behind such practices was Lister, not Pasteur.

The Pasteur Institute immediately became identified with microbiology, which was not taught at the Faculty of Medicine but became the principal line of research at the Institute. Even though Pasteur's initial success with the anti-rabies vaccine had great publicity value, it had only a limited effect on physicians, since few patients contracted rabies. Only in 1894 with the introduction of diphtheria serotherapy, did Pasteur's popularity peak. The 'Pasteurians' became a distinct community with a different pattern of recruitment and training, establishing a new tradition of medical education different from the traditional clinical track. Pasteurians were recruited mainly from the ranks of military physicians and veterinarians who were sent to the Pasteur Institute for practical training.

Despite widespread receptivity to Pasteurian ideas by Parisian physicians, clinical medicine remained separate and distinct from bacteriological research before the First World War. The relatively late incorporation of Pasteurism into clinical medicine may be attributed to the preference of Parisian physicians for appropriating the prestige of the new science without becoming researchers themselves. Following a short period of synthesis during the 1890s, bacteriology and clinical medicine went their separate ways in France until after the Second World War. The short-lived and fragile synthesis began to break down, causing the second generation of Pasteurians (even further removed from clinical medicine), to turn their attention to the dissemination of Pasteurian ideas and practices in the French colonies, where the internal contradictions afflicting French medical culture and French society – between liberalism and public health policies carried out by a state bureacracy – were absent. Pasteurism, like so many other aspects of French medical culture, exemplified the dichotomy between practitioners and researchers, between clinical and laboratory medicine, between élite Paris medicine and ordinary practitioners.

The outsider's view of French medical culture is essential for arriving at a balanced account of that culture and for assessing the impact of the French model outside France. No single recognizable

French medical model existed. The English and the Americans, for example, defined Paris medicine within the context of their own national traditions, using different components of the model to serve their own professional needs. Thus, American and British medical students in Paris took back not only specific medical innovations such as the stethoscope or clinical statistics, but a much broader image of French medical culture tailored to their specific needs, intended to serve reformist trends at home. Americans wished to transform medical practice by incorporating the empirical and technical tools of French medicine. In contrast, the British were more interested in the organization and policies of French medicine, articulating, therefore, a very different interpretation of the French model.[22]. Although Edwin Chadwick never studied in Paris, his career makes this point clear. Chadwick was very impressed with French bureaucratic centralization, and he sought to use it as a model for British public health reform. With a view to such an end, he constructed an idealized model of French medicine, eloquently extolling, for example, the organization of Parisian hospitals with their central admitting office, central bakery, and central pharmacy, and hoping that the British system would follow suit. French medical culture was made to fit different images according to varied national and institutional contexts.[23]

Joy Harvey considers the case of one of these American medical students, Mary Putnam Jacobi. Putnam Jacobi received her MD from the Women's Medical College of Pennsylvania and travelled to Paris in search of clinical experience not readily available in the United States, especially to a woman. She studied in Paris from 1866 to 1871, where she became the first woman to be admitted by the Faculty of Medicine. For a foreign physician, admission to the various hospital clinics was dependent upon social connections, and for a foreign woman, such connections were doubly important. It was owing to the elaborate network of patronage that she established that Putnam Jacobi was able to move freely from one clinic to the next, gaining intimate knowledge of the most advanced practices. Harvey's main argument is found in her use of the word *la visite* in order to recapitulate Putnam Jacobi's educational experience and the manner in which she gained entrance to Parisian medicine. This term, with its double meaning of clinical rounds and social visits, encapsulates the double nature of her introduction to Paris medicine. Without her social visits to prominent Parisian women who provided her with introductions to influential men, such as Danton, the secretary to the Minister of Public Instruction,

Victor Duruy, she would not have been able to overcome the opposition of some of the medical faculty to her admission.

Harvey's paper illustrates one obvious characteristic of nineteenth-century French medical culture. Until the 1870s it was a culture that routinely excluded women, except as patients or nursing sisters. American women had begun to resolve the problem of exclusion from medical schools by founding their own schools, such as the New England Medical College and the Women's Medical College of Pennsylvania. It was the infiltration of foreign women physicians into the French medical school that paved the way for French women as well. Putnam Jacobi's training in French hospital clinics could not be repeated when she returned to teach in the New York Women's Medical College, for she underestimated the difficulty of importing the French clinical experience and planting it on American soil. This clinical experience, highly dependent upon the centralized French medical and institutional structure, was not capable of importation.

Although Putnam Jacobi went to Paris later than most American male medical students, (who were in France from the 1820s through the 1850s), she still sought that which had animated her predecessors – clinical experience. But by this time, male American medical students had already begun substituting Germany and Vienna for Paris, where since the 1850s clinical access had become more restrictive. In addition, as suggested by John Harley Warner, Paris was not as exciting as it used to be, since much of the French medical world that had attracted American men before 1850 had become incorporated into the American medical experience. But if Paris no longer drew American men, it still attracted Putnam Jacobi, a pioneer in the history of women's medical education.[24]

One conclusion emerging from this volume is that élite Parisian medical culture did not characterize French medicine as a whole. Consequently, Parisian medicine must be seen as one strand of a richly textured culture. Others are the community of provincial physicians, patients' perceptions of both physicians and medical therapy, popular responses to medicine, and foreign perceptions of French medicine. Only an integrative approach that takes cognizance of the crucial distinctions between Parisian and provincial medicine and that seeks to locate the intersections between the medical, social, political, and literary spheres, can uncover such richness.

Professionalization was the broader context within which medical culture was defined. Throughout the century the medical profession was in the throes of seeking an identity, with some physicians advocating liberal medicine and others championing social medicine. Both models, inherited from the Revolution, persisted into the twentieth century. Physicians were also unevenly distributed throughout the nation. In Paris and parts of southern France, the supply of physicians exceeded patient demand, and consequently, physicians in these areas felt a greater pressure to expropriate new areas such as pediatrics and obstetrics and to increase their social and professional status by claiming science as their territory.[25] Ultimately they sought to establish their exclusive authority and expert status by asserting what Paul Starr termed the 'legitimate complexity' of medical knowledge.[26] A widening gulf between patients and physicians was also becoming evident by the end of the century. Physicians and patients no longer spoke the same language, as had been the case with Geoffroy and his elite patients in the early eighteenth century. It is hardly surprising, therefore, that concomitant with the transformation of medicine was a growing popular fear of science as being intrusive and disempowering, a repercussion widely reflected, as Hildreth demonstrates, in contemporary theatre.

Various attempts made throughout the century to accomplish a synthesis between clinical medicine and research – whether in the case of medical microscopy or the Pasteurian microbiological programme – remained elusive. And although the dichotomy between the two domains was largely ideological, as many studies of the actual practice and research by physicians demonstrate, the repeated failure to integrate publicly the two approaches is a significant theme of French medical culture.

Various papers help us recognize the shifting focus of physicians in their efforts to locate and understand disease. During the eighteenth century a physician like Geoffroy concentrated on the patient's background and social context, and offered individualized therapies. But even then a different approach to the study of disease was emerging – which, for scientific purposes, redefined patients as bodies composed of organs and tissues. Such was the case with Vicq d'Azyr's anatomy and Laennec's organ-based pathological anatomy. As a reaction to such stringent emphasis on the solid parts of the body as the locus of disease, by the 1830s microscopists and research physicians rediscovered 'humours', and began directing their attention to the dissection of body fluids. The focus shifted from the seat of disease to causes of disease and, later still, with Pasteurian micro-organisms and the bacteriological approach, to outside agents of disease. Finally, late in the century, with the advent of hereditarianism, the emphasis again turned to the family. But with each such shift in orientation, further encroachment on the traditional relations between patients and physicians took place. Since medical knowledge was cumulative, the increasing complexity of medical ideas elevated the physician to the position of expert and invested him with increasing power and authority.

Medical culture was not monolithic. If historical research is to come to terms with the various permutations of nineteenth-century French medicine, it will require the careful analysis of the geographical origins of patients and physicians, and the relationship of class, gender, and race (or what some have considered race) to diagnosis and therapy. For example, a comprehensive gender analysis *vis-à-vis* a discussion of disease categorizations, of the doctor–patient relationship, of educational opportunities and more broadly of the notion of medicine as a basically masculine culture, is still a desideratum. And it is the aim of these essays to offer a modest contribution toward this end.

Notes

• Many thanks to Caroline Hannaway and Joy Harvey for reading this introduction and making a number of helpful comments.

1. Jack Ellis, *The Physician-Legislators of France: Medicine and Politics in the Early Third Republic, 1870–1914* (New York: Cambridge University Press, 1990).
2. Honoré Frégier, *Les classes dangereuses de la population dans les grandes villes et des moyens de les rendre meilleures.* 2 vols (Paris: Baillière, 1840); Louis Chevalier, *Classes laborieuses et classes dangereuses à Paris pendant la première moitié du 19e siècle* (Paris: Plon, 1958); Barrie M. Ratcliffe, 'Classes laborieuses et classes dangereuses à Paris pendant la première moitié du XIXe siècle?: The Chevalier Thesis Re-examined', *French Historical Studies* 17 (1991), 542–74. Ratcliffe challenges the utility and validity of the Chevalier thesis and suggests that middle-class perceptions of physicians and social observers did not square with the reality of urban life in early nineteenth-century Paris.
3. Ian Dowbiggin, *Inheriting Madness: Professionalization and Psychiatric Knowledge in Nineteenth-Century France* (Los Angeles: University of California Press, 1991); Robert Nye, *Crime, Madness, and Politics in Modern France: The Medical Concept of National Decline* (Princeton: Princeton University Press, 1984); Jane Ellen Crisler, 'Saving the Seed: the Scientific Preservation of Children in the Third Republic', Ph.D. Dissertation, University of Wisconsin, 1984; Jean-Pierre Goubert, *The Conquest of Water: The Advent of Health in the Industrial Age* (Princeton: Princeton University Press, 1989).

4. Russell Maulitz, *Morbid Appearances: The Anatomy of Pathology in the Early Nineteenth Century* (New York: Cambridge University Press, 1987); John Harley Warner, 'Remembering Paris: Memory and the American Disciples of French Medicine in the Nineteenth Century', *Bull. Hist. Med.* 65 (1991), 301–25.

5. Stephen Jacyna, (ed.), *A Tale of Three Cities: The Correspondence of William Sharpey and Allen Thomson,* (London: Wellcome Institute for the History of Medicine, 1989), xix–xxi; on Bennett, see John Harley Warner, 'Therapeutic Explanation and the Edinburgh Bloodletting Controversy: Two Perspectives on the Medical Meaning of Science in the Mid Nineteenth Century', *Medical History* 24 (1980), 24–58; Ann La Berge, 'Edwin Chadwick and the French Connection', *Bull. Hist. Med.* 62 (1988), 23–41. Othmar Keel, *La généalogie de l'histopathologie. Une révision déchirante. Philippe Pinel, lecteur discret de James Carmichael Smyth (1741–1821)* (Paris, Vrin, 1979).

6. Martha Hildreth, *Doctors, Bureaucrats, and Public Health in France, 1888–1902* (New York: Garland, 1987); Goubert, *The Conquest of Water.*

7. George Weisz is working on a major study of the Academy of Medicine. See his articles: 'The Medical Elite in France in the Early Nineteenth Century', *Minerva* 25 (1987), 150–70 and 'The Self-Made Mandarin: The Eloges of the French Academy of Medicine, 1824–47', *History of Science* 26 (1988), 13–39.

8. Paul Broca, 'Séance de l'Académie de Médecine', *Moniteur des hôpitaux* 3, 23 January, 1855, 73.

9. *Ibid.*

10. Caroline Hannaway, 'The Société Royale de Médecine and Epidemics in the Ancien Regime', *Bull. Hist. Med.* 46 (1972), 257–73; Weisz, 'The Self-Made Mandarin'.

11. Virginia Berridge and Griffith Edwards, *Opium and the People: Opiate Use in Nineteenth-Century England* (New Haven: Yale University Press, 1987).

12. Itard, 'Rapport général sur les remèdes secrets', *Mémoires de l'Académie royale de Médecine* 2 (1833), 24–31.

13. Matthew Ramsey, *Professional and Popular Medicine in France, 1770–1830: The Social World of Medical Practice* (New York: Cambridge University Press, 1988); George Sussman, 'The Glut of Doctors in Mid-Nineteenth-Century France', *Comparative Studies in Society and History* 19 (1977), 293–303. On the French public health movement, see Ann F. La Berge, *Mission and Method: The Early Nineteenth-Century French Public Health Movement* (New York: Cambridge University Press, 1992).

14. Hildreth, *Doctors, Bureaucrats, and Public Health;* Ramsey, *Professional and Popular Medicine.*

15. Ramsey, *Professional and Popular Medicine;* on the patient's point of view, see Roy Porter, 'The patient's view: doing history from below',

Theory and Society 14 (1985), 175–98.

16. Stanley Reiser, *Medicine and the Reign of Technology* (New York: Cambridge University Press, 1978). Michel Foucault, *The Birth of the Clinic: An Archaeology of Medical Perception*, trans. A. Sheridan Smith (New York: Vintage Books, 1973).

17. Erwin Ackerknecht, *Medicine at the Paris Hospital, 1794–1848* (Baltimore: Johns Hopkins University Press, 1967), 163–80.

18. La Berge, *Mission and Method*; Jan Goldstein, *Console and Classify: The French Psychiatric Profession in the Nineteenth Century* (New York: Cambridge University Press, 1987); Dowbiggin, *Inheriting Madness*.

19. Harry Paul, 'The issue of decline in nineteenth-century French science', *French Historical Studies* 7 (1972), 416–50.

20. Reiser, *Medicine and the Reign of Technology*.

21. Bruno Latour, *The Pasteurization of France*, trans. Alan Sheridan and John Law (Cambridge, MA: Harvard University Press, 1988), 127–9.

22. Warner, 'Remembering Paris', 306–7, 313–14.

23. La Berge, 'Edwin Chadwick'.

24. Warner, 'Remembering Paris', 318–20.

25. George Sussman, 'The Glut of Doctors'.

26. Paul Starr, *The Social Transformation of American Medicine* (New York: Knopf, 1982), 134–44.

1

Academic Medicine and Medical Industrialism: The Regulation of Secret Remedies in Nineteenth-Century France

Matthew Ramsey

The history of the trade in 'secret', or proprietary, remedies, and of the efforts of the medical profession and the state to control it, offers a particularly revealing glimpse into the medical world of France in the eighteenth and nineteenth centuries. Over the space of several generations, the regulatory mechanisms brought representatives of the medical élite into a dialogue with a wide range of remedy owners, both laymen and professionals, who made a living from the sale of these specialties. The campaign to police the remedy trade long received more consistent state support than the programme, equally dear to physicians, to regulate medical practice, because dangerous medications seemed a more immediate threat to life than inept advice, and because the offence was easier to define and prosecute. It suffered, however, from the inherent conflict between the claims of public health and of property – both rights proclaimed by the French Revolution – and between the professional ethos defended by medical reformers, the self-styled *médecins éclairés,* and the reality of the commercialization of the medical field, captured in the title of Roy Porter's recent book on English quackery, *Health for Sale.*[1]

This paper forms the third panel of a triptych. The first article focused on the innovations that the Société Royale de Médecine introduced, with limited success, in the late 1770s and 1780s. The Society reformed and systematized the police of the remedy trade at the national level and imposed strict standards for the authorization of remedies. And yet, quite apart from the practical difficulties of enforcing the ban on the sale of unauthorized remedies, its work fell short of the ideal of the *médecins éclairés,* because the remedies it approved would remain secret, the formula known only to the proprietor and to the Society's examiners.[2] The second article recounted the hopes and disappointments of the Revolutionary and Napoleonic era. The Revolution, which for the *médecins éclairés* initially promised an end to the abuses of the Old Regime, led, instead, to the abolition of the Société de Médecine and to a period of national deregulation, which the efforts of local officials committed to public health could only partly counteract. The Consulate brought new legislation on pharmacy in 1803, which dealt with secret remedies but left major loopholes. The Empire, in 1810, excited expectations of a definitive solution, with the creation of a special Imperial Commission charged with examining all secret remedies (including those with existing privileges, which were now abrogated), publishing the good ones, and outlawing the rest; its failure revealed the pitfalls awaiting any programme that would, in effect, have expropriated the owners of unacceptable compositions without compensation and indemnified the rest in a lump sum at a rate below market value: property rights triumphed over the right to health.[3]

The present study examines the end result of the Enlightenment campaign to control secret remedies.[4] After an interregnum stretching half a dozen years into the Restoration, the new Académie Royale de Médecine resumed the work of the Société Royale and the commission of 1810. The Academy's commission on secret remedies had a firmer institutional base than its Napoleonic predecessor and, unlike its Old Regime counterpart, it was committed in principle to transparency in the medical domain, to publishing the secrets it approved. Unlike the earlier Imperial Commission, however, it did not propose a complete review of existing remedies, and in practice it proved nearly as ineffectual as its predecessors. The Academy gave lasting institutional form to the earlier compromises: it would accord its seal of approval to only a limited number of preparations and would inveigh against those that posed a threat to public health, but without seriously challenging what the academicians would have called 'medical industrialism' – a loaded term that inextricably associated the ideas of commercialization and quackery. This liberal settlement, it might be argued, was both too lax and too strict: too lax in that it made no adequate provision for curtailing the sale of worthless or harmful remedies (and hindered the development of more effective regulatory legislation and agencies in the phar-maceutical field, which came later to France than to many other industrialized countries); too strict, in its narrow assumption that all formulas not in the standard pharmacopoeia would have to be acquired by the government or relegated to the sphere of illicit secret remedies. This legal framework provided only the shakiest foundation for the rapidly growing number of genuinely innovative specialties developed by the new pharmacology and marketed in the second half of the nineteenth century by a large-scale pharmaceutical industry, which transformed the artisanal pharmacist of old, compounding in his laboratory, into a retailer of commercial products.[5]

The regulatory regime that the Restoration monarchy inherited from the Empire suffered from legislative confusion and lacked a suitable institutional base. The law on pharmacy of 21 Germinal Year XI (11 April, 1803), corresponding to the law on medicine of Ventôse of the same year, primarily concerned education; article 32 barred pharmacists from selling 'any secret remedy', while article 36, which proscribed the distribution of remedies from stages in public squares, fairs and markets, also banned 'all printed advertisements and posters that promote secret remedies, under whatever name they may be presented' – a provision seemingly aimed chiefly at itinerant charlatans. A supplementary measure of 29 Pluviôse Year XIII (18 February, 1805) later prescribed penalties for violations of article 36 (a fine of 25-600 francs, plus 3-10 days in prison for a second offence) but left in doubt the penalty for selling secret remedies.[6] This legislation neither outlawed secret remedies altogether nor made new provisions for regulating them; in practice, the holders of Old Regime privileges still exploited them, and the government, represented by the Ministry of the Interior, continued to issue authorizations and police the trade.

The prevailing practices were codified in a decree of 25 Prairial Year XIII (14 June, 1805), which exempted from the restrictions contained in the legislation of Germinal both those preparations that had previously received official privileges, and those that the government might subsequently approve following the advice of 'schools or societies of medicine or of physicians appointed for this purpose'; proprietors could sell their remedies themselves, or through agents, though not, paradoxically, at pharmacies, since the ban on the sale of secret remedies by pharmacists remained in effect.[7] As the vagueness of the Prairial decree would suggest, responsibility for assessment remained highly diffuse, even if loosely coordinated by the Ministry of the Interior; Napoleon never established a successor to the old Société Royale de Médecine.[8] The government depended primarily on the counsel of the Paris School (later Faculty) of Medicine, which relied, in turn, on the work of a Société de l'École [later Faculté] de Médecine, composed of a commission of professors and 32 associates from outside the

Faculty.[9] But the Paris Faculty enjoyed no monopoly; the provincial faculties at Strasbourg and Montpellier advised local authorities, as did the medical societies that had begun to emerge at the end of the revolutionary decade, the Conseil de Salubrité of the department of the Seine, and the 'medical juries' set up under the medical practice law of 1803, whose primary responsibility was to examine candidates for admission to the lower tier of medical practice, the *officiat de santé*, but which were also charged with inspecting pharmacies and sometimes assumed a more ambitious role in policing the medical field.[10]

Napoleon's decree of 18 August, 1810 was intended to bring order to the regulatory process and, more broadly, to 'spread enlightenment' and 'discourage charlatanism'.[11] All earlier authorizations would be annulled; remedy owners, old and new, who wished to sell their preparations would have to submit their formula to the Minister of the Interior, who would consult a five-member special commission, including three professors from the faculties of medicine. On the commission's recommendation, the state would purchase and publish the formulas of novel and useful remedies; the commission was to determine fair compensation. This legislation, then, repudiated the old system of privileged secret remedies: henceforth no approved remedy could be kept a secret. 'Violators' (evidently those persons who continued to sell unauthorized secret remedies) would be duly prosecuted; a police circular issued the following month enjoined the prefects to use the new legislation as the basis for a renewed campaign against quackery. Subsequent decrees, however, postponed until the summer of 1811 the date on which earlier permissions were to be annulled and, to the commissioners' chagrin, exempted from examination those remedies that an earlier commission (presumably of the Faculty of Medicine or the old Société Royale) had pronounced harmless.[12]

The Imperial Commission on Secret Remedies received and responded to petitions from 418 proprietors concerning more than 800 remedies, including two formerly authorized by the Société Royale de Médecine (Belloste's mercurial pills and Laffecteur's antisyphilitic 'rob'). Its members, who considered the commission the Society's continuator, proved as severe as their model, rejecting outright as unoriginal, useless, or even harmful all but those two remedies (no longer novel, but deemed worthy of an indemnity), Mettemberg's 'antipsoric water' (a remedy against scabies, approved with significant reservations), and a handful of others. These included Pradier's poultice for the treatment of gout (the commission approved an indemnity, although it harboured many doubts about the originality of the formula and Pradier's exaggerated claims); Villette's purgative electuary containing guaiacum, used in treating rheumatism, arthritis, and gout; and, a 'universal machine' that supposedly cured gout, rheumatism, paralysis, and other chronic conditions (it was, in fact, an ingeniously constructed device that could be filled with hot water and used to apply heat to various parts of the body).[13] None of these remedies represented a therapeutic breakthrough; the most deserving were variants of well-known formulas or techniques, and the commission could not bring itself to give full credence to the claims of any of the petitioners.

For all its rigour, however, the commission did not propose to emulate the Society's active effort to police the remedy trade. One of its first decisions, in keeping with the language of article 2 of the decree of 18 August, (proprietors would submit their formulas 'if they deem it appropriate'), was to examine only remedies whose owners actually wanted an opinion; the great bulk of remedies on the market remained unexamined. At most, the commissioners encouraged the authorities to suppress remedies submitted for their approval that they deemed dangerous, such as the so-called 'grains of health of Dr Franck' developed by the physician Joseph-Marie Audin-Rouvière (1764–1832), a remedy whose name implied a connection with the celebrated Viennese physician Johann Peter Frank (which Frank denied).[14] Despite the commission's warnings and Frank's disclaimers, Audin-Rouvière emerged as one of the most prominent pill merchants of early nineteenth-century France, touting his remedy in *La Médecine sans médecin* and other popular publications.[15]

The government's solicitude for the property rights of remedy owners, reinforced by pressure from the Conseil d'État, effectively reinstated the tolerance for established products evinced by the decree of Prairial. The Commission itself disbanded in the summer of 1813, returning the regulation of secret remedies very nearly to the *status quo ante*. The 1810 legislation, however, remained on the books. Its chief effect was to establish the formal procedure for future government authorizations: a formula would have to be approved by a medical advisory board and then immediately published. It could also be invoked in prosecutions of vendors of unauthorized remedies. With only one, relatively minor, modification in 1850, the 1810 decree, together with the law of Germinal (as modified by the Prairial decree), remained the fundamental French law on the remedy trade until 1926.

With the failure of the 1810 commission, primary responsibility for examining secret remedies reverted to the Paris Faculty of Medicine, acting as consultant to the Ministry of the Interior, which continued to receive and process petitions for special approbations. In one typical case, a German named Schirvel wrote in early 1820 to the 'Minister of Interior Relations' to boast of his specific against scabies, which an old peasant near his native Aachen had used to cure him in 1802, after the physicians and surgeons of Paris had failed to provide relief. Like many other proprietors of secrets, he refused to divulge his recipe – no one else, he said, could use it successfully – and insisted on clinical trials. He was willing to come to Paris, however, to demonstrate it in the hospitals, 'où je me mettrai en Otage, jusqu'à ce que l'Examen en ait été fait par le Juré [sic] Médical, et que celui-ci ait prononcé sur l'Ex ou la non-Existence de l'Infaillibilité de mon Remède'. Long-established rules of procedure, however, precluded clinical trials unless a review of the exact formula, together with well-authenticated reports, suggested that such tests would be worthwhile.[16]

If the Paris Faculty had had its way, it would have consolidated the right to examine secret remedies with other advisory functions and served in fact if not in name as a national medical academy; its critics, drawn chiefly from the ranks of the independent medical societies (as well as court circles that distrusted the faculty's liberal politics), hoped to restore something like the old Société Royale de Médecine. The creation of an Académie Royale de Médecine, through an ordinance of 20 December, 1820, went far towards resolving this long-simmering dispute. The Academy inherited the functions of the old Société Royale as learned society and public health agency, including the promotion of research and dissemination of new knowledge, coordination of the campaign against epidemic disease (notably vaccination against smallpox, introduced at the beginning of the century), and the regulation of secret remedies and mineral waters; article 2 of the Academy's charter expressly charged it with 'examination of new remedies and secret remedies'. The Society of the Faculty of Medicine was dissolved. The functions of Napoleon's Commission on Secret Remedies, together with many of its papers, now passed to a special commission within the new Academy;[17] the oversight of mineral waters was entrusted to a separate commission.[18]

Unlike the legislation on the Société Royale and the Imperial Commission, the Academy's charter did not expressly empower it to re-examine existing remedies. Nor did the Academy benefit from a reform of pharmaceutical legislation. The Restoration had contributed only one major innovation to pharmaceutical regulation, the first 'French Codex', authorized by a royal ordinance of August, 1816 and published in 1818; the ordinance, which required every pharmacy to keep a copy of the Codex and follow its guidelines, provided a clearer legal basis for defining standard remedies than the 'Parisian pharmacopoeias' of the Old Regime, the last of which had appeared in 1758.[19] The Academy was obliged to work within the legal framework of Germinal, Prairial, and 1810.

Most contemporaries assumed that the Academy, like the Société Royale before it, now enjoyed the exclusive right to examine and approve remedies; its charter said that it had been 'specially instituted' to advise the government on questions relating to public health. In practice, local authorities continued to solicit the expert opinion of provincial medical institutions and to issue permissions to distribute remedies in their jurisdictions. The professional bodies, for their part, behaved inconsistently. In the summer of 1822, for example, the dean of the Faculty of Montpellier advised the prefect of the department of the Hérault that the Faculty could not evaluate a remedy for the government, since this was now the exclusive province of the Academy. Yet almost exactly two years later a commission of four Montpellier professors readily reported to the prefect on a purgative tisane, which they warned should be administered only by a physician.[20] Over the next several decades, as dissatisfaction with the Academy's regulatory activities mounted, provincial institutions increasingly assumed the task of trying to contain the proliferation of unauthorized remedies; at Toulouse, for example, the Society of Medicine, Surgery and Pharmacy boasted its own commission on secret remedies.[21] Only on the Academy's recommendation, however, could the national government purchase and publish the formula of a secret remedy.

Under the legislation and jurisprudence generally recognized at the time of the Academy's inception, several categories of remedies might legally be sold (in addition to 'magistral' remedies that a pharmacist prepared following a physician's prescription for a particular patient): (1) those included in the Codex and the formularies of the faculties of medicine; (2) those which the government had purchased, following the decree of 18 August, 1810; (3) those subsequently approved by the Academy and published, in accordance with the ordinance of 20 December, 1820; (4) those formerly authorized, whose cases had not yet been decided (and which in practice benefited from the extended application of the decree of Prairial).[22] A more ambiguous status attached to a fifth category, comprising remedies whose authors had obtained a patent, in accordance with the revolutionary law of 7 January, 1791; as physicians had long argued, and as the Academy later stressed in a communication of 1829 to the Minister of Commerce, the patent did not confer a privilege but only recognized priority.[23] An even more vexed question was how to define a 'secret' remedy, to which the prohibitory legislation of Germinal expressly applied, as opposed to some conceivably licit category of 'new' remedies. The Imperial Commission had adopted the commonsensical view that a remedy whose composition was publicly announced was not a secret remedy, and many proprietors, who had found that a widely advertised trade name was worth more than a trade secret, argued strenuously that remedies whose formulas had been published (or simply divulged to a medical society), or which were essentially based on formulas contained in an official pharmacopoeia, should not be considered secret. The courts, however, with increasing consistency, came to define a secret remedy as any officinal preparation (one not specially formulated according to a physician's prescription) that did not appear in the Codex and had not been acquired under the terms of the decree of 1810.[24]

In theory, good secret remedies were to be published, so that their benefits could be made available to all, while dangerous or ineffective ones would be proscribed. In practice, as attempts to implement the decree of 1810 had revealed, this programme was unrealizable; the Academy in its early years accepted that useful innovations might be tacitly approved for sale as secret remedies and harmless products tolerated. In 1828, a police ordinance, noting that the existing laws were not enforced, and that secret remedies continued to be widely advertised and sold, recalled the terms of the law of Germinal, which barred pharmacists from selling secret remedies and all persons from advertising them, and the penal measures imposed by the law of 29 Pluviôse Year XIII; it did not, however, renew the total ban on secret remedies implicit in the decree of 1810.[25] One indication of the lenity of government policy was that where article 36 of the Germinal law stated that pharmacists were not allowed to sell any secret remedy, the 1828 ordinance prohibited them from selling 'aucun remède secret, dont le débit n'auroit point été autorisé dans les formes légales'.

Although the Academy could not eliminate secret remedies, it was free to set the standard for according its approbation. Under the protocol it adopted, no remedy would be considered for authorization and publication unless it were a truly novel formulation, or applied in a new way, and its efficacy had been confirmed by clinical observation (though very few remedies reached this stage).[26] The Academy made it known that it would peremptorily refuse approval not only to remedies that proved to be already known but also to bizarre combinations of inert or not very active ingredients, contradictory combinations of active ingredients, and certain dangerous arcana. Like the Société Royale, which had rejected the purely empiricist argument that a remedy's worth could be known only by its effects on patients, the Academy insisted that the formula make at least rough pharmacological sense on paper.

The Academy's commission applied these criteria as stringently as its predecessors had.[27] In a general report of 1827, its chairman, J.-M.-G. Itard (better remembered as the tutor of the wild child of Aveyron), noted that during the academic years 1825–26 and 1826–27, the commission examined 60 remedies whose proprietors had asked the government to reward them for their valuable discovery, grant them the exclusive right to sell it, or purchase the secret. The commissioners condemned all but three harmless preparations, two cosmetic and one dental, which it agreed to tolerate but not endorse. Many of the remedies, Itard observed, were for incurable or shameful diseases, especially cancer and syphilis; these were the ancestral territory of the empiric. One petitioner thoughtlessly wrapped a sample in a flyer that offered a description of his remedy very different from the one he gave the Academy. Another sent in half-ounce pills the size of a macaroon, which the patient was supposed to chew. Still another proposed, as a remedy for rabies, a magic formula written on a piece of paper, which the patient was to swallow; the Academy renewed, under the Restoration, the dialogue of enlightened with traditional popular medicine begun in the 1770s by the Société Royale. Recognizing that the therapeutic properties of an unfamiliar remedy could not necessarily be deduced from its formula, the commission tested eight preparations and found that three were ineffective, while five possessed the same properties as remedies that were already known and therefore deserved no special approbation. Only Sency's powder (also spelled Senci or Sancy), prepared by a certain Bazière from a mixture of marine plants and used to treat goitre, won the commission's unstinting approval.[28]

By the end of the Restoration, the list of remedies approved by the commission had reached a grand total of two, with the addition in 1829 of Dr Ollivier's antisyphilitic biscuits.[29] The commission also proposed paying an indemnity to buy out the old privilege for Belloste's pills, without, however, endorsing them.[30] Although the Academy formally recommended that the government acquire each of these remedies (Belloste's pills in 1830, Sency's powder in 1831, and Ollivier's biscuits in 1832), no action followed, and the proprietors continued to exploit them as approved secret remedies, as they might have under the Old Regime, while boasting of the Academy's endorsement.[31] Unable to collect his hoped-for indemnity, the unfortunate Bazière entered into several disastrous partnerships to market his powder; by 1843, in severely straitened circumstances, he was forced to appeal once more to the government, offering two new remedies and a modified formula and novel application for his old one.[32]

An informal survey of the remedies rejected during the Academy's first decade suggests that the corpus was not markedly different from that with which the Société Royale had to deal. Many simply replicated familiar formulas; it is likely that most derived from a written compendium rather than original inventions or oral tradition. One balm proposed in 1827, which the commissioners described as similar to ointments possessed by every municipality and perhaps every family, was produced by boiling for six hours a mixture of ingredients that included apples, grapes, wax and unwashed butter.[33] A petitioner from Strasbourg proposed a water of walnuts, a remedy against dropsy, which, among its other virtues, could also cure plague and restore wine that had turned. The commissioners noted drily that this water would be truly miraculous if it produced even a fraction of the effects attributed to it; but it was in fact only a well-known preparation called *l'eau des troix noix*, which could be found in several pharmacopoeias.[34]

Another proprietor, a certain Perret, submitted an elixir of long life in 1828 that included brandy, rhubarb and saffron, but also theriac, the old blunderbuss antivenin and panacea. Perret insisted that he had found the recipe not in a published formulary but in the papers of a medical doctor, Jornette, who had died at the age of 104 as the result of a fall from a horse. This secret was said to have been preserved in his family for several centuries; a grandparent had lived to be 130, his father to the age of 112, his mother to 102. This remedy, apart from its virtue as 'un véritable contre poison, le sincère et parfait ami de l'homme et des femmes', had numerous wonderful properties: it restored nerves, relieved indigestion, calmed diarrhoea (but also gently purged), induced menstruation (suggesting its possible use as an abortifacient), killed worms, and cured dropsy, intermittent fevers, smallpox, and many other diseases besides. It could also be used in cases of drunkenness and as a tonic for the old and infirm. One of the agreeable things about his remedy, Perret added, was that it could do no harm, whatever the dose; the only precaution the patient must observe was not to consume milk products or any raw foods while using it. The Academy's commission, ignoring Perret's more fanciful claims, recorded the matter-of-fact comment that his remedy was very close to the elixir of long life found in the Codex – an oblique comment on the traditionalism of the official pharmacopoeia itself.[35]

Many petitioners, including the great majority of those without medical training, not only proposed banal remedies but also, in the commissioners' view, did not understand how to formulate them and could not be trusted to apply them safely and effectively. One such proprietor, Delrieu of the department of the Tarn, proposed a version of another standby of the old polypharmacy, orvietan, which he said he had inherited from his father-in-law, the chevalier Henri Toscan (an active empiric who, under the Old Regime, had secured many local authorizations to peddle his remedy). The inhabitants of the Tarn, he assured the Academy, used it for many ailments of man and beast, and he enclosed a batch of testimonials, including two signed by witnesses who claimed medical credentials. The commissioners discounted the testimonials, not on principle but because the illnesses were not carefully described. As for the recipe itself, the commissioners noted that 'pour la perfectionner, ce chevalier Toscan l'a augmenté d'une quarantaine de drogues. C'est à peu près le nombre de celles que nos pharmaciens plus éclairés ont ôté à la préparation de la thériaque.' The remedy might help in some cases, but not in others, and it could be dangerous, especially in Delrieu's hands.[36] Similar considerations led the Academy to proscribe a remedy for ulcers that included an astringent powder made from 'dragon's blood' (a resin, so called because of its dark-red colour) hammered into thin sheets of lead, which were applied to the affected parts. The petitioner, a 57-year-old man, sadly but unavailingly pointed out that after long services he was left with a net pension of only 114 francs, 66 centimes. The commissioners, ignoring this *ad hominem* plea, judged that the remedy was not a secret, was not always effective, and could be dangerous.[37]

Other remedies – elaborations from the traditional corpus, borrowings from folk medicine, fanciful innovations – the Academy rejected out of hand. It dismissed, for example, the remedy of a

Mlle. Blin as a hodgepodge and 'a ridiculous exaggeration of polypharmacy'.[38] Another report, on the fox grease that a certain Blondé had proposed as an astringent for hernias (although it had once been praised as an emollient and relaxant), belittled all the miraculous properties attributed to healing substances and objects in popular medicine:

> L'observation et l'expérience ont depuis longtemps montré ce qu'il y a de chimérique dans ces vertus toutes spéciales attribués par les crédules partisans des amulettes, des signatures, et de tant d'autres superstitions thérapeutiques, à la plupart des produits animaux, notamment aux dif[f]érentes graisses des quadrupèdes. Les découvertes de la chimie moderne, en confirmant ces résultats, ont fait voir, que toutes ces graisses sont essentiellement formées des mêmes principes immédiats, et que ces principes, moins médicinaux qu'alimentaires, peuvent avoir leur utilité comme excipients, comme intermèdes, mais ne constituent pas à proprement parler des agents médicamenteux.[39]

Organic chemistry, by reducing elaborately derived concoctions of dungs, greases, and oils to their constituents, sounded the death knell of the old polypharmacy – though it died a slow death. The Academy, like the Société Royale in the Old Regime, moved more quickly than the official pharmacopoeia, which long conserved traditional concoctions; the Codex of 1818 did remove from a mercurial plaster such ingredients as human saliva, frogs, earthworms and viper grease, but it retained oil of earthworms and snail syrup, which lasted until the Codex of 1884, and spirit of hartshorn, which survived until 1908, as did theriac, although viper meat had by then been eliminated as an ingredient.[40]

In the case of one of the more baroque remedies submitted to the Academy, the boluses for treating madness proposed by Sarta, a merchant of Perpignan, the commission spelled out its reasons for summarily rejecting it. (These were the large pills singled out for ridicule by Itard in his 'Rapport général'.) The Academy could have refused to judge on the grounds that Sarta had not provided the recipe, but such a response would have kept the petitioner in a false state of hope (and kept the examiners, it was implied, in fear of another importunate petition). The commission condemned the notion of applying a single remedy to a whole class of disorders due to different causes, especially in the case of mental illness, which was least likely to be cured by empirical arcana; mental patients, moreover, would be the most likely of all to resist chewing up a huge pill each morning, as Sarta's directions required. Psychiatrists, as Jan Goldstein has shown, might take lessons in moral treatment from laymen,[41] but the medical profession seems to have drawn the line at secret remedies.

What was this extraordinary therapy, which the petitioner hoped to demonstrate on two patients from Bicêtre? Sarta set forth his ideas in a soberly worded manuscript entitled 'Avis important pour l'humanité souffrante: manière de prendre le remède contre la folie, ou aliénation d'esprit et accidens des vapeurs; composé de trente pillules ou tablettes rondes, et d'une de forme longue et carrée, d'une bonne odeur et d'un bon goût.' His method included, first of all, the medicament of unidentified composition, whose enormous size may have conferred on it a certain symbolic efficacy (studies of placebos have suggested that very large or small pills work best, since patients believe that they are getting a lot of medicine in the first case and a very potent one in the second).[42] The remedy was to be taken in conjunction with a regimen that included a special diet and enjoined the patient from getting wet (though he might wash his hands with tepid water). Sarta even made allowances for moral therapy; during the course of treatment, he wrote, the patient required distractions and was not to be contradicted. He attempted to justify his method not only by invoking successful outcomes but also by explaining its physiological action as he understood it. Even if not completely cured, any patient would be much relieved by taking his remedy, 'et s'il plaît à Dieu, les deux mouvemens de son cerveau, l'un qui répond à celui du coeur, et l'autre à celui des poumons, ainsi que le désordre qui existait dans ses fibres, rentreront dans leur ordre naturel, parce que ce remède améliora le moral et le physique.' As an afterthought, Sarta noted that his remedy might also be administered to '[les] femmes enceintes devenues sottes'; but he modestly conceded that he did not purport to cure hereditary insanity and claimed only to have found the answer to accidental insanity, which was unfortunately all too frequent in this day and age. Some readers other than the Academy's commissioners might have conceded the remedy's possible effect on the imagination, a standard point among apologists for unconventional therapies (had not Fodéré suggested that physicians could learn much from empirics about the power of the imagination?)[43] But the examiners' brief was narrow, and they had no option but to give short shrift to the boluses.[44]

The commissioners heard Sarta out and dealt with him gently. Other petitioners suffered much sharper rebukes, particularly those who had received some medical training, which, in the commissioners' view, ought to have taught them the worthlessness of the remedies they proposed; in 1825, for example, the examiners expressed astonishment at the ignorance or charlatanism of an *officier de santé* who had proposed a specific.[45] In 1823, the commissioners harshly condemned three remedies submitted by Pradel of Ferney-Voltaire, all of them reminiscent of the empirical medicine of the seventeenth and early eighteenth centuries: a vinegar intended as a preservative against the plague; a perfume for the same purpose; and a balm for use against plague and scurvy. The last, like many baroque remedies of the early modern period, contained a powdered precious stone (sapphire, in this case). The commissioners, after perusing the certificates that detailed the remedy's triumphant exploits, observed that it was not even clear whether Pradel meant to treat the diseases of man or beast; the certificates indicated that one of his remedies had been used against the epizootic of 'contagious typhus' that raged among cattle in 1814. The second remedy, they added, could be dangerous when thrown on a fire (the usual practice when fumigating against the plague) because it contained flowers of sulfur, which would produce noxious fumes. They concluded: 'l'annonce du S.r Pradel est, pour votre commission, l'annonce d'un charlatan qui a abusé de la bonne foi et de l'ignorance de quelques personnes pour en tirer des certificats'.[46]

Like its predecessors, the Academy's commission insisted on making the pharmacological properties of a remedy the basis for its decision, ignoring claims to special address in applying it as well as other, more personal appeals. A farrier from Bourbon-Vendée proposed an empirical cure for cancer but feared rejection if the examiners evaluated only the composition of his remedy, since the outcome depended as much on the technique of treatment as on the ingredients; the Academy demanded the recipe.[47] The proprietor of a medicinal syrup described, in touching tones, how he had suffered an illness 'par suite des chagrins que lui occasionnèrent la perte de son bien-être'. A physician of Lyons had given him the recipe for a specific, telling him that he could cure himself with it and then give it to his friends. He had decided to sell the syrup because he was, alas, 'sans état et chargé de famille'.[48] His eloquence left the commissioners unmoved.

As the Academy interpreted its charge, it might pass beyond the narrow consideration of a remedy's efficacy only in those rare cases when it advised the government to acquire a formula and was obliged, like the Imperial Commission, to recommend the compensation due the proprietor. Here, in addition to the remedy's medical value, the commissioners were to take into account the profits that the inventor or owner had already derived from it and might hope to receive in the future; in practice, they weighed the petitioner's personal circumstances, arriving in the end at a moral calculation of retributive justice more than a hard computation of market worth.

The best illustration is the case of Belloste's mercurial pills, which confronted the Academy in 1830 as it had the Imperial Commission two decades earlier and the Société Royale a full half-century before.[49] In a damning paralepsis, the commissioners declined to pronounce a formal judgement on the remedy but added that if they had judged it anew, they would say that it was an unimportant modification of a well-known formula recognized before, during, and after the putative inventor's lifetime. All the previous examiners had overlooked very similar formulas, blending mercury and purgatives, that had appeared in various compendia published in 1537, 1615, 1626, and 1632 – well before Augustin Belloste's supposed discovery of 1680. What was more, the previous examiners had overlooked an error in the formula given to the Société Royale by Augustin's grandson; his French translation from Augustin's German inadvertently doubled the dose of honey, significantly altering the potency of the preparation. It was on the basis of this superficial examination that the remedy had been prepared and sold for 72 years under various official privileges. Nonetheless, the commissioners believed that they could not turn a deaf ear to their petitioner, the son of the Belloste heir who had petitioned the 1810 Commission on the subject of this remedy and had only recently died.

> C'est qu'appuyé de l'approbation des Geoffroy, des Andry, des Lassone, des Vicq d'Azyr de la Société royale de médecine, et de celles plus récentes de la commission de révision [an appeals board set up to review contested cases from the Imperial Commission of 1810] et de la faculté de médecine, la famille Belloste a dû voir un moyen d'existence dans la vente de ses pillules; et particulièrement, le seul et dernier possesseur de la formule a pu avec confiance et justice, se reposer sur l'autorité de nos sommités médicales, pour croire que cette ressource ne lui manqueroit pas à la fin de sa carrière. Irions-nous donc aujourd'hui, qu'il touche bientôt à l'âge où de simples soins deviennent une nécessité, lui ravir, sans aucune compensation, peut-être son seul moyen d'existence? Cette grande rigueur seroit une souveraine injustice.

Since the surviving Belloste, who had once hoped to receive a lump sum of 24,000 francs, now asked only an annual pension of 600 francs, the Academy agreed that the government should pay it, on condition that Belloste renounce all further claims by any heirs of Augustin, that he no longer prepare or distribute any remedy, and that the formula of the pills be published immediately.[50]

The formula seems not to have been announced by the Academy; Maurice Bouvet, who published a long and learned article on the history of the remedy in 1928, without having been able to consult the dossier in the Academy of Medicine, was not certain what it was. Bouvet also speculates that the indemnity was never paid.[51] In any case, the Belloste remedy, even if it had been dethroned from its position as an original invention, remained among a limited number of seemingly harmless and (according to the prevailing wisdom) effective remedies, which the Academy believed it could well tolerate. This specialty subsequently declined as a proprietary medicine, although a similar officinal formulation, which differed only slightly from the secret remedy, remained a standard part of the *armamentarium* until mercurial preparations gave way to antisyphilitics based on arsenic or bismuth. The case illustrates the continuing sensitivity of the bureaucracy to the property rights of remedy sellers and the willingness of the enlightened physicians to recognize the vendors' economic needs, provided that their own cardinal principles were not compromised: publication of valid remedies; suppression of dangerous ones; no sale or administration of remedies by unqualified persons.

In addition to assessing the remedies submitted to it, the Academy, like the Société Royale before it (though on a less ambitious scale), assumed a police function in the 1820s, helping to enforce the laws regulating the remedy trade – even though a strict construction of its charter suggested, as Itard noted in his 1827 report, that 'l'Académie n'a pas mission de proscrire les remèdes secrets, mais de les juger quand ils lui sont déférés par le gouvernement.'[52] In Paris, it took over to some extent from the Conseil de Salubrité of the Seine the surveillance of remedy vendors, working in collaboration, as the Council had, with the prefect of police.[53] Although the Academy did not actively track provincial remedy vendors, the Ministry of the Interior regularly transmitted to it the cases reported from the *départements*. As Itard observed, 'les autorités locales poursuivent [les] colporteurs de remèdes illicites, et c'est par suite de cette battue générale (permettez-nous l'expression) qu'ils arrivent eux ou leurs oeuvres dans les bureaux du ministre, et de là dans le sein de l'Académie pour y être jugés.'[54] These defendants, as they might be called, swelled the ranks of the petitioners who actively sought official approbation for their remedies. In August 1828, for example, the prefect of police sent to the Academy, together with copies of the recent ordinance calling for stricter enforcement of the laws against secret remedies, three requests from pharmacists who wished to advertise in newspapers, and copies of 19 journals and prospectuses containing publicity for various remedies that had appeared since the promulgation of the ordinance. Which cases, he asked, deserved to be prosecuted? The Academy noted that one case involved (among other advertised remedies) mustard seed, which could be sold by anyone authorized to retail simples; five involved cosmetics (which the Academy's commissioners called potentially as dangerous as remedies); and two involved refreshing syrups, which *confiseurs, droguistes,* and *épiciers* as well as pharmacists might sell, although the physicians feared that the former group might be led to market truly medicinal syrups. The other products were unambiguously medicinal preparations, promoted in violation of the law of Germinal.[55]

When public safety seemed at stake, the Academy asked that a drug be suppressed, as it did, for example, in the case of a remedy for rabies used by a primary school teacher, a preparation of rue, sage, and clover steeped in white wine and flavoured with clove and orange peel when given to humans, with the marc to be kept in reserve to apply to the wound. More rigorous than the Imperial Commission, a report by François-Joseph Double made a similar recommendation in the case of Mettemberg's water.[56] In its campaign against dangerous remedies, the Academy enjoyed the assistance of local medical societies and health councils, and in particular of certain departmental medical juries. An exceptionally activist jury at Nantes, for example, urged banning all advertising for secret remedies and pressed the prefect to act against individual vendors, such as a certain Turquant, who maintained a local distribution centre for a type of vermifuge manufactured in Angers.[57]

In practice, however, the remedy vendors and their customers proved a stubborn lot; prosecutions were difficult to set in motion, and convictions hard to win and sustain on appeal. One pharmacist, for example, convicted in May, 1830 by a *tribunal correctionnel* for selling a *sel désopilant* (whose putative function was to open or relieve the spleen or liver) won a reversal of the judgement on the grounds that the formula had been divulged and could not be considered a secret remedy under the terms of the law of Germinal (the contrary principle was not firmly established in French jurisprudence until mid-century).[58] The available sanctions were not in any case strong enough to act as serious deterrents to the remedy merchants, who seemed to accept them as a necessary cost of doing business. The Academy vented its frustration in 1828 in a message to the Paris prefect of police. Secret remedies compromised both health and morality (the latter by promising a sure cure for venereal disease, thereby removing 'un puissant moyen de défense contre les séductions du vice').

> Le charlatanisme a franchi toutes les barrières qu'on a voulu lui opposer. Votre commission des remèdes secrets, qui, par la nature des travaux dont vous l'avez chargé, devrait contribuer à rendre vains ses efforts, est presque réduite à être témoin de ses succès; et trop souvent elle a éprouvé une pénible surprise en trouvant annoncé sur nos murs la même préparation dont elle vous avait fait reconnaître la veille l'inutilité ou le danger.[59]

In any direct contest between medical industrialism and academic medicine, the former was left in possession of the field.

No case better illustrates the failure of police measures and the continued appeal of proprietary remedies, whatever the evidence accumulated against them by the medical profession, than that of the drugs known as the purgative and vomi-purgative of Leroy.[60] Originally developed by a Norman *officier de santé* named Jean Pelgas (1732–1804), promoted by his son-in-law, the surgeon Louis Leroy (1766–1842), who gave the remedies their name, and manufactured in Paris by the pharmacist Cottin, Leroy's son-in-law, these preparations were the best known and probably the most destructive pharmaceutical specialties of early-nineteenth-century France. The definitive formulas were said to have been established by Pelgas and Leroy in 1795; when the remedies were first sold in Paris in 1798, the purgative was dubbed *le remède populaire*.[61] The purgative, available in several 'degrees' (strengths), was described as a tincture of scammony, turpeth root, and jalap root; the vomi-purgative contained senna extract, tartar emetic, and white wine.

The appeal of these drastics to people of all social ranks, not only in France but throughout Europe and in many parts of the New World, bears out the argument, developed in a classic article by Charles Rosenberg, that such aggressive therapies won wide acceptance because they demonstrably worked in the sense of producing visible results (purges really purged), and because their actions made sense within a shared system of explanation.[62] The explanatory framework was humoralist – purges and vomits

42

evacuated corrupted humours – though it was an idiosyncratic version of humoralism that Pelgas and Leroy propounded in the various French and foreign-language editions of their *Médecine curative, ou la purgation dirigée contre la cause des maladies....*[63] (Leroy and his associates also churned out innumerable pamphlets, brochures, and other ephemera, including a periodical, which went through 47 weekly numbers in 1823–24.)[64] Leroy always distinguished between his own curative medicine and official medicine, which was merely palliative. His therapeutics rested on the notion that every person carried within himself from birth a germ of innate corruption; this germ, developing in varying degrees at certain epochs of life, vitiated the blood and humours and was responsible for all diseases. Every patient was like a cask whose lees had gone bad, and which needed to be rinsed several times. Hence medicine and purgation were practically synonymous; Leroy made much of the fact that in French a purgative was commonly called *une médecine.*

Leroy's humoralist pathology and therapeutics resembled in their broad outlines those of other patent-remedy vendors of the first half of the nineteenth century, including such prominent figures as Audin-Rouvière and James Morison, founder of the 'British College of Health' and promoter of Morison's pills, which won a wide market in France in the middle decades of the century. (Morison also preached the doctrine of the single origin of disease, impurity of the blood caused by acrimonious humours, which could be cured with a single remedy, his vegetable purge.)[65] These writers all sharply criticized, as dangerously depletive, the common practice of repeatedly bleeding patients, promoted by François Broussais; their denunciations of the hecatombs attributable to heroic bloodletting oddly mirror the rhetoric of their opponents on the victims of reckless purging. Broussais's solidist emphasis on localized lesions ran counter to the humoralism of the pill merchants, and his tendency to attribute disease to lesions of the gastrointestinal tract made him and his followers particularly wary of drastic remedies that irritated and even corroded its lining; but his insistence on a single cause of disease and essentially a single remedy (bleeding, supplemented by special diets) ironically parallels the doctrines of his contemporary, Leroy. The latter's positions, and the controversy they provoked, must be appreciated within the larger context of early-nineteenth-century debates on pathology and therapeutics.

The Leroy remedies first came to the attention of the government in the interregnum between the active years of the 1810 commission and the foundation of the Academy of Medicine. In October 1817 the prefect of the Loiret passed on to the Minister of the Interior a report by the departmental medical jury on the effects of the preparation in Montargis. The symptoms of patients who had taken the remedy were said to include anxiety, trembling, vomiting, suffocation, weakness, diarrhoea, pains in the joints and abdomen, paleness, and even Hippocratic facies, prodrome of death. The physicians of the town had responded with elaborate counter-measures: opiate antispasmodics to calm the bowels, and wine of quinquina; in some cases, they prescribed aromatic sitz baths, or leeches applied to the anus as an anti-inflammatory measure, 'pour faire cesser une phlegmasie inquiétante du thorax et de l'abdomen'. Despite the physicians' intervention, the jury reported, some victims had scarcely regained their health after six to eight months. The Minister asked the Paris Faculty to inform him whether Leroy's preparation was a secret remedy; if so, he wished to stop its sale until an assessment had been completed. Even if the formula were published, and the remedy therefore not secret, he would still like the Faculty's opinion.[66]

The sale of Leroy's remedies continued, however, and new reports of its ravages arrived over the next several years. In 1818 the prefect of the Rhône notified the Minister of Police of a death ascribed to the vomi-purgative and noted that a member of the medical jury had informed him of other complaints in the region. [67] In the summer of 1819, according to a communication from the psychiatrist Esquirol, a physician employed by the secretariat of the Conseil d'État took one of Leroy's remedies to counteract a feeling of malaise aggravated by overwork and died from its effects.[68] In March, 1820, the Bureau des Secours et Hôpitaux within the Ministry of the Interior reported another case to the Faculty: a brewer at Beauvais, denounced to the royal procureur for violating the law of Germinal, had administered Leroy's vomi-purgative, in one case with fatal consequences.[69]

Notwithstanding these alarming accounts, no thorough investigation of Leroy and his remedies appears to have taken place until 1821. On 12 February of that year, Leroy submitted to the Minister of the Interior the recipes for his remedies and a letter of justification. He identified himself as a former *maître en chirurgie* and *chirurgien consultant*; citing his book, *La Médecine curative*, which gave the formula for his remedies, he argued that his purgative and vomi-purgative were not, strictly speaking, secret remedies and that, therefore, the legislation on the sale of secret remedies did not apply to him. He requested not approbation under these laws but a simple certificate indicating that his recipe had been duly received.[70]

On 21 February the Conseil de Salubrité de la Seine denounced Leroy to the prefect of police as a mere 'illiterate *officier de santé*'. His *Médecine curative* it dismissed as a 'monument of ignorance and ineptitude'; as for his purgative, it was identical,. except for one ingredient, to the commonly known *eau de vie allemande*, an active remedy that could be extremely dangerous if used without caution.[71] The Council urged the prefect to take repressive measures. Prosecution, however, offered little hope of success, since Leroy was an authorized *officier de santé*, and his remedy, as he constantly maintained, was not a secret.

Through the spring and summer of 1821, the remedy continued to wreak havoc in the provinces as well as Paris. At the end of July, the acting mayor of Fontenay-le-Comte in the Vendée asked several *officiers de santé* to prepare a report on the death of a local midwife, Mme Barbarde, who had succumbed after taking one of Leroy's remedies. The victim, they reported, had expired in agony, although she found that eating currants seemed to alleviate somewhat the 'fire' in her oesophagus and stomach. The devasting effects of this drastic recalled to the authors the action of one of the most notorious proprietary remedies of the Old Regime, the *poudres d'Ailhaud*. In view of the preparation's obvious toxicity, they could only wonder at Leroy's claims; his writings asserted, for example, that his daughter had been purged with his remedy the day after her birth, and that by the age of ten she had taken it 2,000 times. Elsewhere, they noted hopefully, the local authorities had taken steps to control such dangerous remedies; Lausanne, for example, had banned them.[72]

In September, Baron Capelle, the Conseiller d'État chargé de l'Administration Générale des Hospices et Établissements de Bienfaisance, appealed to the Academy of Medicine for advice. Although the recommendation of the Conseil de Salubrité to prosecute Leroy could not be put into effect, since his activities apparently came within the letter of the law, it did seem desirable, as the use of the remedies spread rapidly through the provinces, either to ban them outright or at least to warn the public against them. He sent along the recipe and a batch of documents, including the report on the fatality in the Vendée.[73] The Academy appointed a special commission of seven, consisting of four physicians (Bourdois de la Mothe, Chaussier, Double and Récamier), two pharmacists (Boullay and Vauquelin), and the physiologist Magendie, to prepare a report.[74]

In the meantime, the vogue for the remedies knew no bounds. A pharmacist in Bordeaux reported to a Paris colleague that they were all the rage, despite the victims attributed to them; everyone was talking about them.[75] At Nantes, Dr Guillaume Laennec reported with even-handed contempt, 'on en embarque pour les nègres voire même pour les colons, espèce d'homme presque aussi sotte, aussi crédule, aussi superstitieuse, que ses esclaves'.[76] In Guadeloupe, the captain of a ship used the purgative to treat himself and three sailors. In Point-à-Pitre, a lieutenant colonel, the local commandant, treated himself with the purgative and survived; encouraged by his friends, though, he persisted in taking the remedy and died. November brought a further report of victims in Martinique.[77]

As the list of reported victims mounted, and the Academy's deliberate investigation proceeded, a furious controversy over the remedies divided French public opinion; it was to continue with scarcely diminished vigour well into the July Monarchy. Leroy was attacked both for his theory[78] and for the charlatanical way in which he flogged his remedies. In the well-established genre of antiquackery literature, a special place was now reserved for his exploits, and sceptics (chiefly medical professionals) cranked out articles and pamphlets denouncing their errant colleague.[79] An *officier de santé* named J.-B. Dupont published a series of articles in the *Écho du Nord* highly critical of the remedies and of their promoter, whom he called a charlatan; when Leroy published the testimonials of satisfied patients, he neglected 'd'y joindre une pièce indispensable; c'est la liste nombreuse, immense, des individus que son remède a envoyés dans l'autre monde'. According to Dupont, the periodical received a stream of rejoinders, including a letter from one of the remedies' most passionate defenders, 'écrite en mauvais français, remplie d'invectives et d'ordures, résultat des nombreuses évacuations que l'auteur venait de se procurer'.[80] When Dupont published his critique in book form and advertised it in the *Écho du Nord* at the highly affordable price of 50 centimes, a champion of curative medicine challenged him to donate 100 sous (5 francs) to the poor for each published testimonial that he questioned and offered to pay him 100 francs apiece for any that proved to be spurious.[81]

At Lyons, a group of physicians sent a petition to the Minister of the Interior denouncing the remedy. They were answered by an eccentric Leroy apologist, Charles-Henri Curchod, a former Prussian artillery officer, who submitted a memoir defending both the remedy and his own right to use and promote it, in the name of individual liberty.[82] Curchod was also the author of several similar polemical pieces, including an open letter to Leroy in which he claimed to thrive on repeated doses of the purgative, publicly urged it on others (not as a physician, he said, but as a 'philanthropist' unaffected by medical practice legislation), and drove home the standard arguments offered by Leroy and his defenders against accusations of medical industrialism and violations of the legislation of 1803. Leroy's remedies could not be called secret, since he had published them; indeed, since the government had allowed his *Médecine curative* to run through a dozen printings, the formulas had in effect become official. Moreover, they were legal in that Leroy 'prescribed' them in his book. It was as unreasonable to expect every prescription (*ordonnance*) to be handwritten as to say that one should not obey royal ordinances (*les ordonnances du roi* – there is also, perhaps, a crude pun on the surgeon's name) without having before one a copy in the king's own hand.[83]

Curchod was particularly quick to identify with Leroy as the victim of official power; a paranoid streak had already emerged in some of his earlier writings on his own messy divorce case in the canton of Vaud, dating back to 1806, which left him feeling terribly ill-used by an arbitrary political system.[84] But he was not alone in seeing Leroy's professional critics as self-serving defenders of monopoly. The master himself, despite his unwavering faith in the ultimate triumph of his cause, was tormented by the nagging fear that in the short term he would fall prey to *un coup d'autorité*,[85] and he wrote repeatedly about enemies, persecutions, and plots. Like the proverbial paranoid who has real enemies, Leroy did, indeed, face a growing network of dedicated opponents, including local medical organizations and officials. In January, 1823, the Société de Médecine, Chirurgie, et Pharmacie de la Ville de Douai denounced Leroy's vomi-purgative in a report addressed, with possibly a hint of nostalgia, to the 'Société royale de médecine'. In Metz, the mayor banned the sale of the remedy by anyone but pharmacists.[86]

The Academy's report to the Minister of the Interior, which it finally presented in May 1823, offered not only a judgement on Leroy's arcana but also a more general statement of its position on the subject of secret remedies.[87] In principle, the Academy was still willing to sanction new remedies whose efficacy had been demonstrated through clinical trials. It would, for example, have approved morphine, strychnine and quinine, if the 'inventors' had kept the composition secret and had wished to exploit it.

47

Mais lorsque l'Académie est appelée à prononcer sur des combinaisons plus ou moins bizarres de substances inertes ou de peu d'efficacité, conseillées cependant contre les maladies les plus graves, elle les repousse sans un examen bien approfondi. L'expérience des siècles passés a suffisamment fait justice de ces prétendus spécifiques, qui ne trompent guère que ceux qui veulent en faire le trafic.

D'un autre côté, si l'on soumet à l'Académie des médicamens actifs dans lesquels les substances unies en plus ou moins grand nombre tendent à se détruire les un les autres, et à former des composés variables par leur nature autant que par leurs effets; si on lui adresse des recettes dont les élémens se trouvent portés à des doses assez élevées pour alarmer la prudence éclairée du médecin et compromettre la santé des malades, l'Académie les rejette aussi par la seule force des ses lumières et de sa conviction.

Unoriginal formulations would be rejected in a similarly peremptory fashion. In addition,

il existe encore des arcanes que la confiante crédulité du peuple s'est en quelque sorte appropriés, et dont elle abuse d'une étrange manière. Ces arcanes, parce qu'ils n'ont pas toujours eu des effets funestes, ou bien parce qu'ils ont été et qu'ils peuvent réellement être utiles dans certains cas que le médecin seul peut calculer et prévoir, sont universellement prônés. On les conseille contre toutes les maladies, on les emploie dans toutes les circonstances, on les livre de toutes mains, et le mal qu'ils produisent est à peine calculable. L'Académie croit devoir poursuivre ces arcanes de toutes la force de sa raison, de tout l'ascendant de son opinion, de toute la puissance de son crédit.

The Leroy remedies belonged to this last category.[88]

The Academy also reported the result of its analysis of Leroy's purgative and vomi-purgative, in two forms: the preparation supplied by the pharmacist Cottin, Leroy's regular distributor in Paris, and a second batch prepared independently according to Leroy's directions. The purgative, it said, was composed of 'drastics' macerated in alcohol and then disguised with molasses; the vomi-purgative included sal ammoniac and tartrate of potassium in white wine and water. Several procedures, including tests on animals, led the academicians to suspect that the actual composition of the remedies sold to the public differed from the formula supplied by Leroy.

Since an abundant literature existed on the physiological insults to the gastrointestinal tract produced by violent irritants, the Academy's commissioners were able to provide a well-documented discussion, including specific case histories of patients who had taken drastics supplied by empirics. Evidence against Leroy could be gathered from his own book, and from accounts of patients who took his remedies and later consulted physicians. One case had been reported of mass poisoning of soldiers in a barrack, who presented symptoms including headaches and mental alienation. Other complaints had arrived from prefects and medical juries, or had been published in medical journals. Tests on animals confirmed the clinical descriptions. When the preparations were introduced into the stomach of two animals by means of a syringe and catheter, they did not vomit but displayed clear malaise; an autopsy revealed local lesions. In two other cases, the preparation was injected into the rectum. All four subjects exhibited inflammation *(phlogose)*.

The continued commercial success of such preparations, despite their manifestly noxious effects, could be attributed to the visible evidence of their operation – essentially the argument invoked by Rosenberg:

> Les faits de ce genre sont d'autant plus nombreux, que, de toutes les médications, la purgation est celle dont on abuse le plus dans la médecine populaire. Aussi est-ce sûrement à cette cause qu'il faut attribuer le grand nombre des maladies chroniques qui affligent l'espèce humaine et qui désolent les médecins, et le nombre bien plus considérable encore des maladies aiguës dégénérées en chroniques, toujours au détriment des malades. Comme l'action primitive des purgatifs parle immédiatement aux sens, chacun croit en pouvoir déterminer justement l'efficacité, en la calculant d'après la quantité des résultats matériels. C'est par les sens que le vulgaire se laisse le plus facilement surprendre, parce que c'est précisément par-là qu'il pense ne pouvoir être trompé.[89]

In the Academy's view, small doses of such drastics could be used appropriately in certain cases – to treat mental alienation, the sequelae of apoplexy, and some forms of dropsy, and to dry up milk in the breasts. But Leroy's remedies were dangerous in the extreme.

The conclusion was inescapable: the remedy should be suppressed, so far as possible. Already certain mayors, including those of Metz and Rennes, had warned local residents against the remedies, and other alarms had issued from the health councils of the Seine and of Pointe-à-Pitre in Guadeloupe. Several cases were now before the courts, although Leroy's guilt had not yet been established before any tribunal. To alert officials and the general public, the Academy asked that its report be printed and distributed, and it was duly published in July, 1823. An extract appeared in a regular circular of the Ministry of the Interior.[90]

Rather than lay the matter to rest, the official report inflamed the controversy over Leroy's remedies. His defenders, Curchod among them, denounced the Academy as biased and doctrinaire, as did the master himself.[91] A physician-ally, Claude-Pierre Martin, argued that the preparations were much less violent than the Academy suggested (they had worked with the fourth-degree purgative, reserved for the most stubborn cases, rather than the second degree normally administered to adults); the commission's animal studies had failed to replicate the effects produced in a human patient taking the normal dose. (Other professionals then excoriated Martin as a turncoat who had no doubt been corrupted by a material interest in Leroy's enterprise.)[92] Subsequently, when Étienne Pariset, the Academy's permanent secretary, denounced secret remedies in a report on the Academy's work between 1821 and 1824, he singled out Leroy's for special condemnation; Leroy replied in a pamphlet that attacked Pariset as a bad physician, orator and citizen and suggested that he could not even speak for the Academy, since he had been appointed by the state rather than elected by his peers.[93] As adviser to the the government, the Academy might have the last word, but it could not dominate the free market of public discourse any more than the remedy trade.

The prefects took advantage of the ministerial circular of 1823 to ban distribution of Leroy's remedies, except by pharmacists (since the formula was public knowledge, it was held that the prohibition against their selling secret remedies contained in the law of Germinal did not apply).[94] The most prominent laymen who distributed the drugs were prosecuted under the law of Germinal.[95] The remedies' continued notoriety, however, prompted another ministerial circular calling for stricter enforcement and reminding the prefects that although pharmacists could fill a prescription for the remedies, they were not allowed to keep in stock any preparations not listed in the Codex.[96] Leroy and his followers continued to defy such injunctions, although the government did succeed in suppressing Leroy's periodical, after an ordinance of 15 August, 1824 reestablished the censorship of periodicals.[97]

Without Leroy's financial records we cannot measure the effects of the Academy's intervention of 1823 on sales of the purgative and vomi-purgative, but the surviving evidence clearly indicates that official censure did not end their widespread use; at most, it drove the traffic underground. In 1826, the Conseil de Salubrité of Nantes reported that the Leroy purgative and vomi-purgative were still sold clandestinely; an implacable enemy of secret remedies, it

50

called for revoking the decrees that tolerated the sale of such arcana and objected to the continued presence of a commission on secret remedies within the Academy of Medicine.[98] In December of that year, the physician Martel, in the department of the Loire, informed the prefect of a case of fatal poisoning caused by one of Leroy's remedies (despite a decree issued in August 1823, following receipt of the Academy's report) and supplied him with a copy of the report on the post mortem he had performed on the victim.[99] In another case of the same year, events took a more bizarre turn. A woman at Saint-Étienne took a Leroy remedy and then, in agony from its effects, summoned a physician; notwithstanding his ministrations, she died, and his autopsy report, communicated to the authorities and published in the local newspaper, attributed her death to the remedy. This publication offended those who believed in Leroy and his remedies; they thought that 'l'esprit de corps [avait] présidé à la rédaction du Rapport de l'Académie Royale de Médecine sur le remède de Le Roy', and attributed the woman's horrible intestinal symptoms and ultimate death to cholera morbus. An increasingly *ad hominem* exchange of correspondence in the pages of the newspaper led to a duel in which the physician killed one of Leroy's champions, a student in the mining school at Saint-Étienne.[100]

In 1827, in response to fresh pleas from the Conseil de Salubrité at Nantes, the prefect of the Loire-Inférieure sought authorization from the Minister of the Interior to ban the sale of Leroy's vomi-purgative; once more, the response affirmed that it was possible to prevent pharmacists from stocking it, but that problems arose whenever the procureurs attempted to apply the penal provisions of the law. In the prefect's view, new legislation was needed.[101] Despite renewed prohibitions the trade continued as before, in France and overseas. In January 1827 the governor of Martinique received a warning from an unusual source, the inspector of the book trade, who announced the shipment of 37 cases of Leroy's remedies, together with a set of his promotional books.[102] (As in the Old Regime, censorship and the police of the remedy trade sometimes overlapped.) In 1828, finally, the Minister of the Interior issued his circular asking for stricter enforcement of the legislation on secret remedies; Leroy, although not mentioned by name, was clearly implicated. In the Loire-Inférieure, the then prefect circularized his subprefects and mayors, reminding them of the legislation, as the Minister had directed, and of his predecessor's decree on the sale of Leroy's purgative.[103] More than this he could not do.

If this most scandalous of early-nineteenth-century proprietary remedies could not be suppressed, it is hardly surprising that more innocuous ones, particularly those that had enjoyed some form of official sanction, flourished as they did, even without the Academy's sanction. This was true, for example, of the celebrated antisyphilitic known as the *rob Laffecteur* – a thick syrup (though technically not a 'rob' produced by boiling down fruit juice) prepared from vegetable extracts. Controversy surrounded both the origins and composition of the remedy (some charged that it contained hidden mercury), but the Société Royale, after performing many clinical trials, issued a warrant for it in 1778 to a partnership headed by the physician Pierre Boyveau (who claimed to have discovered it in 1764) and his father-in-law, the marquis de Marcilly. According to most accounts, they chose to market it under the name of Denis Laffecteur, an employee of the Ministry of War, so as to avoid connecting themselves publicly to the remedy trade; Laffecteur, who was to serve as their agent, received both monetary compensation and a share in the business.[104] After the remedy had proved hugely successful, Boyveau, in an apparent reversal of his earlier *pudeur*, began calling himself Boyveau-Laffecteur. In 1793, the principals in the partnership, Boyveau and Laffecteur, split up; each party continued to sell the specialty, Laffecteur as the *rob Laffecteur* and Boyveau as the *rob Boyveau-Laffecteur*.

The rob remained a subject of controversy in the first decades of the nineteenth century, more because of disputes over proprietorship and the legal implications of the Old Regime warrant than because of the drug's composition and pharmacological properties (it was widely accepted by then that the rob contained no mercury and was effective against syphilis, though not necessarily against scrofula or gonorrhoea, as was claimed for modified versions).[105] Boyveau and Laffecteur reciprocally denounced each other, Laffecteur maintaining that the recipe was his own family secret and that Boyveau had not contributed capital to the partnership, while Boyveau insisted that Laffecteur had served only as a front for the actual inventor and backers. Both complained of counterfeiters; both claimed the privileges granted by the warrant of 1778, including the right to distribute the remedy through a network of private agents.[106] When the Imperial Commission summoned proprietors of previously approved remedies to resubmit them for evaluation, neither Boyveau nor Laffecteur responded. The commissioners did hear, however, from Boyveau's partner Hoffmann (also known as Hoffmann-Laffecteur) and from yet another claimant, a certain Gouzil of Bordeaux. The latter asserted that he had acquired the remedy from the true original proprietor, Develuos, who had introduced it to France from Arabia and later sold it to de Marcilly, Boyveau, and company for 50,000 livres in promissory notes that became worthless when the partnership declared bankruptcy. The Commission suggested an indemnity of 30,000 francs, to be divided among the legitimate claimants, including Gouzil; it was never paid.[107]

Laffecteur's remedy declined after his death in 1821, but Boyveau's was vigorously promoted after his death in 1813 by his heirs, chiefly his older son, who assumed the name Boyveau-Laffecteur; the Boyveaus insisted that they were the exclusive beneficiaries of the warrant of 1778, that their retail outlets remained legal, and that the recipe was still secret, despite published assertions that it was indistinguishable from standard formulas and had, in effect, entered the public domain.[108] Starting in the late 1820s, the Boyveau-Laffecteur operation encountered determined competition from another supplier of an antisyphilitic rob, a young physician named Jean Giraudeau (1802–1861), or Giraudeau 'de Saint-Gervais' as he began to call himself, after a town, Saint-Gervais-les-Trois-Clochers, located near his birthplace of Châtellerault. Boyveau-Laffecteur announced that Giraudeau's version of the rob was worthless, consisting of almost pure molasses, and that Giraudeau, despite his medical credentials, was an unscrupulous hawker of secret remedies, continually in trouble with the law, whereas he, Boyveau, continued to enjoy the privileged status conferred by the warrant of the Sociéte Royale.[109] On Giraudeau's legal difficulties, Boyveau was undoubtedly correct; in 1829, the *tribunal correctionnel* of the Seine sentenced him to pay a fine of 600 francs (the maximum possible penalty) for the illegal sale of secret remedies, and he suffered further convictions in the two decades that followed.

Giraudeau, however, proved the more gifted promoter, writing a series of medical self-help books and publishing a *Journal de médecine usuelle*, all to advertise his remedies; the journal ultimately appeared in English, German, Dutch, Spanish, Italian, Greek and Russian editions. Giraudeau also diversified more skilfully than his rival, developing new versions of the rob, regenerative as well as antisyphilitic, and promising that his blood purifiers would cure a variety of disorders, especially skin diseases; cholera joined the list after its arrival in France in 1832.[110] Despite his conviction in 1829, which drove him to seek refuge in the provinces, and subsequent prosecutions, Giraudeau refused to give up the rob and mounted a tenacious legal defence of his activities, arguing that his medical degree exempted him from the police regulations on pharmacy, and that his remedies, whose formulas he had fully published after his first brush with the law in 1829, were not secret.[111] Like many such entrepreneurs, Giraudeau saw himself as a persecuted innovator, the victim of professional élitism – 'les académies et les sociétés savantes, en général, sont disposées à croire que nul n'a d'esprit hors eux et leurs amis' – though he also craved official recognition; he boasted of nonexistent medical appointments, called himself the author of a dissertation approved by the Faculty of Medicine (which was in fact his very routine thesis for the Paris medical doctorate), and liked to cite a letter he had received in 1827 from Pariset complimenting him on a work he had written on the treatment of syphilitic diseases.[112] (According to Boyveau, Giraudeau had altered the letter to make it appear that Pariset endorsed his remedy.)[113] In 1836, Giraudeau won a minor victory when Martin du Nord, a former *procureur-général* of the Paris court, became Minister of Commerce and scandalized the Academy of Medicine by awarding him an inventor's patent valid for 15 years. But whether such a patent could legitimate the sale of a remedy remained a subject of dispute, and Giraudeau was still not shielded from prosecution.

Giraudeau's fondest hope was to enter into a partnership with Boyveau-Laffecteur that would allow him to shelter under the warrant of 1778, an arrangement he had requested since 1828, only to meet with indignant refusals and condemnations; he responded to Boyveau's animadversions by suing him for defamation, all the while urging the merits of a partnership. But financial pressures took their toll on the Boyveau family, and in 1842 Giraudeau succeeded in acquiring the share of the business belonging to the younger brother, then practising medicine in Paris, for 20,000 francs; his remaining rival charged that he cut the price of the rob from 25 to 15 francs a litre and substituted an inferior product for the genuine article. This disloyal competition produced the intended effect, and in 1849 Giraudeau purchased the remaining share in the Boyveau estate for 70,000 francs.[114] Despite the increasing hostility of the medical establishment, his business continued to grow; even the conservative *Gazette médicale de Paris* carried an advertisement for the rob in 1847 promising a discount for soldiers, sailors and persons sent by physicians, and it was not alone.[115] Giraudeau later acquired the languishing *rob Laffecteur* as well and became sole heir to the privilege of 1778, which was not finally invalidated by the courts until 1866, five years after his death.[116] The specialties subsequently passed into the hands of a certain Jules Ferré, and when Maurice Bouvet studied the history of the rob not long after the First World War, they were still being marketed by H. Ferré et Cie., though as *dépuratifs végétaux* rather than antisyphilitics. In all of this, the Academy of Medicine, which never gave its formal approval to any version of the rob, was at most a keenly interested bystander.

Many other instances could be cited of remedies and remedy-sellers prospering in the face of prohibitions and police measures emanating from Paris.[117] In the end, the Enlightenment project of reforming the trade in proprietary remedies fell far short of its aspirations. On paper, the programmes of the Imperial Commission and the Academy came closer than that of the Société Royale to realizing the hopes of the *médecins éclairés*, who had opposed secrecy in therapeutics. In its assessments, the Academy's commission was arguably the most rigorous of all, as its analysis of the Belloste remedy would suggest, and the Academy continued in principle to oppose medical secrets. In practice, however, it tolerated the continued sale of approved secret formulas, and its commissioners always scrupulously respected the principle of confidentiality. The Academy, moreover, proved less fully committed than the Société Royale to policing the remedy trade and to an overt war on charlatanism; even its comprehensive report on Leroy's preparations, it should be noted, came in response to an initiative from the government. It was partly that the academicians saw their institution differently, essentially as an advisory body on questions relating to public health rather than as an active public health agency. But all efforts to suppress medical industrialism confronted the continuing vitality of the medical market-place, the practical difficulties of enforcement, and the tendency of the state to avoid massive intervention where property rights were at stake.

For some members of the medical élite, the work of the Academy's commission on secret remedies embodied a contradiction; after the legislation of 1810, how could secret remedies be both legally abolished and legally regulated? Like the Société Royale before it, the Academy, though congratulated by many for the firmness with which it upheld professional and scientific standards, was accused of encouraging the very abuses it sought to contain. The pharmacists of Nantes, for example, expressed dismay in 1841 that the Academy's charter had empowered it to examine secret remedies, which had no legal existence, and suggested that the Academy, despite its initial declarations, actually stimulated charlatanism by welcoming new nostrums. A little more than a decade later, the author of an antiquackery tract similarly concluded that the Academy helped empiricism more than it hindered it. Was it now, he asked, 'de la dignité de l'Académie de Médecine de conserver dans son sein une commission dite des remèdes secrets?'[118]

The criticisms of the Academy's activities point to a shift in emphasis in the long-standing debates over secret remedies. In the early nineteenth century, as in the eighteenth, most physicians remained sceptical of claims for a remedy's special efficacy, whether against one or many diseases; many also opposed secrecy as a form of mystification. The prevailing assumptions of neo-Hippocratic medicine emphasized that each case required a complex course of treatment finely adjusted by an experienced physician to the patient's particular constitution, temperament, and changing constellation of symptoms. To suppose otherwise was a popular error. 'Pour l'ignorant', M.-J.-M. Richard wrote in an 1833 medical thesis, 'la médecine n'est que le bonheur d'avoir une recette convenable pour chaque maladie'.[119] For the Société Académique de Nantes, in 1831, 'ce n'est que l'ignorance la plus grossière, ou le charlatanisme le plus déhonté qui puissent prétendre à imposer un remède applicable à tout un ordre de maladies'.[120] A related consideration militated against keeping a formula secret, for physicians would then be handicapped in their efforts to adapt its use to the individual case. In the Hautes-Alpes, during the interregnum between the Imperial Commission and the Academy, a member of the medical jury, who continued to embrace the neo-Hippocratic medicine of the Enlightenment, deplored the effects of the existing legislation as he understood them: 'une loy a fait acheter tous les remèdes secrets, quoi qu'il ne doive point exister de secrets pour le médecin instruit et qui a toutes les productions de la nature pour ressource en les adaptant au tempérament, à la maladie, aux lieux, aux eaux et au climat où est le malade'.[121] More generally, the prudent physician needed to understand the pharmacological activity (and possible risks) of the remedies he prescribed, and scientific progress demanded the widest possible dissemination of information.[122]

Even more than the eighteenth-century *médecins éclairés*, the nineteenth-century critics of secret remedies underscored their links to the old and now largely discredited empirical *armamentarium* that had accumulated since Antiquity: they were emblems of the terrible hold of tradition on therapeutics. For a committee of the Société Académique de Médecine at Marseilles, in 1829, 'les remèdes secrets sont pour la médecine un point de contact avec les siècles d'ignorance', something like alchemy, astonishing to behold in a *siècle positif*.[123] Another commentator drew a parallel both with alchemy and with Druidism and recalled the many rules and rituals surrounding the preparation of remedies in prescientific medicine, such as injunctions governing which garments one was to wear while gathering plants, or whether the right or left hand was to be used to pick them. Other remedies, he pointed out, embodied the outdated approaches of a more recent past, including some preparations (like the *rob Boyveau-Laffecteur*) that the government still tolerated because of warrants and authorizations issued under the Old Regime. 'N'est-il pas ridicule de voir l'efficacité de substances médicamenteuses basée sur des rapports datant du XVIIIe siècle, époque où l'anatomie se bornait à la description grossière des organes?'[124]

Such critics dismissed as self-defeating and archaic the practice of making a group of eminent academicians patiently work through masses of petitions, knowing in advance that almost all of them proposed remedies that they would reject as unoriginal or worthless, while at the same time accepting that a few genuine discoveries might occasionally emerge that deserved official sanction. As the commissioners of the Société Royale had quickly discovered, most formulas submitted for examination resembled those contained in published compendia, and nearly all the rest resulted from random observation and trial-and-error experimentation, usually with combinations of familiar ingredients. Already, in the Old Regime, some *médecins éclairés* had criticized as unproductive the Society's project of sifting through the corpus of empirical remedies, and they had looked forward to an era when new therapies would be derived from the application of scientific principles. Now, in what their early-nineteenth-century counterparts hailed as the dawn of a science of pharmacology,[125] the Academy seemingly remained wedded to the older model.

As the new pharmacology adopted standardized procedures and proved itself by developing new drugs, and as the concept of specificity of disease and treatment gained wider acceptance, this argument came to form the core of the radical critique of the old approach to regulating secret remedies developed by a militant minority within the medical elite. The most important innovations of early-nineteenth-century French pharmacy, such as the isolation of strychnine (1818) and quinine (1820), derived from the systematic work of medical scientists (of whom several of the most prominent, such as the physiologist Magendie and the chemist Pelletier, sat in the Academy) rather than the efforts of private practitioners and inspired laymen. They characteristically involved the introduction of novel or newly refined substances, and the study of their specific physiological action, rather than the recombination of familiar (and usually impure) ingredients that yielded the 'recipe' for a secret remedy. The work of Caventou and Pelletier in isolating quinine from cinchona bark provided the model.

Moreover (the critics argued), the researchers who contributed to the major advances of scientific pharmacology never presented their discoveries as secret remedies or attempted to profit from them in the manner of their medical colleagues Leroy and Giraudeau.[126] As in the Old Regime, some voices (chiefly those of proprietors) continued well into the nineteenth century to defend proprietary remedies in the name of the inventor's property right in his discovery and on the grounds that confining production and distribution of a remedy to the owner, who would put his name on the product and stand behind it, was the best form of quality control.[127] For want of an effective patent system applicable to medicines, illicit secrecy remained the only means for the inventor of a therapy to derive a financial return from his contribution. But a strong current of professional opinion rejected the idea of a novel remedy as a property to be exploited. Not only did *l'industrialisme* run counter to a widely shared ideal of *l'homme de l'art* as disinterested philanthropist, but as a practical matter it seemed increasingly difficult to determine ownership of a treatment developed by chemists, physiologists, research pharmacists and physicians, all performing specialized tasks; it would make almost as much sense, one commentator suggested, to claim a legal property interest in a surgical operation.[128]

This prejudice against proprietorship is one factor that helps us understand why, for more than a century after the founding of the Academy of Medicine, France did not accommodate to changes in the pharmaceutical field by abandoning the entire legal framework associated with the secret remedy and substituting a modern patent system for pharmaceutical innovations. In the absence of fundamental reform, the regulatory system under the July, Monarchy and subsequent regimes became increasingly paradoxical, marked on the one hand by ever more rigorous jurisprudence and an Academy devoted to maintenance of the highest scientific standards, and on the other hand by lax enforcement, a declining practical role for the Academy in the assessment of pharmaceuticals, and an unending chorus of complaints about the harm caused by secret remedies and the deficiencies of French pharmaceutical legislation.

In principle, the law of 1803, as reinforced by the decree of

1810, had outlawed the sale of secret remedies, and by the late 1830s, France's highest court, the Cour de Cassation, leaned towards the strict interpretation that any preparation was *ipso facto* a 'secret remedy' if it did not fall into one of three categories: formulas listed in the Codex; those acquired and published under the law of 1810; and magistral remedies composed by a pharmacist for a particular patient following a physician's prescription. Exceptions would be made only for preparations that were more foods, hygienic products, and the like, than medicines. A decision of 9 November, 1840 clearly affirmed this interpretation.[129] Many proprietors, as has been seen, tried to cover themselves by taking out a *brevet* under the patent law of 1791, despite the argument, made by the Academy and many legal commentators, that patents simply documented an inventor's claim to priority and had in any case been superseded in the field of pharmacy by the legislation of 1803 and 1810.[130] New patent legislation adopted on 5 July, 1844 definitively resolved the question by explicitly providing that no further patents would be awarded for remedies.[131]

Some local courts, it is true, continued to find in favour of defendants whose remedies had been published, or had been approved by the government for use in hospitals or other institutions (without having been acquired under the decree of 1810), as well as those, like the *rob Boyveau-Laffecteur,* that enjoyed privileges conferred under the Old Regime. As late as 1856, a judgment of the appeals court of Metz overturned the conviction of Giraudeau de Saint-Gervais in part on the grounds that the rob derived a kind of prescriptive legitimacy from many decades of toleration.[132] But the judicial decision most often taken as a model in the later nineteenth century, issued at Metz in 1857 by the same court that had shown indulgence toward Giraudeau the year before, essentially affirmed the definition of a legal remedy applied earlier by the Cour de Cassation. The court did allow the pharmaceutical industry some further leeway, making exceptions not only for remedies that were less medicines than foods, cosmetics, or hygienic products but also for those that were essentially the same as, or improvements on, formulas given in the Codex.[133] Anything else, however, was technically a secret remedy and therefore illegal. So strictly was this interpretation applied that a pharmacist could be convicted of violating article 32 of the law of Germinal for dispensing, on a physician's prescription, a pure chemical compound whose uses were well established in clinical medicine, but which was not an officially approved remedy.[134]

So rigorous a system placed a heavy burden on therapeutic innovation; although contemporaries increasingly distinguished between new 'special remedies' or 'pharmaceutical specialties' and old-style 'secret remedies', both suffered equal restriction under existing legislation and jurisprudence. A new remedy had to be sold to the government, which seemed unwilling to pay, or at least listed in the Codex, which might take years (the second edition appeared in 1837, and subsequent editions in 1866, 1884 – with a supplement in 1895 – and 1908). To allow manufacturers more latitude, on the recommendation of the Minister of Agriculture and Commerce, a decree of 3 May, 1850 provided that they might legally sell remedies approved by the Academy and the Minister, and published in the Academy's bulletin, while awaiting incorporation in the Codex;[135] in implementing the decree, the Academy treated such 'new' remedies as a category distinct from secret remedies and not subject to the principle of confidentiality.[136] Remedy makers undoubtedly benefited from a measure allowing them to market their remedies legally, but they paid a heavy price, since they were obliged to divulge a trade secret with no prospect of compensation.

The Academy, moreover, did not fully assume the role now assigned to it; as one commentator noted in a celebrated case of 1906 involving a widely used drug substance, the Academy had not published a remedy in more than 30 years.[137] After an extraordinary burst of energy in the 1820s, the activities of the commission on secret remedies appear to have slowed, in two stages. The initial change of pace reflected a diminishing case load after the first decade. In his annual report on the Academy's activities for 1833, its secretary, Pariset, observed that the number of petitions addressed to its commission on secret remedies was declining; part of its task in its first years had been to deal with the accumulated backlog of remedies whose owners hoped for official authorization.[138] The commission nevertheless continued to meet regularly as before, and to judge submissions with much the same alacrity and severity.[139] In 1843 Pariset could still offer his assurance that only two remedies, Sency's powder and Ollivier's biscuits, had received the Academy's formal approbation, and that the Academy had never actually authorized the sale of secret remedies.[140] In the 1830s and 1840s, it favourably judged only a few other products, without urging acquisition and publication, and in the same period it rejected many hundreds of remedies.[141]

In the second half of the century, however, the Academy's zeal diminished, and towards its end the academicians seem gradually to have withdrawn from the assessment of new therapies. It is possible, too, that manufacturers declined to submit new remedies for evaluation, either because they justifiably feared an unfavourable outcome, or because they wished to preserve a trade secret; this question deserves further investigation. The Academy continued to publish reports but did not sustain its systematic review and ritual denunciation of secret remedies; the reports, typically confined to an enumeration of rejections, concerned only a small number of preparations and suggested a certain scepticism and weariness.[142] One can find in the archives the usual recipes for medical secrets, their wax seals still unbroken and their contents unread. Where Enlightenment medicine had conducted a dialogue of the deaf with empiricism, academic medicine seems to have broken off the dialogue altogether. Nor did it attempt to keep pace with the progress of scientific pharmacology. As George Weisz has argued, by the early twentieth century the Academy's emphasis had shifted from technical discussions of disease and therapies to larger questions of policy and public health; as the division of labour proceeded in medical science and practice, the Academy had less of a role to play in appraising and disseminating new contributions from throughout the field of medicine, functions increasingly relegated to specialized societies and journals.[143] In retrospect, the busy first decade of the commission on secret remedies seems like the opening, not of a new medical era, but of the last phase of an older project.

The vast majority of pharmaceutical specialties therefore remained unapproved and technically illegal. This is not to say that they were suppressed; laxity of enforcement continued to match legislative rigour. With the Academy playing an increasingly marginal role, coordination from the centre was limited, confined to occasional exhortations along the lines of the ministerial circular of 1828, calling for systematic action against violators. Local authorities dragged their feet, in part because prosecution was often difficult (particularly before the 1850s, while jurisprudence was still uncertain, notably on the question of penalties for the unauthorized sale of secret remedies),[144] but also because the very severity of the law made its wholesale application unthinkable. Prosecutors tended to single out cases involving dangerous preparations, dispensing accidents, or fraud or other grossly deceptive practices, but to many observers the way in which repression occasionally punctuated a general pattern of inaction made the law seem arbitrary as well as harsh.

France thus found itself without any effective mechanism for regulating the remedy trade, and the problem of secret remedies remained, into the twentieth century, an obsessive concern of the medical and pharmaceutical professions. For much of the nineteenth century the complaints emphasized the harm done by dangerous or ineffective preparations, and the loudest protests came from pharmacists, who could not themselves sell secret remedies and saw in the trade a direct threat to their livelihood. The question preoccupied local professional societies as well as the Academy and was regularly debated at medical and pharmaceutical conventions;[145] at the great national medical congress convened in Paris in 1845, the section on abuses and illegal activities in medicine and pharmacy devoted particular attention to secret remedies.[146] Unhappy professionals exhorted the government to institute reforms, characteristically demanding the publication of all useful new therapies, combined with a strict ban on the sale and advertisement of secret remedies. At Marseilles, a commission of the Société Académique de Médecine called in 1829 for complete proscription, 'sans avoir égard aux droits des propriétaires, qui doivent se taire devant les intérêts de la santé publique.'[147] Subsequent proposals rang changes on the same theme.

As many reformers recognized, most of their goals were already expressed in existing legislation, and the basic problem was one of application. Some, convinced that only a professional institution would take enforcement seriously, advocated a stronger role for the Academy as a kind of national medical 'chamber of discipline', on the model of the local agencies proposed under the Restoration to implement the laws on medicine and pharmacy and to police the conduct of the health professions from within.[148] In an address to the Academy in 1842, Hippolyte Royer-Collard, professor of hygiene at the Paris Faculty of Medicine, suggested that the Academy elect each year a commission to apply medical and pharmaceutical regulations.[149] Such a transformation of the Academy's function, however, would have led it well beyond the responsibilities specified in its charter and would have required far greater support in both the Academy and the government than the proposal ever enjoyed. No other institution had the legal standing to coordinate execution of the law of Germinal at the national level. In the provinces, public health councils, medical schools, and professional associations helped keep pressure on local authorities, compensating for the abolition of the medical juries in 1854, but their efforts were largely confined to the major urban centres.

In the later nineteenth century, as the manufacture of pharmaceutical specialties increased, pharmacists came to see that their interest lay in being allowed to sell them, while physicians (particularly those in public programmes of medical assistance, who were most closely bound by legislative restrictions) chafed at the constraints placed on the legally recognized *armamentarium*. Although the dangers of quack remedies remained a familiar topos in the medical literature, and the pharmaceutical *syndicats* that emerged at the end of the century were vigilant in denouncing them, the emphasis began to shift towards the regulatory regime's inability to accommodate genuinely useful innovations. By the early twentieth century, even the government found it difficult to sustain the remarkably expansive conception of the illicit secret remedy that prevailed in French law; finance legislation adopted in 1916 that placed a tax on *les spécialités pharmaceutiques* was taken by many as an oblique legitimation of secret remedies, despite the vigorous denials of jurists.[150]

This unforgiving and paradoxical regime was finally reformed only in 1926, on the recommendation of a commission on pharmaceutical specialties established by the Minister of Labour and Hygiene, motivated in part by the wish to make modern drugs legally available to the state medical assistance programme. Henceforth, following a presidential decree of 13 July, 'remedies prepared in advance for sale to the public' would be allowed, provided that the exact ingredients were listed on the package and container, together with the name and address of the responsible pharmacist (still the only legally recognized manufacturer).[151] The old ban on secret remedies remained in force, but in a sense it hardly mattered. France had entered a much more liberal pharmaceutical regime, in which the introduction of new remedies did not ordinarily require the approval of the Academy of Medicine or the government, and the modern drug industry could flourish unhindered by ambiguous legal status. The one major exception involved biologicals, such as serums and vaccines; a law of 1895 had provided that they could not be marketed without the authorization of the Academy and the Comité Consultatif d'Hygiène Publique (as the national health council was then called).[152]

The presidential decree gave *de jure* recognition to the long-established pattern of *de facto* toleration. Characteristically, the legislation of 1926 created no new institution to police the remedy trade; indeed, it embodied the classically liberal principle of substituting informed free choice (based on the information disclosed on the label) for regulation. The contrast with the decree of 1810 is instructive. On the one hand, the Napoleonic measure required government approval for new remedies (in principle all useful preparations would be acquired and published while useless or harmful ones would be proscribed), whereas the decree of 1926 imposed no such restriction and did not discriminate between good and bad remedies. On the other hand, the later measure insisted that any remedy offered for sale to the public had to include a clear description of its composition, whereas the decree of 1810 had demanded only official – not necessarily accessible – publication of the formula of approved remedies.

In the end, the history of the regulation of secret remedies in postrevolutionary France is in large part the history of toleration, a pattern not confined to the pharmaceutical realm. Though we still often think of modern France as the land of centralization, heavy-handed bureaucracy, and the strong state, we would do better to think of the state, in Stanley Hoffmann's classic formulation, as centralized but limited, authoritarian but noninterventionist.[153] Industrial and labour legislation came relatively late to France; so did effective public health legislation, in part because of the tension between public hygiene and political economy, so ably documented by William Coleman.[154] The Revolution had proclaimed both a right to health and the sanctity of property rights; when they conflicted, as the experience of the 1810 commission demonstrated, it was the former that generally had to yield. The remedy trade remained part of the liberal economy already emerging at the end of the Old Regime and only confirmed by the Revolution's definitive destruction of the guild system. Long after the United States, in the Progressive Era, had created a Pure Food and Drugs Administration and mounted a campaign at the federal level against proprietary remedies (with mixed results, it is true), France in the interwar period remained to a large extent the land of the open pharmaceutical market, its drug industry restrained chiefly by voluntary self-regulation based on the expertise of its own Laboratoire National de Contrôle des Médicaments. It took the corporatism of the Vichy regime to impose a new legal order on pharmacy, in 1941, regulating the ownership of pharmacies and establishing a new registration system for remedies. Even then, despite restrictions on pharmaceutical advertising dating back to the law of Germinal, France, as any visitor could attest, was still a place where hyperbolic health claims could be made for products ranging from liver pills to chlorophyll chewing gum, at least until a decree on pharmaceutical publicity introduced by Simone Veil as Minister of Health in 1976 set stricter limits on advertising both to the public and to the medical profession.[155] *De jure* rigour, *de facto laissez-faire,* the Academy an island of enlightened disapprobation in a sea of commercialism: this framework emerged nearly two centuries ago and proved, like many things in French society, remarkably resistant to change.

Notes

1. *Health for Sale: Quackery in England, 1660–1850* (Manchester, 1989).

2. Matthew Ramsey, 'Traditional Medicine and Medical Enlightenment: The Regulation of Secret Remedies in the Ancien Régime', *Historical Reflections/Réflexions historiques* vol. 9 (1982), nos 1–2, 215–32 (special number republished as *La Médicalisation de la société française, 1770–1830,* Jean-Pierre Goubert (ed.) [Waterloo, Ontario, 1982]).

3. Ramsey, 'Property Rights and the Right to Health: The Regulation of Secret Remedies in France, 1789–1815', in William F. Bynum and Roy Porter, (eds), *Medical Fringe and Medical Orthodoxy* (London, 1986), 79–105.

4. For overviews of the regulation of the remedy trade in the nineteenth century, see André Narod Narodetzki, *Le Remède secret: Législation et jurisprudence de la loi du 21 germinal an XI au décret du 13 juillet 1926* (Paris, 1928); Maurice Bouvet, 'La Législation de la spécialité pharmaceutique sous le régime de la loi de germinal', *Pharmacie française* 28 (1924): 2–9, 25–34, 51–62; and Alex Berman, 'Drug Control in Nineteenth-Century France: Antecedents and Directions', in John B. Blake, (ed.), *Safeguarding the Public: Historical Aspects of Medicinal Drug Control* (Baltimore, 1970).

5. We do not yet have an adequate history of nineteenth-century French pharmacy; for a prospectus, see Olivier Faure, 'Officines, pharmaciens et médicaments en France au XIXe siècle', *Bulletin de la Société d'Histoire Moderne,* 16th ser., no. 44 (1989), 31–8. Some older surveys of pharmaceutical history provide useful overviews; see, for example, André Pontier, *Histoire de la pharmacie* (Paris, 1900); L. Reutter de Rosemont, *Histoire de la pharmacie à travers les âges,* 2 vols (Paris, 1931); and Maurice Bouvet, *Histoire de la pharmacie en France des origines à nos jours* (Paris, 1937). Much can also be gleaned from the best local and regional studies, notably Guy Thuillier, 'Pour une histoire du médicament en Nivernais au XIXe siècle', *Revue d'histoire économique et sociale* 53 (1975): 73–98. On the *materia medica* of the first half of the century, see also Paul Delaunay, *D'une révolution à l'autre, 1789–1848: l'évolution des théories et de la pratique médicale* (Paris, 1949), 78–84.

6. Text of Germinal law in *Bulletin des lois,* 3d ser., 5 (Year XI), no. 2676, 121–9. On the Pluviôse law see Adolphe Trébuchet,

Jurisprudence de la médecine, de la chirurgie, et de la pharmacie en France (Paris, 1834), 366; text in *Bulletin des lois*, 4th ser., 3, no. 552.

7. Text in *Bulletin des lois*, 4th ser., 3 (Year XIII), no. 813, 227; quotation from article 1.

8. An extensive set of files on secret remedies, mingled with those involving questions of medical practice, can be found in the F^8 series at the Archives Nationales.

9. On the Paris Faculty's consultative functions and its pretension to assume the role of a national medical academy, see George Weisz, 'Les Professeurs parisiens et l'Académie de Médecine', in Christophe Charle and Régine Ferré, (eds), *Le Personnel de l'enseignement supérieur en France aux XIXe et XXe siècles* (Paris, 1985), 47–65.

10. On the medical societies, see Erwin H. Ackerknecht, *Medicine at the Paris Hospital, 1794–1848* (Baltimore, 1967), ch. 9; on the Conseil de Salubrité, see Ann Fowler La Berge, 'The Paris Health Council, 1802–1848', *Bulletin of the History of Medicine* 49 (1975): 339–52.

11. Text in *Bulletin des lois*, 4th ser., 13 (1811), no. 5874, 152–5.

12. On the legislation and on the Imperial Commission's work, see Ramsey, 'Property Rights', 92–100.

13. The commission's records of its work can be found in Académie Nationale de Médecine, MS 43, 'Registre servant à la transcription des rapports faits à la Commission [des Remèdes Secrets] sur la présentation des remèdes secrets', and 'Délibérations de la Commission des Remèdes Secrets' (register). The first entry is dated 30 November, 1810, the last, 14 August, 1813. On the remedy owners for whom the commission recommended compensation, see reports nos 54, 134–5, 223, 361, 362, and 463. In addition, Lafay's gentle vomi-purgative seemed promising as a replacement for ipecac but required more tests (no. 133).

14. *Ibid.*, no. 345.

15. Audin-Rouvière, *La Médecine sans médecin . . .* (Paris, 1823, and later editions. On the use of popular medical literature to promote proprietary remedies, see Matthew Ramsey, 'The Popularization of Medicine in France, 1650–1900', in Roy Porter, (ed.), *The Popularization of Medicine, 1650–1850* (London, 1992), 118–19.

16. Archives Nationales F^8 165, Schirvel file, his letters of 6 January, and 14 February, 1820.

17. On the origins of the Academy and its relation to the Paris Faculty of Medicine and the earlier medical societies, see George Weisz, 'Constructing the Medical Elite in France: The Creation of the Royal Academy of Medicine, 1814–20', *Medical History* 30 (1986): 419–43, and 'The Medical Elite in France in the Early Nineteenth Century', *Minerva: A Review of Science, Learning and Policy* 25 (1987): 150–70. The text of the ordinance of 20 December, 1820 is in Trébuchet, *Jurisprudence*, pt 3, ch. 1, no. 23.

18. On the work of this commission, see George Weisz, 'Water Cures

and Science: The French Academy of Medicine and Mineral Waters in the Nineteenth Century', *Bulletin of the History of Medicine* 64 (1990): 393–416.

19. *Codex medicamentarius, sive Pharmacopoeia gallica . . .* (Paris, 1818); see Marcel Delépine, 'Les Transformations des Pharmacopées Parisiennes et Françaises', *Revue d'histoire de la pharmacie* 19 (1931): 181–96, 241–53.

20. Archives Départementales de l'Hérault 106 M 1: dean to prefect, 24 July, 1822; commission report, 21 July, 1824.

21. See Société de Médecine, Chirurgie, et Pharmacie de Toulouse, *Rapport de la Commission des Remèdes Secrets, lu dans la séance du 17 septembre 1850,* copy in Bibliothèque Nationale (henceforth BN), T⁷ 268.

22. Trébuchet, *Jurisprudence*, 404.

23. On this question see Adolphe Trébuchet, 'Des brevets d'invention délivrés pour remèdes secrets', *Annales d'hygiène publique et de médecine légale* 29 (1843): 203–11.

24. On subsequent regulations and jurisprudence, see Narodetzki, *Le Remède secret.*

25. Text in Trébuchet, *Jurisprudence*, pt 3, ch. 3, no. 7; see also *Journal général de médecine* 104 (1828): 373–83 (includes commentary by the pharmacist L. J. Lebouidre Delalande on the ordinance and the law of Germinal).

26. See Trébuchet, *Jurisprudence*, 369–71, on criteria to be applied.

27. On the work of the commission, see archives of the Académie Nationale de Médecine (henceforth AM), *liasse* 26, *feuilles de présence et procès-verbaux,* 1823–1885. Dossiers on particular cases are in the following boxes (which will not be cited individually in the notes that follow): 65, materials inherited from the Napoleonic commission and work of the Academy through 1824 (lacuna for 1822); 66, 1825/6; 67, 1827/8; 68, 1829/30, 69, 1831/2. The remaining boxes (through no. 100) include dossiers from the period 1833–1940, with several lacunae; no. 101 contains registers covering the period from 6 June, 1882 to 1 March, 1927.

28. Itard, 'Rapport général sur les remèdes secrets', annual public session of 1827, in *Mémoires de l'Académie Royale de Médecine*, vol. 2, pt 1, *historique* (1833), 24–31.

29. By 1833 the Academy had still approved only these two remedies, according to a report by the Academy's permanent secretary, Étienne Pariset, 'Compte-rendu des travaux de l'Académie pendant l'année 1833', *Mémoires de l'Académie de Médecine,* 4 (1835): 31–2. See also *Archives générales de médecine* 21 (1829): 134, on Ollivier's biscuits (strongly defended in the Academy by Orfila), and *ibid.,* 22 (1830): 418, on Belloste's pills.

30. *Archives générales de médecine* 22 (1830): 418–19.

31. Bouvet, 'Législation', 31, cites report by Gueneau de Mussy,

Academy's session of 28 November, 1843, which notes that the three
purchases had been approved but the funds never budgeted. (See
'Rapport de M. Gueneau de Mussy, sur la poudre de Sency [contre le
goître]', *Bulletin de l'Académie Royale de Médecine* 9 [1843–4]:
226–30.) Bouvet also notes that at the beginning of the July,
Monarchy the list of authorized preparations, in addition to the
poudre de Sancy and Ollivier's biscuits, included Belloste's pills, the
rob Boyveau-Laffecteur (an avatar of the *rob Laffecteur* originally
approved by the Société Royale de Médecine), Dr Franck's grains of
health, the *poudre d'Irroë*, the *pommade antiophtalmique* of the widow
Farnier, and Kunckel's dermatological preparations, together with
such nonmedical products as Mme Botot's mouthwash and
Regnauld's cough drops. (The source is a statement issued in 1831
by d'Argout, Minister of Commerce and Public Works, reproduced
in Adolphe Laugier and Victor Duruy, *Pandectes pharmaceutiques*
[Paris, 1837], 304–5). None of these, however, won the Academy's
approbation as novel and effective remedies; the first four essentially
enjoyed extensions of earlier privileges (that of the *poudre d'Irroë*
dated back to the reign of Louis XV). Kunckel's preparations, as
Bouvet notes, received only provisional authorizations in 1819 and
1821. After a series of further experiments, the Academy decided in
1831 to tolerate their sale, without conferring its approbation; in
1836 it formally rejected them (*Bulletin de l'Académie Royale de
Médecine* 1 [1836]: 952). On the eight 'approved' remedies, see also
Eugène Soubeiran, 'Discours sur les remèdes secrets, autorisés par le
gouvernement', *Journal de pharmacie et de chimie* 22 (1852): 416–40.
Many essentially cosmetic products, such as Boulet's *pommade
cutanée* were simply tolerated, on the model of the Old Regime
permission tacite (on Boulet, see *Archives générales de médecine* 22
[1830]: 417); the Academy similarly recognized Regnauld's *pâte
pectorale* as a commonplace product similar to cough drops described
in pharmacopoeias, and as much a candy as a remedy.
32. Gueneau de Mussy, 'Rapport'.
33. AM, Courante file, 1827.
34. AM, Lavalle file, 1828.
35. AM, Perret file, 1828.
36. AM, report by Itard, 1 April, 1826.
37. AM, Collet to Minister of the Interior, 26 December, 1826;
commission's report, 6 February, 1827.
38. AM, Blin file, 1823; Academy's report, 21 May.
39. AM, 1825, Blondé file; report, 18 October.
40. Delaunay, *D'une révolution*, 78. See also Alex Berman, 'The
Persistence of Theriac in France', *Pharmacy in History* 12 (1970):
5–12, and Delépine, 'Transformations des Pharmacopées'. The
codex of 1908 was the first to include systematic assays for identity
and purity.

41. Goldstein, *Console and Classify: The French Psychiatric Profession in the Nineteenth Century* (Cambridge, 1987).

42. See Arthur K. Shapiro, 'A Contribution to a History of the Placebo Effect', *Behavioral Science,* 5 (1960): 119, citing A. Leslie, 'Ethics and Practice of Placebo Therapy', *American Journal of Medicine* 16 (1954): 854.

43. François-Emmanuel Fodéré, *Traité de médecine légale et d'hygiène publique, ou de police de santé, adapté aux codes de l'Empire français, et aux connaissances actuelles,* 6 vols (Paris, 1813), 6: 411.

44. AM, 1827, Sarta file.

45. AM, 1825, Piaget file.

46. AM, Pradel file, commission's report, 16 December, 1822.

47. Archives Nationales F⁸ 162, Percheron file, 1830/1; Percheron to Minister of the Interior, 14 December, 1830.

48. AM, 1824, Alix file.

49. See Ramsey, 'Traditional Medicine', 230–1 (which gives the recipe), and 'Property Rights', 97–9.

50. AM, Belloste file, report of commission on secret remedies, approved 9 March, 1830; see also AM MS 43.

51. Maurice Bouvet, 'Les Pilules de Belloste', *Bulletin des sciences pharmacologiques* 35 (1928): 246–59, 297–312. For a contemporaneous report on the Academy's investigation, see *Archives générales de médecine* 22 (1830): 418–19.

52. 'Rapport général', 27.

53. V. de Moléon, (ed.), *Rapports généraux sur la salubrité publique, rédigés par les conseils ou les administrations,* pt 2, *Rapports généraux sur les travaux du Conseil de Salubrité de la ville de Paris,* 2 vols (Paris, 1828–41), 1: 328–9.

54. 'Rapport général', 30.

55. AM, 'Rapport sur la lettre de Mʳ le Préfet de Police en date du 16 août 1828', 2 September, 1828.

56. AM, Arnault-Bion file, petition to Minister of the Interior, with recipe, 9 November, 1824; request for suppression, 4 January, 1825. Double, report of 28 November, 1824, summarized in *Archives générales de médecine* 6 (1824): 618.

57. Archives Communales de Nantes I 5 8, dossier 6, prefect of Loire-Inférieure to mayor on jury's report, 29 December, 1820.

58. Delaunay, *D'une Révolution,* 90.

59. AM, report on prefect's letter, 2 September, 1828. The prefect had written to the Academy on 16 August, enclosing copies of the ordinance of 21 June, on secret remedies that denounced abuses and called for better enforcement.

60. Except as noted, this account is based on documents in the archives of the Académie Royale de Médecine.

61. These and other details of the remedies' history, together with a bibliography of writings on Leroy's formulas and methods, can be

found in *Méthode purgative de Le Roy: faits de pratique et guérisons* (Paris, 1886).

62. Charles E. Rosenberg, 'The Therapeutic Revolution: Medicine, Meaning, and Social Change in Nineteenth-Century America', in Rosenberg and Morris J. Vogel, (eds), *The Therapeutic Revolution: Essays in the Social History of American Medicine* (Philadelphia, 1979), 3–25.

63. 5th edn, (Paris, 1817). Titles of the earlier edns varied, e.g., *La Médecine naturelle, curative et populaire, contenant l'exposé de la cause des maladies et celui des moyens propres à opérer sciemment et sûrement la guérison des maladies, découverts ou approfondis par J. Pelgas . . . ,* 3rd edn, (1812). The last edition in the BN dates from 1836. Leroy also published two editions of a rejoinder to critics of this work and of his remedies, *Le Charlatanisme démasqué, ou la Médecine appréciée à sa juste valeur, par un ami de la vérité et de l'humanité* (Orléans, 1819); the second edition (Paris, 1819), is described in its subtitle as *[Un] ouvrage composé pour repousser les injures et calomnies qui ont été dirigées ou qui pourroient l'être contre la 'Médecine curative du chirurgien Le Roi'. . . .* Successive editions of *La Médecine curative* also devoted an increasing number of pages to Leroy's running polemical battle with his critics, as well as to testimonials for his remedies.

64. *Gazette des malades, ou recueil des faits-pratiques de médecine, de chirurgie et de chimie.*

65. See William H. Helfand, 'James Morison and His Pills: A Study of the Nineteenth Century Pharmaceutical Market', *Transactions of the British Society for the History of Pharmacy*, 1974, 101–35. Morison's writings were translated into French, and his disciples across the Channel produced an abundant literature; see, for example, Morison, *Nouvelles Vérités médicales, ou Connaissance des causes des maladies* (Paris, 1839), and V.-C. Charles de Saint-Félix, *Morisoniana français, ou Nouvelle Doctrine de l'hygeist Morison . . .* (Paris, 1836). Cf. the case of Félix-Louis-Auguste de Bourla, who resented suggestions that his remedy was the same as Leroy's but in fact espoused a nearly identical system (Bourla, *Mémoire pour faire triompher la vérité qui se rattache le plus au bonheur général de la société* [Bordeaux, 1830]). Bourla, who described himself as a former military surgeon, argued that the cause of disease was not in the blood but in the humours, and that putrescent humours could be expelled through repeated use of his purgatives. Since 'la vie est dans le sang' (22), bleeding was generally to be avoided; the leeches favoured by the Broussais school were simply 'la saignée déguisée' (34–5).

66. Minister of Interior to Faculty, 15 October, 1817.

67. Archives Nationales F⁷ 9292, no. 11543, 2 October, 1818.

68. Ms note by Esquirol on physician Guiton. Chaussier added the comment: 'Faut-il donc donner le nom de remède à un poison

horrible?'

69. Interior Ministry, Bureau des Secours et Hôpitaux, to Paris Faculty, 17 March, 1820.

70. Leroy to Minister of Interior, 12 February, 1821.

71. Report, 21 February, 1821.

72. Report by *officiers de santé* to Bréchard, mayor of Fontenay-le-Comte, 29 July, 1821.

73. Baron Capelle to Academy, 14 September, 1821.

74. AM, 2 October, 1821.

75. Pharmacist Chavoix to Boullay, 15 October, 1821.

76. Archives Départementales de la Loire-Inférieure 4 X 231, 1 January, 1822, quoted in Jacques Léonard, *Les Médecins de l'Ouest au XIXe siècle* (Paris, 1978), 617.

77. AM, Ministère de la Marine et des Colonies, extract of reports by Conseil de Santé, Point-à-Pitre, 3 October and 1 November, 1821; extract from letter of Dr Noverre, Martinique, 7 November.

78. In the long line of anti-Leroy tracts, see, for example, Cazaugran, MD, *Lettre à Monsieur J. M. M.* (Toulouse, n.d. [1825]), which attacks the idea that blood cannot be superfluous, and F. J. Lebout, *La Vraie Médecine aux prises avec le charlatanisme, ou Examen critique de plusieurs doctrines médicales dangereuses pour le peuple, et particulièrement de la médecine dite curative de M. Leroy* (Paris, 1837), a satirical dialogue, which suggests that excretion serves a normal physiological function, not that of expelling superfluous or impure humours (166).

79. One example, among several attacked by Leroy in his *Médecine curative*: F.-P. Émangard, *Du charlatanisme en général et de quelques remèdes secrets en particulier* (L'Aigle, 1823). Much of the polemical material on Leroy is presumably now lost, but a substantial collection, including many of Leroy's own publications and pamphlets such as Émangard's, is conserved at the BN; see its *Catalogue des sciences médicales*, vol. 2 (Paris, 1873), 737–9. A particularly clever and well-informed anti-Leroy tract in the collection is the anonymous *Pot-pourri sur la médecine prétendue curative du chirurgien Leroy . . . , par un vosgien valétudinaire* (Paris, 1823), BN Te^151 1151; it contains an extended parallel between Leroy's remedy and medical system and the eighteenth-century counterparts promoted by the empiric J.-P.-G. Ailhaud. For a typical tit-for-tat exchange, see *Médecine curative panchymagogue de Monsieur Le Roy: Du syrmaïsme, ou de la purgation par haut et bas, par un vétérinaire, ami de l'humanité* (Montbrison, 1826), BN Te^151 1171, and *Réponse à l'écrit intitulé Du syrmaïsme . . .* (Lyons, 1826), BN Te^151 1172.

80. Dupont, *Examen critique des ouvrages et des purgatifs du Sr Leroy* (Paris, 1824), 14, 15.

81. Renard (described as the holder of a Paris medical doctorate), letter

in L. Bernard, comp., *Réponse à l'erreur, à l'ignorance et à la mauvaise foi de ces gens qui veulent intimider, effrayer et terroriser; qui veulent faire des dupes et non pas des amis* (Lille, 1824), 3.

82. 'Les tribunaux d'Orléans, respectant la liberté individuelle & les principes de la charité chrétienne, ont déclaré "qu'il est à chacun d'avoir recours à tous les moyens curatifs, bons ou mauvais, auxquels il a confiance, qu'il peut en faire usage, qu'il peut même, lorsqu'il est persuadé d'en avoir éprouvé les bons effets, en recommander l'usage sans contravention aux lois"'(Archives Nationales F⁸ 152, Curchod to Minister of Interior, 'Mémoire . . . tendant à réfuter la pétition de MM. les Médecins de Lyon relative aux médicaments du chirurgien Le Roy', June 1822); Curchod borrowed the quotation from Leroy's *Charlatanisme démasqué.* Cf. Curchod, *A M. R. de La Prade, Médecin de l'Hôtel-Dieu à Lyon* (Lyons, 1822).

83. [Curchod], *Lettre adressé à M. Leroy, chirurgien consultant à Paris* (Lyons, 1825), 8–9. Cf. *idem, Avis aux amis de l'humanité souffrante* ([Lyons], 1822) and *Le Remède dit Leroy est-il réellement un poison? ou Observations d'un philanthrope sur les principales objections des antagonistes de la médecine curative, dédiées aux amis de la vérité et de l'humanité* (Lyons, 1823).

84. See, for example, Curchod, *Le Cri de l'opprimé, dédié aux pères de la Patrie* (Geneva, 1810).

85. This expression, which Leroy attributed to his enemies, occurs in *La Médecine curative* (Paris: imprimerie de Nicolas-Vaucluse, 1823), 9.

86. AM, 6 January, 1823.

87. *Extrait d'un rapport présenté à s. exc. M⁸ʳ le Ministre secrétaire d'état de l'intérieur, par l'Académie Royale de Médecine* (Paris, 1823).

88. *Ibid.,* 3.

89. *Ibid.,* 11.

90. Archives Nationales F⁷ 9292, no. 11543, Administration Générale des Communes des Hospices, des Établissements de Bienfaisance, des Hospices, et des Établissements Sanitaires, Division des Hospices, 2ᵉ bureau, circular no. 40, 19 July, 1823.

91. [Curchod], *Réfutation du rapport de l'Académie Royale de Médecine, adressée à son Excellence le Ministre de l'Intérieur, relatif aux remèdes de M. Leroy; Leroy, Un petit mot à l'oreille de l'Académie Royale de Médecine, au sujet du rapport présenté par elle à S. E. le ministre de l'Intérieur, concernant les médicamens indiqués dans la 'Médecine curative' du chirurgien Le Roy, par l'auteur du 'Charlatanisme démasqué . . .* (Paris, 1824). Cf. Bernard, *Réponse à l'erreur,* 27, n. 1, which calls the Academy's report exaggerated at best, adding that 'l'on pourrait même dire, à celui qui l'a rédigé, et à ceux qui l'ont approuvé, qu'ils ont surpris la religion du ministre'.

92. Martin, *Examen critique de l'extrait d'un Rapport, présenté à S. Exc. le ministre-secrétaire d'État de l'Intérieur, par l'Académie Royale de Médecine . . .* (Paris, n.d. [1823]). For a response to Martin, see

Dupont, *Examen critique*, 47–8.

93. Lettre à M. Pariset . . . (Paris, 1826).

94. On the response in one department, the Charente, and its failure to halt widespread sales of the drugs by tavern-keepers, chair-makers and others, alone or in league with medical men, see Jacques Planty-Mauxion, *Appel sur la répression des abus introduits dans l'exercice de l'art de guérir.* . . , 3 parts in 1 vol. (Angoulême, 1826–9), *Complément de l'appel,* 65–6, 75–6, 138.

95. See, for example, *Plaidoyer de M. Duclos, dans le procès qui a été intenté par le ministère public devant le tribunal de police correctionnelle de Provins, le 12 novembre 1823* . . . (Provins and Nogent-sur-Seine, 1824). Duclos was convicted and fined; the decision of the Minister of the Interior, he wrote, 'basée sur un rapport mensonger de l'Académie de Médecine', had provided '[une] belle occasion pour MM. les Docteurs et Pharmaciens, de mettre en exécution un projet conçu depuis long-temps de me faire un procès'.

96. Archives Nationales F⁷ 9292, no. 11543, Ministry of the Interior, Division des Hospices, 2ᵉ bureau, circular no. 44.

97. Leroy, *Aux abonnés de la Gazette des malades* (Paris, 1824).

98. Archives Départementales de la Loire-Atlantique 1 M 1358, no. 326, 30 October, 1826.

99. Archives Départementales de la Loire 38 M 9, no. 5, 21 December, 1826; autopsy report dated 15 December.

100. On the events leading to the duel, see Archives Nationales F⁻ 9292, no. 11543, prefect, Loire, to Minister of the Interior, 9 August, 1826. On the polemics, see *L'Ermite de Saint-Étienne, ou son opinion sur la petite guerre qui s'est élevée à Saint-Étienne (Loire), entre les partisans et les antagonistes de la méthode du chirurgien Le Roy* (Paris, 1826); quotation, 38.

101. Archives Départementales de la Loire-Atlantique 1 M 1358, no. 323A, prefect to Conseil de Salubrité, 18 April, 1827.

102. Archives Nationales F⁷ 9292, no. 11543.

103. Archives Départementales de la Loire-Atlantique 1 M 1358, no. 318, 18 June, 1828.

104. For an overview of the rob's history, see Maurice Bouvet, 'Un remède secret du XVIIIᵉ siècle: le Rob Boyveau-Laffecteur', *Bulletin de la Société d'Histoire de la Pharmacie* 39 (1923): 264–72, and Étienne Michelon, *Histoire pharmacotechnique et pharmacologique du mercure à travers les siècles* (Tours, 1906), 187–98. On the rob in the Old Regime, see also Ramsey, 'Traditional Medicine', 227–9.

105. On the rob's medical uses, see Nicolas-Philibert Adelon *et al.*, *Dictionnaire des sciences médicales par une société de médecins et de chirurgiens,* . . . , 60 vols (Paris: 1812–22), s.v. 'Rob antisyphilitique de Laffecteur' (by François Fournier de Pescay).

106. See, for example, Boyveau-Laffecteur's flyer, *Question de propriété soumise au Conseil d'État* (n.p., n.d.); the copy in Archives

Départementales de l'Hérault 106 M 1 has a handwritten notation at the bottom giving the address of Boyveau's agent in Montpellier.

107. AM MS 43, nos 133 (Gouzil) and 134 (Hoffmann). The commissioners, while disclaiming any responsibility for deciding *questions de droit*, recognized Develuos's priority on the basis of his publications dating from the 1760s and a warrant granted in 1768 by the Commission Royale de Médecine (a special agency that regulated secret remedies before that function passed to the Société Royale in 1778). They seem to have based their conclusion that Gouzil's claims had at least some merit on the close resemblance of the formula he provided to those of both Develuos and Boyveau.

108. The BN has a collection of advertisements and prospectuses for the remedy, put out by the various distributors between 1778 and 1856 (Te[151] 1300); see, for example, *Communication à MM. les préfets, sous-préfets et maires des départemens, relative à la légalité des dépôts du rob anti-syphilitique de Laffecteur* (n.d. [no earlier than 1829]). See also *Précis historique et observations sur les effets du rob antisyphilitique de Boyveau-Laffecteur . . .* , new edn, (Paris, 1821).

109. Boyveau-Laffecteur's arguments against Giraudeau can be found in his *Notes supplétives à ma demande adressée à M. le préfet de police contre le Sr Giraudeau de St-Gervais* (Paris, 1845). The quarrel of the two champions of the rob Laffecteur was a notorious one; see, for example, Lucien Dupont, *Du charlatanisme médical en France: Considérations philanthropiques* (Lille, 1838), 24–5.

110. See, for example, Giraudeau de Saint-Gervais, *L'Art de se guérir soi-même, ou Traitement des maladies vénériennes sans mercure . . .* (Paris, 1827); *Art de guérir les dartres en détruisant leur principe par une méthode végétale . . .* (Paris, 1828). The collections of the BN include numerous editions and variations of these and other overlapping works, as well as of the *Journal de médecine usuelle.* For Giraudeau's ambitious claims for his remedies, see, for example, the *Journal de médecine usuelle*, no. 101, 30 March, 1850, 1. The remedy was said to cure various skin diseases, together with 'les accidents provenant des couches, de l'âge critique et de l'âcreté héréditaire des humeurs. Comme dépuratif puissant, il préserve du choléra, convient pour les catarrhes de vessie, les rétrécissements et la faiblesse des organes provenant d'abus d'injections ou de sondes . . . .'

111. See, for example, *A Monsieur le président et à Messieurs les conseillers à la Cour de Cassation* (n.p., n.d. [no earlier than 1847]).

112. *Ibid.*, 4, 22.

113. Boyveau-Laffecteur, *Notes supplétives*, 3.

114. See 'Vente de la propriété du Rob de Boyveau-Laffecteur, à M. Giraudeau de Saint-Gervais', appendix to Giraudeau, *A Monsieur le président.*

115. Léonard, *Médecins de l'Ouest*, 617.

116. Narodetzki, *Le Remède secret*, 94.

117. See, for example, Thuillier, 'Pour une histoire du médicament', who writes of pharmaceutical 'anarchy' in the Nivernais in the first half of the nineteenth century and 'un certain désordre' even in the second (78, 94).

118. *Observations soumises à la Cour royale de Rennes par les pharmaciens de Nantes, appelants à un jugement rendu par le tribunal de police correctionnelle de Nantes, le 22 mai 1841;* Piogey, *Du charlatanisme*, 26. For a contrasting view of the Academy's sense of mission, see Victor Meurein, *De l'influence fâcheuse des remèdes secrets et des remèdes spéciaux sur la médecine et la pharmacie au point de vue scientifique et professionnel; jurisprudence française en matière de remèdes secrets et spéciaux* (Toulouse, 1852), ii.

119. Michel-Joseph-Marie Richard, *Sur les erreurs populaires relatives à la médecine et leurs dangers,* published Paris medical thesis, 1833, no. 36, 6.

120. Société Académique de Nantes, 1831 report, quoted in 'Rapport sur les voies et moyens proprosés pour réprimer le charlatanisme . . .', *Annales de la Société Royale Académique de Nantes et du département de la Loire-Inférieure,* 2d ser., 2 (1841): 394–5.

121. Archives Départementales des Hautes-Alpes 141M, nos 123–4, Reinoard to prefect, 5 October, 1817.

122. See, for example, Planty-Mauxion, *Appel sur la répression des abus,* 142, n. 1.

123. E. Féraud *et al., Rapport fait à la Société Académique de Médecine sur les questions relatives au projet de loi sur la médecine* (Marseille, 1829), 27–8.

124. Piogey, *Du charlatanisme,* 20.

125. On the new pharmacy, see, for example, *ibid.,* 20–1.

126. Planty-Mauxion, for example, in *Appel sur la répression des abus,* 142, n. 1, cites Portal, Magendie, Caventou, Pelletier, Chaptal, Vauquelain, and Broussais as great innovators who never attempted to make trade secrets of their discoveries.

127. See, for example, *Appel en Cour royale: Atteinte à la liberté individuelle des médecins et des pharmaciens; examen de la question des remèdes secrets* ([Paris], 1829), and *Quelques observations relatives à l'annonce et aux remèdes secrets* (Paris, 1845), whose anonymous author, a champion of pharmacists' freedom to advertise and sell remedies, identified himself as a member of the great national medical congress held in Paris in 1845.

128. Piogey, *Du charlatanisme,* 25.

129. Quoted in Meurein, *De l'influence,* 2.

130. See, for example, Cornac *et al.,* 'Project de lettre à M. le ministre des travaux publics et du commerce, touchant la concession de brevets d'invention pour remèdes', *Annales d'hygiène publique et de médecine légale* 19 (1838): 226–31, and Trébuchet, 'Des brevets d'invention'.

131. See Bouvet, 'Législation', 53.

132. Text in Narodetzki, *Le Remède secret*, 134–5, n. 1.
133. Text of judgment in *ibid.*, 35–40.
134. See, for example, *ibid.*, 54–74, on a notorious case of 1906 involving urotropin, used to treat bladder infections; the remedy could not be considered magistral, despite the prescription, because the pharmacist had ordered it from a commercial laboratory instead of 'compounding' this simple drug substance following the physician's express directions.
135. Text in *ibid.*, 29.
136. See Gaultier de Claubry, report of the Commission des Remèdes Secrets et Nouveaux, on the implications of the decree of 3 May, *Bulletin de l'Académie Nationale de Médecine* 15 (1849–50): 1017–19.
137. Albert Legris, deputy *avocat-général* of the Cour de Cassation, quoted in Narodetzki, *Le Remède secret*, 67; this is the case mentioned above in n. 134.
138. Pariset, 'Compte-rendu . . . 1833', 31.
139. The commission's findings were reported at regular intervals in the *Bulletin de l'Académie*, whose first volume covered the academic year 1836/7 (when all proposed remedies were rejected). See also AM *liasse* 26, for the commission's minutes.
140. 'M. Pariset, au nom de l'Académie de Medecine, à M. Sauçon, pharmacien', 30 March, 1843, quoted in Meurein, *De l'influence*, 71–2.
141. The remedies that were favourably received included Vallet's pills of iron carbonate (used in the treatment of chlorosis, 1838), Rogé's *limonade* (a purgative solution of magnesium citrate, 1847), a preparation of cusso (the brayera plant, used against tapeworm) brought back from Africa by the explorer Rochet d'Héricourt (1847), and Belloc's charcoal for digestive disorders (1849), together with preparations of ferrous lactate by Gélis and Conté. Report on Vallet: *Bulletin de l'Académie Royale de Médecine* 2 (1837–8): 706–14; on Rogé and Rochet d'Héricourt: *ibid.*, 12 (1846–7): 684–96. Each of these three individuals had submitted a paper on his remedy, and in all these cases, the Academy, on the basis of the positive results of clinical tests, voted to thank the author for his contribution – an endorsement, to be sure, but less than a formal approbation. The Academy also urged Rochet d'Héricourt 'à nous procurer du Cousso à un prix raisonnable par tous les moyens qui sont en son pouvoir' and called for chemical analysis of the plant (694); but its committee's report also noted that pomegranate root was more effective (even if less gentle). To the list of approved remedies could be added the *pains ferrugineux* of Derouet-Boissières, cited in a circular of 2 November, 1850 from the Minister of Agriculture and Commerce, Dumas, to the prefects, quoted in Narodetzki, *Le Remède secret*, 30–1. See also Bouvet, *Le Remède secret*, 33, and Delaunay, *D'une révolution*, 89.

142. The reports concerned 44 remedies in academic year 1864/5, for example, 21 in 1890, and still fewer in 1920, when the commission received at least 14 submissions but presented its report to the Academy in secret session. See *Bulletin de l'Académie Imperiale de Médecine*, vol. 30, and *Bulletin de l'Académie Nationale de Médecine*, 3rd ser., vols 23–4, 83–4.

143. Weisz, *The Medical Mandarins: The French Academy of Medicine in the Nineteenth and Twentieth Centuries*, forthcoming. This development may also be seen as part of a secular and more general transformation of France's national academies from the scientific institutions of the Old Regime, with a relatively young membership actively engaged in research and practice, to the essentially honorific institutions of the late twentieth century, in which membership normally crowns a long and illustrious career.

144. The dimensions of the problem are apparent, for example, in the trials involving the Leroy remedies; see *Médicamens Le Roy: Jugement du tribunal de Rouen et arrêt de la cour royale de la même ville* (Paris, 1842), and *Jugement et arrêts concernant la médecine de Le Roy* (Paris, 1844), BN Te[151] 1177–8. In the absence of explicit penal provisions in the law of Germinal or other modern legislation, the courts turned to Old Regime regulations, chiefly an *arrêt* of the Parlement of Paris of 23 July, 1748, which required apothecaries in the capital to follow the formulary of the Medical Faculty of Paris. In 1867, the Cour de Cassation definitively sanctioned the view that the law of Germinal had extended these provisions to all of France (reversing its earlier position that the law of Germinal had completely superseded earlier legislation), but this interpretation remained controversial. See Narodetzki, *Le Remède secret*, 105–18.

145. See Bouvet, 'Législation', 54–5, 58–9. Féraud *et al.*, *Rapport*, was the work of a committee of a medical society of Marseilles; Meurein, *De l'influence*, was a prize-winning essay for a contest sponsored by the Société de Médecine, Chirurgie et Pharmacie de Toulouse in 1852 on the triple subject, 'De l'influence des remèdes secrets sur la médecine et la pharmacie au double point de vue scientifique et professionnel; des remèdes dits spéciaux, considérés au même point de vue; de la jurisprudence française en matière de remèdes secrets et spéciaux.'

146. *Actes du Congrès médical de France, session de 1845, section de médecine* (Paris, 1846), 213–15; Bouvet, 'Législation', 55.

147. Féraud *et al.*, 'Rapport', 28.

148. See, for example, Planty-Mauxion, *Appel sur la répression des abus*, 3.

149. Royer-Collard, *Proposition faite à l'Académie Royale de Médecine, dans la séance du 31 mai 1842, dans le but de réprimer le charlatanisme en médecine . . .* (Paris, 1842); reprinted from *Bulletin de l'Académie*, 7.

150. Narodetzki, *Le Remède secret*, 121–8 (text of law, 121–2).

151. Text of decree of 13 July, 1926 in *ibid.*, 203–4; Narodetzski's ch. 3, 187–216, is devoted to the background and implications of this legislation.

152. Law of 25 April, 1895 (text in *ibid.*, 138–9, n. 2); the most widely used vaccine, for smallpox, was exempted.

153. Stanley Hoffmann, 'Paradoxes of the French Political Community', in Hoffmann *et al.*, *In Search of France* (Cambridge, Mass., 1963), 1–117.

154. Coleman, *Death is a Social Disease: Public Health and Political Economy in Early Industrial France* (Madison, Wisc., 1982).

155. See Leigh Hancher, *Regulating for Competition: Government, Law, and the Pharmaceutical Industry in the United Kingdom and France* (Oxford: 1990), chs 4 and 8, and, on the American experience, James Harvey Young, Jr., *The Medical Messiahs: A Social History of Health Quackery in Twentieth-Century America* (Princeton, 1967). Cf. Young, *The Toadstool Millionaires: A Social History of Patent Medicines in America before Federal Regulation* (Princeton, 1961). The French legislation of 1941 awarded 'visas' to drugs that could demonstrate therapeutic value, safety, and novelty – the last provision a *de facto* patent, at a time when French law still did not formally permit patents for medicines (a special type of patent for drugs was introduced following an overhaul of the system of registration in 1959).

2

Consultation by Letter in Early Eighteenth-Century Paris: The Medical Practice of Etienne-François Geoffroy[1]

Laurence Brockliss

Introduction

A substantial part of élite medical practice in seventeenth- and eighteenth-century Europe consisted of giving consultations by letter. Patients, or their representatives, would approach the leading physicians of the day through a written communication which would provide details of the nature, history and treatment of the malady for which advice was sought. The consultant would then prepare a written reply wherein he would outline his own diagnosis of the disease and suggest a suitable cure. At no stage would the consultant necessarily see the patient, even as was often the case, he or she lived locally.

In part, the practice reflected the limited diagnostic tools in the hands of contemporary physicians. Before the invention of the stethoscope and the widespread medical use of the thermometer physicians had few objective means of studying illness: primarily they relied on the patient's description of his malady which could be just as conveniently conveyed by letter as by word of mouth.[2] Even in the early–modern period, however, some form of hands-on medical investigation took place. Urinoscopy, so favoured by medieval physicians, definitely went out of fashion but the ritual of taking the patient's pulse was never abandoned.[3] More importantly, the practice of consulting by letter was encouraged by the contemporary concept of status. In the seventeenth and eighteenth centuries those who made their livings using their heads rather than their hands were more highly honoured. Given this fact the status of the medical physician was potentially ambiguous. Medicine was one of the three 'higher' sciences taught in Europe's universities and, like its sisters theology and law, was deemed an intellectual, not a practical, discipline devoted to the study of causes. On the other hand, medicine had an obvious practical dimension which continually threatened to transform it into an art, and consequently placed it at the bottom of the hierarchy of sciences.[4] The obvious way for physicians to emphasize their status was to touch their patients as little as possible. Seeing patients, of course, was generally inevitable, especially in a period when home visits were frequent.[5] Consulting by letter, however, conveniently removed the patient from sight altogether. The physician would offer his advice on a written request as a learned man of science whose knowledge stemmed from his wide reading as much as, if not more than, his personal experience. Thereby, he would only confirm his status the more in that he was aping the behaviour of his brother professionals. Learned theologians and lawyers also consulted by letter in response to demands for solutions to moral dilemmas and legal problems.[6]

The practice of consulting by letter, it must be said, was established in late medieval Europe. It was not an invention of the early–modern period. Indeed, as early as 1150 the abbot of Cluny, Peter the Venerable, wrote to a *medicus* called Bartholomeus (perhaps of Salerno) seeking advice on an upper-respiratory problem.[7] However, it seems likely that before 1500 the practice was only well established in Italy, where it was commonplace from the thirteenth century for town councils as well as prominent individuals to demand a consultation in writing. Whereas the archives contain many medical *consilia* from Renaissance Italy, I have encountered none in France before the 1620s.[8] Obviously, for the practice to flourish more widely a variety of conditions needed to be fulfilled. There had to be a reasonably well-organized and reliable postal network, a high level of literacy among the élite, and a contemporary medical discourse common to both patients and practitioners. All three conditions pertained in most parts of Western Europe by the end of the seventeenth century.[9] Significantly, the Scientific Revolution had had little effect on medical vocabulary. Athough Galenism had been re-placed by chemical or mechanical explanations of physiological change, the medical philosophers of the Enlightenment still deployed a traditional qualitative vocabulary based largely on culinary metaphors which was easily assimilated by a lay audience.[10] Not surprisingly, then, the Age of the Enlightenment was also the age of consulting by letter *par excellence*. There is no better testimony to the popularity of the genre at the turn of the eighteenth century than that it was patronized by the greatest princes of Europe. Thus William of Orange in 1702 sought consultations from all the leading medical practitioners of the continent, including (albeit incognito) the chief physician of his arch-enemy Louis XIV.[11]

In the Age of the Enlightenment consultation by letter also played an important part in intra-professional evaluation. For a provincial physician to seek advice from the leading lights of the profession was a mark of deference, a way of acknowledging the superiority of a handful of medical stars. In an age of patronage it was the means whereby a junior doctor could place his foot on the first rung of the medical ladder. In 1731 the young François Boissier de Sauvages, a practitioner in the small town of Alès near Nîmes consulted the great Boerhaave on the malady of one of his lady patients. At the same time, he sent the Leiden physician a copy of his recently published essay on nosology implicitly hoping for Boerhaave's approbation.[12] In contrast, less deferential and ambitious medical men used the practice to demonstrate (to themselves at least) that the reputation of such medical stars was overblown. In the mid-eighteenth century the most famous practitioner in Montpellier was Antoine Fizes (1690–1768), supposedly a great expert on venereal disease. When Tobias Smollett visited the town in 1763 he could not resist testing Fizes's reputation by seeking a consultation on his own pulmonary condition. Needless to say, the Scottish doctor found Fizes's consultation inadequate. Not only did the Montpellier physician mis-diagnose Smollett's complaint by ignoring what Smollett had written. Furthermore, even if Fizes's diagnosis had been correct, his suggested treatment was unacceptable: 'his remedies savour strongly of the old woman'.[13]

Given the importance of consulting by letter it is peculiar at first sight that the practice has been largely ignored by early–modern medical historians. Moreover, as consulting by letter was an eighteenth-century art form and the efforts of several physicians, such as the French vitalist P. J. Barthez (1734–1806), were published, material for a study of the phenomenon would seem to be readily available.[14] On the other hand, studying the practice is much more difficult than it might seem, for the collections of printed consultations only tell one half of the story. They provide the physician's response to the request for advice but never the original letter. Hence, it is always hard to tell whether the consultations are literary fictions. In the age of the epistolary novel, physicians might well have used printed collections of consultations as a way of showing off their knowledge in an elegant and popular fashion. Unfortunately, it is also difficult to study the original correspondence in manuscript, for in-coming letters seem to have been largely destroyed. However, in the course of my researches into seventeenth-

and eighteenth-century French medical practice, I have discovered a cache of manuscript consultations in the Paris Bibliothèque de la Faculté de Médecine which actually does tell both sides of the story. This is a collection of some 400 cases which were submitted to the judgement of the early-eighteenth century Parisian physician, Etienne-François Geoffroy (1672–1731). The earliest consultations were composed in the early 1700s but the large majority of the correspondence dates from the 1720s, especially the six years 1724–1730. Admittedly, the record is not complete but by and large the collection contains both the original request and Geoffroy's subsequent reply in the form of a draft (often much corrected).[15]

In the light of the remarks above, the value of this collection cannot be exaggerated. The present chapter uses the Geoffroy correspondence to examine the phenomenon of consulting by letter in early–modern France for the first time.[16] However, the chapter has a deeper purpose, for the collection also provides an important insight into the realities of French seventeenth- and eighteenth-century medical practice *tout court*. In the case of England a great deal has been done in recent years to map the history of medical practice in this period, especially through the efforts of Roy Porter and his colleagues in the Wellcome Units in Great Britain.[17] In the case of France, however, our knowledge is still in its infancy. This in part reflects the problems of locating the source material from which the map can be constructed, once an attempt is made to go beyond the printed textbooks and polemics published by prominent practitioners.[18] In particular it is difficult to study medical practice from the patient's point of view, quite rightly a central concern of current medical history. The Catholic French, unlike the Calvinist English, were not usually given to committing the intimate details of their physical and spiritual health to paper. There are no French diarists, like Josselin and Pepys, and memoir writers seldom provide information about their diseases.[19] The Geoffroy correspondence, therefore, is a privileged source. As a result, the present chapter also aims to provide a novel insight into patient–practitioner relations in early eighteenth-century France and further fuel the debate as to whether medicine in the early–modern period was patient-led.[20]

Etienne-François Geoffroy

Geoffroy was born in 1672 into a dynasty of Parisian apothecaries.[21] His father, Matthieu-François Geoffroy, was an enthusiastic devotee of the experimental philosophy whose home was used for demonstrations and lectures. From an early age, therefore,

Etienne-François rubbed shoulders with *académiciens*. He was intended to follow his father's profession and in 1692 was sent to Montpellier to prepare for his Paris *maîtrise* which he obtained in 1694.[22] Geoffroy himself, however, expressed the wish to become a physician and he never practised the art of pharmacy. On his return to Paris he turned his attention to the new science, becoming a pupil of the chemist, Willem Homberg (1652–1715), one of his father's scientific friends. At the same time, he must have studied medicine at the Paris faculty and the Jardin du Roi,[23] for in 1698, although not yet qualified, he went to England as the personal physician of the French ambassador. In England Geoffroy pursued his scientific interests. Armed with a letter of introduction to the secretary Hans Sloane from the botanist Joseph Pitton de Tournefort (*c.* 1655–1708), he quickly showed off his experimental prowess before the Royal Society and was elected a candidate member.[24] Once more in France a similar honour was accorded him by the Académie des Sciences. He was made an *élève chimiste* in January 1699 and an *associé chimiste* in the following December, eventually becoming a *pensionnaire chimiste* in 1715. In the next few years he must have decided to take his medical degree, for in 1702 after a trip to Italy he became a bachelor in medicine at the Paris faculty. Two years later, after sustaining the stipulated three dissertations, he became a doctor in medicine and gained the right to practise as a physician in the capital.[25]

The rest of Geoffroy's life was passed in four different guises. In the first he was a leading light in the Paris scientific community. Between 1700 and 1720 Geoffroy contributed 17 articles to the *Mémoires de l'Académie des Sciences*. The most famous was a paper published in 1718 which pioneered the study of chemical affinity. In it Geoffroy explored the different tendencies of substances to unite with one another and formulated the law that when two substances are united, one or other will in preference unite with a third that is introduced where there is a greater rapport (his word). Geoffroy also played an important role in the popularization of Newtonian optics in France. Having received a copy of the 1704 English *Opticks* from Sloane, Geoffroy immediately translated it into French. Although the translation was never published, he did read a précis of the *Opticks* before the Académie des Sciences in 1706–7. Geoffroy also helped Père Sébastien replicate Newton's colour experiments for the first time in France in 1719.[26]

In his second guise, Geoffroy was a teacher. From 1707–30 he held the post of 'démonstrateur de l'intérieur des plantes et professeur en chimie et pharmacie' at the Paris Jardin du Roi, first as substitute for the king's chief physician, Gui-Crescent Fagon (1638–1718), and then from 1712 in his own right. From 1709–31 he also held a chair at the Paris Collège Royal. This was a college independent of the University of Paris which provided quality teaching in the traditional sciences.[27] Geoffroy gave a course on *matière médicale* and his lectures were posthumously published.[28] In addition, for one year 1714–15, Geoffroy taught botany at the Paris faculty as well.[29] He seems to have been an extremely assiduous lecturer, purportedly teaching for four to five hours at a time without a break. He was also very interested in perfecting the teaching resources of the Jardin du Roi. Many of his letters to Sloane concern building up the natural history cabinet and the collection of plants in the botanical garden. Thus in May 1715 Sloane promised to forward duplicate examples of plants in his own possession which were lacking at Paris. Geoffroy was profoundly grateful:

> Elles [the plants] rendront les demonstrations des Drogues que que [sic] je suis obligé de faire tantôt au jardin du Roy et tantôt au College-royal beaucoup plus curieuses et plus instructives, et elles m'eclairciront en meme temps sur bien des doutes que les descriptions ou les figures que nous en avons nous laissent encore.[30]

Thirdly, Geoffroy was a staunch and prominent member of the Paris medical college. This was a body some hundred strong of Paris MDs, which ran the faculty and monopolized medical practice in the capital. Geoffroy made an impact on the corporation even before he graduated in that the dissertations he sustained before its representatives were penned by his own hand and not by the hand of the president of the *soutenance*. Once a member of the corporation, he kept a high profile by using the *soutenance* to promote outlandish views. A few months after his graduation he presided over a *soutenance* where a bachelor promoted the spermatozoist reproductive theories of Leeuwenhoek and Hartsoeker.[31] Geoffroy's contribution to faculty life was recognized in 1726 when he was elected dean for two years, and then in 1728 unprecedently for a further two-year term. This proved an onerous task and may well have undermined his health, for he was required to defend the faculty's traditional right to organize surgical teaching in the face of the foundation of a college of surgery run by the Paris surgeons themselves.[32]

Finally, Geoffroy was a medical practitioner. Immediately on graduation he seems to have shown little interest in plying his profession, and it is possible that it was only in the last ten years that it really became an important part of his life. Nevertheless, the sheer number of patients that consulted him by letter in the 1720s is testimony to his reputation as a practitioner. This was presumably built on the twin foundations of his work as an *académicien* and his prodigious learning. Few other members of the Paris college could hold a candle to him in either respect. The weight of his learning is attested to by the size of his library, one of the largest medical libraries in France in the eighteenth century. On his death his library contained 2,090 works, of which a half were on medical subjects.[33] In contrast, when the contemporary Paris physician, P. J. B. Chomel (1671–1740), died he left only 49 books altogether. One of the few other early-eighteenth century members of the Paris college with a similar collection must have been the iatromechanist Philippe Hecquet (1661–1737), who in the course of his life purportedly gave 1,300 volumes to the Paris faculty in order to help start the faculty's library.[34]

Geoffroy's Patients

The *mémoires* sent to Geoffroy essentially provide histories of his patients' illnesses. Unfortunately, they contain only limited information about the patients themselves, especially as many clients remained anonymous for reasons which will be discussed below. However, enough biographical details can be gleaned from the in-coming letters to construct a reasonably detailed account of the social constituency from which Geoffroy's practice was drawn.

Geoffroy was consulted by both men and women in virtually equal proportions, but his patients were predominantly in their forties and fifties. Interestingly, hardly any consultations were demanded for children. A notable exception was a letter of 19 September, 1728 seeking Geoffroy's advice in the case of one Croville *fils* of Mantes who had broken his thigh in a fall the year before.[35] Older patients were just as rare, although a handful of Geoffroy's patients were extremely venerable. In October 1723, for instance, he received a letter from an 80-year-old asthmatic called Frère Louis de l'Asseré. The aged monk was suitably apologetic:

> quoy que je sois d'une condition qui ne doit pas avoir de l'attachement a la vie; cependant n'en estant pas le Maistre on le doit conserver autant que faire se peut.[36]

The social and professional background of Geoffroy's clients was inevitably fairly exclusive. The majority were drawn from the rural nobility, the *noblesse de robe*, and the great mercantile families of northern France, such as the Danse of Beauvais.[37] A significant proportion of his clients was drawn from the Church, especially from members of the regular clergy. Many of his clerical patients must have been equally well-born for they were often heads of religious houses, but some were evidently relatively indigent curés. One such was the *abbé* de Morfontaine who in 1723 fell victim to an erysipelas of the stomach. The *mémoire* sent to Geoffroy on his behalf warned the Paris physician:

> que le Malade est reduitt à un si modique Revenu qu'il est obligé de s'epargner sur tout; ainsi il suplie Monsieur Geoffroy de luy marquer un Regime qui ne coute pas beaucoup, à moins que le contraire ne soit absolument necesssaire, pour sa vie et sa santé.[38]

Nevertheless, if Geoffroy had an exclusive clientele he did not have an *entrée* into the highest echelons of French society. Although Geoffroy ministered to a number of titled noblemen and women, he was never patronized by the cream of Versailles society. His aristocratic clients tended to live in the countryside, like the Marquis de Brichanteau and his sister who lived at Donnemarie-en-Brie (presumably Donnemarie-Dontilly near Provins).[39] No prince of the blood, nor even a duke consulted him. Nor did Geoffroy have an international reputation. Only one case has come to light of a foreigner who asked his advice. This was an Irish lady who approached him, probably in late 1728, about a breast ulcer which had appeared in November 1727 and failed to improve despite three operations. Even she, though, did not write to Geoffroy from her native land, but from Boulogne (or perhaps Paris) as she set out on a visit to France.[40] In the main Geoffroy's clients were French men and women residing north of the Loire.

But Geoffroy's failure to attract the custom of Europe's princes and aristocrats is not surprising. Although an *académicien*, he was never a court physician, in contrast to Fagon who was both.[41] Moreover, his standing at the French court may have been tarnished by his Jansenist proclivities, even if these were not vocally paraded. Jansenists were austere Counter-Reformation Catholics whose quasi-predestinarian theories of grace were deemed heretical by a series of popes. In early-eighteenth century France they were to be found in large numbers among members of the lower clergy and the lay professions. Geoffroy was one of the 46 members of the Paris faculty who in 1718 supported the University in its appeal to a General Council against the anti-Jansenist Bull *Unigenitus*.[42] He also had Jansenist patients. In May 1730 he was asked to consult on behalf of a widow of Rheims, a Mme L'Espargnol. The lady in question, according to the correspondence, was a close relative of the Parisian *robe* family, Pâris. This was a leading Jansenist family in the capital which had recently lost its most notorious member, the deacon François de Pâris. The deacon's tomb in Saint-Médard had immediately become a Jansenist thaumaturgical shrine. In that the correspondent had no hesitation in referring to the odour of sanctity in which the good deacon had died, Geoffroy's allegiance was clearly public knowledge.[43]

Only a handful of Geoffroy's clients approached him directly. Most chose to do so through intermediaries. Those who wrote directly were in the main titled aristocrats or patients with whom he was already in contact. The Comtesse d'Orville who wrote to the Paris physician from her estate near Montdidier in Picardy on 8 May, 1730 had a foot in both camps. She was already undergoing treatment prescribed by Geoffroy for a swollen belly and wrote to the physician complaining that after taking his remedies for ten days she had received no improvement.[44] The small number of patients who wrote personally to Geoffroy would suggest that it was the custom for all but the socially most prominent to obtain a consultation by letter through an intermediary who was already known to the consultant. This made sense, for seventeenth- and eighteenth-century French society largely functioned through patronage contacts. Assistance and information were definitely purchasable, but normally only with a letter of introduction. It would have been surprising if medical advice had been obtainable in a different way.[45] Certainly, there was no other obvious reason why intermediaries were used, provided the patient was capable of wielding a pen. Contemporary medical discourse was common property as has been noted, so there was no problem of communication. Moreover, the *mémoires* and the consultations were written in French, so there was no need, as there had been 50 years earlier, for the patient to seek an expert in Latin to describe his condition.

For the large part, Geoffroy's patients used medical men as their intermediaries. This was usually their ordinary physician but it might equally be an apothecary or a surgeon, such as Hébert an apothecary from Falaise in Normandy who corresponded with Geoffroy on several occasions (once on account of his own daughter).[46] Clearly, Geoffroy did not stand on his dignity as a physician. He did not refuse to provide consultations for patients who were being treated, in theory illegally, by members of the subordinate medical professions.[47] Medical men were the obvious intermediaries in that they were the most likely people in the neighbourhood to know Geoffroy personally. Furthermore, it was commonsense to entrust the composition of the *mémoire* to a doctor. Although contemporary medical discourse was common to both doctor and patient, the doctor had the firmer command over the vocabulary. He had a better knowledge of what information to supply and could set it down in an ordered and literate manner. Lay communications often came in the form of an unorganized stream of consciousness.[48] There can be no doubt that Geoffroy preferred to receive a *mémoire* written by a professional. On several occasions he defended the potential inadequacy of his response on the grounds that he had received insufficient details from the lay correspondent. Indeed, he was often quite brutal, as in a letter of 1724:

> Pour prononcer plus surement sur les remedes qui conviennent à Mademoiselle du Valory il seroit a souhaitter qu'on nous eut envoye un detail exact et bien circonstantié de la malade depuis le commencement jusques a present, qu'on nous eut marqué ce qu'elle a fait jusques a present.[49]

The deployment of medical intermediaries helps to explain the anonymity of many of the patients. It can be assumed that contemporary medical ethics forbade revealing the identity of one's clients to a third party, especially if the patient were a lady. This, of course, would be particularly the case if the intermediary had taken it upon his own initiative to write to Geoffroy.[50] Anonymity seems to have prevailed whatever the malady. Medical men did not just protect the identities of patients with embarrassing complaints. On the occasions when local practitioners did break their silence, then, this often reflected an unusual hostility between patient and doctor (at least on the side of the correspondent). Witness the case of Beauvallon, *marchand du vin* of Rheims, the victim of an apoplectic fit in January 1730. Beauvallon's doctor, who specifically named his 33-year-old patient, evidently loathed the man. Provider of the best champagne in the country, Beauvallon had exploited his good fortune to live a life of total debauchery since the tender age of 15. Every night the merchant had retired in a drunken stupour, often making himself vomit in order to drink the more. Even an attack of jaundice seven or eight years before had not checked his indulgence. Obviously, there could be only one (albeit unstated) conclusion. Beauvallon had been deservedly struck down.[51] So intemperate was the letter, it is difficult to imagine it was shown to the champagne merchant before it was sent. This, though, must have been generally the custom, just as the consultation was normally addressed to the anonymous or named patient via the hands of his doctor.[52] The medical man was definitely only the intermediary.

Professionals, however, were not the only intermediaries. Some patients relied on the good offices of their family and kin; others on the help of friends or even relative outsiders. Often this reflected their poor state of health. The sick would use their husband or wife as an amanuensis because they themselves were too weak to put pen to paper. But sometimes it reflected the patient's isolation, both social and geographical. Living in the countryside, members of the lesser nobility, especially, were understandably out of touch with the professional medical community. Geoffroy's name would be given them by a more mobile member of the local community, a lawyer or cleric, and the latter would then be prevailed upon to contact the famous doctor on their behalf.

A study of the letters written by relatives provides an interesting insight into the intimacies of family life. In an age and in a section of society where conjugal bliss was supposedly absent, it is instructive to discover that a Monsieur Ferrier had a detailed knowledge of his wife's menstrual problems after only four months of marriage.[53] A study of the role of lay outsiders as intermediaries provides equally interesting insights into the solidarity of local communities. The *abbé* de Morfontaine was initially introduced to Geoffroy by a *premier-président* of the Paris Parlement, one Pelletier (probably of the family Le Peletier de Saint-Fargeau), who claimed to be his parishioner. As the *abbé* was too indigent to be a Paris *curé*, he was presumably in charge of a rural parish in the Paris basin where Pelletier owned land. The *abbé* was clearly loved by his flock. A second letter informing Geoffroy of his patient's progress was written (in appalling French) by an extremely worried carpenter, called Delamare.[54]

Lay intermediaries normally limited their communication to listing the patient's complaints and detailing any previous treatment. The occasional intermediary, however, aped the professionals by offering his own considered judgement on the case. In early 1728 Geoffroy was asked to consult for a lady of 28 to 30 years who was suffering from *demangeaisons* in her arms and other parts. Wherever the itch struck, there, it seems, would sprout a tuft of hair an inch long. The anonymous lady was sponsored by a Paris professor of philosophy, Gaspard Poitevin, professor at the University's Collège de Beauvais. Poitevin had his own theories as to the cause of the disease which Geoffroy in his reply unsportingly shot down. In the professor's opinion the disease was caused by the presence of little insects under the skin, a complaint, he maintained, identified by the physician, Ettmuller, *inter alios*.[55]

There is little point in detailing the diseases from which Geoffroy's patients thought they were suffering, for the early eighteenth century was still a pre-nosological age. There was a standard vocabulary of disease used by both patient and doctor which the modern world has largely retained but the terms were used loosely, although admittedly never arbitrarily. A patient's complaint was diagnosed by reference to the most dominant symptom, so that those suffering from chest-pains and breathing difficulties were uniformally classed as asthmatic, even if they had swollen limbs or were spitting blood.[56] As it was, giving the disease a label was irrelevant in the eyes of the physician. What was essential (as we will see) was identifying the internal lesion which had caused the symptoms. A good physician recognized that the same lesion could be the cause of different symptoms in different individuals. All that need be said on this score, therefore, was that the maladies were necessarily chronic. Although Geoffroy was an assiduous correspondant (except when ill himself towards the end of his life),[57] a patient could expect a wait of several weeks between sending the letter and receiving the consultation. Falaise is no great distance from Paris, yet a letter dated 5 November, 1729 was not answered by Geoffroy until 2 December, and this was a standard delay.[58] Many acute, killer diseases in consequence can never have been the subject of consultation by letter. No one wrote to Geoffroy from Marseilles in 1721 asking his opinion on how to cure the plague!

It is more fruitful to examine at what stage of a patient's malady Geoffroy was called in. In some cases, it was only after a matter of days. A letter was written on behalf of a Monsieur Taton on Tuesday 11 May, 1728 who had been suffering from pains in the urethra and stomach only since the early hours of the previous Saturday.[59] In most cases, however, the patient had been afflicted for many years, if not always (except in their own minds) from the same disease. One unfortunate lady, Madame de la Buretiere, who consulted Geoffroy in 1724 was a 60-year-old who had suffered for some 20 years from conjunctivitis. Her physician claimed that the complaint had come with her periods, but the lady herself told a different story. As a child she had suffered from unspecified fluxions (of the chest) but the onset of puberty had alleviated the problem by purging her of the infected humour. For 30 years she had only had to endure a 'pituite douce' which she had expressed through frequent expectoration.

However, her periods had ended when she was 38 and for eight to ten days she had been subject to a continual fit of spitting. The humour had then moved to her leg, only to quit this part of her body in turn and enter her eyes. As a result of this chronic condition, she had eventually become melancholic.[60]

However long the patient's suffering, Geoffroy's opinion was always sought for one or two reasons. Usually it was because the malady had suddenly worsened and the patient, previously reconciled to his or her chronic complaint, had taken fright after failing to respond to a course of treatment advocated by the attendant medical practitioner. Madame de la Buretiere's condition, for instance, had deteriorated four months before the *mémoire* to Geoffroy was written, when her conjunctivitis became suddenly permanent. Initially she had put herself in the hands of an oculist, imagining initially that the problem was surgical rather than physical.[61] Realizing, however, that the problem stemmed from the brain, she had put herself in the hands of the physicians. Over the past months she had been bled, purged, immersed, put on a meat-free diet, and forced to wear a seton, but all to no effect. Her head was full, her eyes poured and she was spitting thick mucous. Exercise, advised by her friends, only made things worse. Finally, she had been advised to take the waters at Bourbon L'Archambauld.[62] At this point, Madame de la Buretiere's will seems to have snapped. Four days before her physician wrote to Geoffroy, she had become convinced that she was going blind. It was at this juncture that the physician, either on his own or his patient's initiative, decided to call in his Paris colleague.

In the main, recourse to Geoffroy was the result of medical failure. Sometimes, on the other hand, it could represent medical success. This was true in the case of Monsieur Taton. The latter had been subjected over the three days of his illness to two phlebotomies and two rectal injections. He had also been given whey and violet honey. Although initially Taton's pain had not diminished, after the second phlebotomy he had evacuated his bowels and was much relieved. His physician, therefore, was not writing to Geoffroy in despair. On the contrary, he was merely writing to seek his support on the best way to prevent the malady recurring. In the physician's opinion, Taton was suffering from nephritic colic and should proceed to take a course of Saint-Amand water (a spa in Flanders). Geoffroy was asked to concur in the diagnosis and restorative treatment. In such cases, it is hard to imagine that the initiative to approach the Parisian doctor came from the patient. Rather, it would seem that Taton's physician was inventing an excuse to write to Geoffroy and demonstrate his therapeutic skill. By writing to Geoffroy on a minor matter he brought to the Paris doctor's attention his name and credentials in a suitably deferential manner. At a later date, he could capitalize on this initial correspondence to seek a patronage favour.[63]

Not surprisingly, cases of this kind only produced a single consultation. Geoffroy replied on 15 May, 1728, and Monsieur Taton disappeared from medical history. It is more surprising that there is also little feedback about the progress of patients whose state was desperate. Nearly always in the collection the correspondence consists only of the *mémoire* and the reply, so the future medical history remains unknown. There could be several reasons for this. It may have been the case that Geoffroy's suggestions proved successful (we are perhaps too hasty to dismiss early–modern medicine). But the more likely reason is that neither patients nor their practitioners felt obliged to stay with the Paris physician if his remedies, after suitable trial, proved ineffective. They presumably just sought another consultation from a different doctor. Indeed, it is quite possible that patients were seeking consultations from Geoffroy and one or two of his colleagues at the very same time.[64] If so, then they presumably chose which course of treatment suited them best.

Significantly, the patients who kept in touch with Geoffroy were generally his titled patients and others who wrote to him directly or through their spouses. As many of these people had doubtless approached Geoffroy without the advice or support of local practitioners they had arguably made him their personal physician (albeit at a distance and for a limited time). How frequently they kept in touch with Geoffroy is impossible to say. Much of the evidence for their existence comes from the chance survival of a single letter *in medias res*. Probably, they only wrote when feeling ill or disgruntled. Equally it is impossible to tell whether they were seeing other practitioners. Obviously, this could not always be avoided. On 21 May, 1730, Geoffroy received a letter from one Madame Dargouges, resident at Fleury near Fontainebleau. Madame Dargouges's husband, it appeared, had contracted a cough and fever after walking in the cold. Madame Dargouges apologized for not contacting Geoffroy at the fever's onset. Her husband was admittedly Geoffroy's patient, but he had required urgent attention. As a result she had summoned a doctor from Etampes who took all day to arrive,[65] and then two days later she had sent for the king's physician, Helvétius, residing with the court at Fontainebleau. As he had not been able to come until the next day her son had sent for a very skilful père de la Charité (i.e., a member of a regular order who practised illegally). Eventually, her husband had been seen by Helvétius on two occasions, and her husband was now on the mend. The letter was therefore really a courtesy note, to which Geoffroy civilly replied linking the fever with her husband's malady that he was already treating; i.e., 'l'humeur d'Eresipel qui etoit sur ses jambes'.[66]

Those who did place themselves in Geoffroy's hands did not always show a readiness to abide by the Paris physician's advice. His personal patients frequently acted on their own intiative. The Comtesse d'Orville who wrote to Geoffroy on 8 May, 1730 gave his treatment less than a ten days' trial. As two days before writing she had begun to spit mucous, she judged the *bouillons* and tisane prescribed for her swollen belly had warmed her chest and should be discontinued.[67] Another patient, one Monsieur Darmesson (perhaps D'Ormesson), took the prescribed remedy but in his own way. Sent to take the waters at Forges in 1717, he stayed four weeks rather than three as ordered and only took seven glasses of water per day against the usual nine to ten. Darmesson, like the Comtesse, was highly disgruntled as he announced his departure to Dieppe (his home town?) Sent to Forges to cure his backache, he was now feverous with pains in his chest. 'Enfin quoyque j'aye toujours bon apetit, je n'oserois dire que jaye receu du soulagement des eaux.'[68]

Some of Geoffroy's patients, on the other hand, were loyal and deferential to a fault. Madame de la Buretiere had sought a consultation for her conjunctivitis in September 1724. In January 1725, she wrote to Geoffroy providing him with a sombre progress report. Her eyes were still running if a little less inflamed, but her vapours were no better. Her head and hands trembled and she was very melancholic, crying over 'bagatelles'. Nevertheless, she was following Geoffroy's advice carefully and was highly appreciative offering him as a present 12 cases of the local Orléans wine. In one respect she had taken her own initiative in that she had found the two *bouillons* a day the doctor had ordered too filling. Thus 'elle a retranché depuis quelque jours le Bouillon de l'aprés midy'. She was, however, alarmed by her own temerity and wanted reassurance that she had done right.[69] Madame de la Buretiere was just as deferential in the letter she wrote to Geoffroy over a year later in March 1726. This time the catalogue of her woes was more heart-felt, their presentation confused, and the tone desperate. Although she had followed the prescribed regime, even when she found it repugnant to do so in the case of drinking whey, she had got no better.[70] For 15 (read 18) months she had been taking Geoffroy's remedies. The Parisian doctor was asked to think what such dedication must be like for a woman of 60. All the same, even now she did not abuse her tormentor or declare their relationship to be over. Rather, the letter began with a pathetic apology for bothering Geoffroy yet again where she reiterated her confidence in his judgement (it seems that she had written an earlier letter to which the Paris doctor had not replied). The letter merely ended with a plea for an honest prognosis. She demanded that Geoffroy tell her the purpose of the purgatory she had undergone and what was the likely outcome if her malady still failed to respond to the treatment. After a year and a half she was still in his hands.[71]

Geoffroy's Medical Practice

In the early eighteenth century most French physicians embraced some form of iatromechanism. Essentially, they all agreed that the body was a hydraulic machine which only remained in good working order as long as the fluids retained their optimum volume, consistency and velocity. At the same time they were pathological reductionists, who argued that all internal diseases, whatever the symptoms, were ultimately caused by a humoral vitiation in a particular part of the body. Contemporary physicians were divided, however, as to the role chemical reactions played in the creation and vitiation of the body's fluids. One group, represented by the Paris physician Philippe Hecquet (1661–1737), insisted that there were no chemical reactions at all in the body. A physiological process such as chilification was dependent wholly upon the mastication, pummelling and sieving to which ingested food was subject as it moved from the mouth to the bloodstream. A malign chilification stemmed from a loss of elasticity or tonus of the solid parts. Others, such as the Montpellier professor Jean Astruc (1684–1766), disagreed and maintained that both normal and pathological changes to the body's fluids were largely the result of chemical processes. The argument had an important effect on therapeutics, for the supporters of trituration tended to promote phlebotomy as the supreme remedy whereby the fluids might be restored to their natural state, while their opponents vaunted the value of chemically-induced purgation.[72]

Geoffroy's allegiance was determined by his background and interests. As an apothecary by training and an experimental chemist by inclination, he was inevitably a supporter of the chemical school, and he made his position abundantly clear in the dissertations that he sustained before the faculty in 1703.[73] Intriguingly, however, his medical consultations give the reader no indication of this chemical bias. His diagnosis simply begins by identifying the nature and location of the humoral vitiation in the light of the symptoms described in the *mémoire*. Perhaps there were professional reasons for this. Geoffroy's own credibility and the credibility of his Parisian colleagues would scarcely have been enhanced had patients been forcibly reminded of the philosophical divisions within the faculty. It was awkward enough for professional authority that the contemporary physiological debate could be easily followed by an interested laity. Too many polemicists compounded the problem of a shared medical discourse by publishing their diatribes in the vernacular.[74]

On the other hand, what does strike the reader forcibly is Geoffroy's reductionism. Even if the symptoms are so diverse as to indicate the presence of various diseases, they are always reducible to a single internal problem. In his reply to the *mémoire* presented by De la Goudonniere of Falaise in 1729 on behalf of an anonymous 40-year-old lady, Geoffroy declared that the patient was suffering from four separate complaints: hypochondriacal melancholy, a bladder problem, scurvy and rhumatism. Nevertheless, he insisted that the complaints were all interconnected and stemmed from a coagulation of the blood in the vessels of the viscera which in turn produced circulatory difficulties.[75] In Geoffroy's opinion the same vitiated humour could not only produce different symptoms, but could also change its location. An asthmatic patient who consulted him in August 1728 had been afflicted by diarrhoea or dysentery (flux of the belly) the previous summer. This, he insisted in his consultation, was no coincidence: the acrid humour in the chest had moved to the stomach. Indeed, the propensity for vitiated humours to shift position made their amelioration difficult: the cure could sometimes be worse than the disease; this was particularly so with gout.[76]

As all Geoffroy's patients were found to be suffering from 'un embarras' of the fluids in the form of a coagulated or acrid humour, the whole thrust of his therapeutics was to thin and sweeten ('adoucir') the blood. Understandably, given his reductionism, the general procedure was the same in every case.

In the first place, his patients were advised to place themselves, if they had not already done so, on a strict regime. All alcoholic beverages and stimulants, such as coffee, were banned. Instead, patients were normally advised to drink nothing but a herbal tisane. This could include a variety of herbs, but the favoured ingredient was couch-grass (*chiendent*). At the same time, the patient was placed on a bland diet which basically comprised clear meat soups (*bouillons*) made from veal and a variety of herbs. If patients were allowed to eat anything heavier, then they were restricted to white meat and fish. Spicy foods, dairy products and vegetables were all banned.

In the second instance patients were given a programme of medication. This invariably began with a phlebotomy, which served as an introduction to a twice-daily course of specialist *bouillons*. These looked suspiciously similar to the *bouillons* which formed the normal diet, except that they were made from calves' feet, the eyes of crayfish,[77] and a grander selection of herbs (though couch-grass was usually included). This course of *bouillons* finished, the patient was instructed next to take a series of (presumably hot) baths of river water. The patient would be required to stay in the bath for as long as two hours and usually expected to drink asses' or goats' milk in the form of whey while immersed. Finally, after the baths, the treatment would be ended by a course of mineral waters, either taken at home or *in situ*.[78] While taking the specialist *bouillons* the patient would frequently be subjected to daily rectal injections (often of purified water) and the course of baths would be prefaced, punctuated and ended by purgative doses of manna and Epsom salts. At the end of the treatment the malignant humour should have been eradicated. The treatment, it should be noted, was slow (it could last months), gentle and cumulative. The patient was only moderately depleted by bleeding, the purgatives were mild, and great emphasis was placed on the healing powers of a draconian diet. Geoffroy, although a chemist, did not usually prescribe *vomitaria*. In this respect, his treatment would have been approved by the arch mechanist, Philippe Hecquet, who accused the chemists of using violent purgatives indiscriminately.[79]

It must not be thought, however, that Geoffroy's therapy was unsubtle for being predictable. While the basic regime and treatment was always the same, the details varied enormously according to the severity of the disease, its previous handling, and the temperament/sex and age of the patient. Geoffroy, then, was very much the Hippocratic doctor: he treated an individual, not a disease entity. In many cases, too, he was careful to suggest alternative therapeutic strategies if the patient did not improve as quickly as expected. Flexibility within a given set of parameters was the hallmark of Geoffroy as a consultant.

Thus, while his central interest was in dietary control, he did not totally ignore the other non-naturals. Admittedly, he showed no interest in the therapeutic value of sexual activity, unlike certain fringe practitioners in eighteenth-century England.[80] But he did approve of physical activity *tout court*, at least in moderation. Indeed, in the case of patients adjudged to be suffering from hypochondria exercise was vital. A lady whose indisposition had been brought on by the death of her husband, suppressed periods and a bad regime, was told in December 1729 that there was nothing Geoffroy could do for her unless she pulled herself together, got out of the house, and sought companions. If she was not going to leave the house, then she had to play shuttlecock.[81] Priests and nuns in this condition were always told to give up their duties. A 42-year-old nun was told in 1727 that she had to give up exercising her mind and exercise her body instead.[82] Changes of air, too, were recommended. Another nun who had been suffering from an asthmatic complaint for many years and had recently found relief on temporarily leaving her convent was advised to seek another house, if after a year's absence the improvement was manifest.[83]

In a similar vein, the standard treatment that Geoffroy advocated was only a skeletal framework which was fleshed out according to the individual case. One part of the treatment might be left out in a specific case, another part lengthened or shortened, yet another subject to a particular refinement. There was no part of the treatment which might not be adapted in some way. Normally, Geoffroy advocated that patients should be bled by the arm. If a greater amount of blood needed to be drawn, then he would further suggest that the foot be bled and sometimes (in dire cases) the neck. This was the treatment advocated in the case of a 32-year-old woman who suffered from chronic headaches and seemed to be threatened by an imminent apoplexy. It was a treatment, however, to be resorted to only if the headaches persisted after she had been initially bled more conventionally. In this case, specifically, Geoffroy suggested that the patient be first bled by the foot and then by the foot and arm. This was because the woman was in the third to fourth month of her sixth pregnancy and bleeding by the arm alone might cause her to go into premature labour.[84]

The specialist *bouillons*, baths, and drinks could all be adulterated to improve their laxative effects. It was commonplace to add Glauber salts (thought to be exceptionally mild), purified nitre, or some other mineral to the *bouillons*. This, though, was never done in an arbitrary fashion. A lady diagnosed as suffering from a melancholic and scorbutic complaint in April 1730 was told to add Glauber salts to her *bouillons* only once she felt better. Geoffroy did not like to promote the continual depletion of the sick.[85]

The mineral waters which Geoffroy recommended were also, it seems, never chosen at random. He stated a preference for the waters of Forges on several occasions, but this was not always his choice. He found Forges water usually preferable because of its mildness. In contrast, he believed that the waters of Bourbon and Balaruc (also much used at this period) too easily over-agitated the blood and could rupture the blood vessels and cause haemorrhaging.[86] There again, this could recommend their use in the case of apoplectic and paralytic patients, such as the Comtesse de Souteron sent to Bourbon in 1727.[87] Nephritic cases, however, could be directed to yet another spring. A lady of Orléans suffering from the stone was told in the summer of 1730 to take the waters of Sainte-Reine at the rate of five to six glasses each morning. These waters, Geoffroy insisted, were exactly right for the lady's condition:

> Cette Eau de Ste Reine est chargé d'un nitre subtil tres propre a diviser la masse de sang, a la temperer, a calmer l'ardeur des Reins, a fondre la (sic) matieres glareuses qui s'arretent dans les reins, qui en s'y dessechant produisent les sables.[88]

In many cases, furthermore, Geoffroy suggested an additional remedy as part of the overall treatment. This was usually either a pill (a bolus) or an opiate taken once a day for a specific period. Such medicines were a significant addition to the standard treatment, for they were both mineral and vegetable based and illustrated Geoffroy's chemical allegiance. They were often prescribed only as a fallback if the initial 'milder' treatment failed. Their prescription indicated an important increase to the cost of the cure. Whereas most *bouillons, lavements*, and purgatives could be concocted by the patient, his family or servants, pills and opiates could really only be obtained from apothecaries. Geoffroy in his consultation carefully detailed how the medicine should be made, and the patient presumably passed the letter to his pharmacist. Typical was the opiate that Madame Pecquet de Sainte-Victoire was asked to take for her suppressed periods in 1729. This was composed from 'safran de mars aperitif preparé à la rosée, ... , racine d'arum, sechée et pulverisée, ... gomme ammoniac choisie en larmes, ... extrait d'absinthe, [and] un gros d'extrait d'elixir de propriétés de Paracelse'. The opiate was concocted by mixing together the ingredients with syrup of Artemisia.[89]

Sometimes, on the other hand, the medicines were specific herbal tisanes. Patients with nephritic complaints, for instance, were asked to take a lithontriptic, based on the star-thistle. This, Geoffroy revealed, was a remedy much in vogue, known as the remedy of Monsieur Barille (presumably after its inventor). Described as 'icy', it had to be taken every month on either the 28th or 29th day of the moon's cycle. While it was taken every other part of the treatment had to be interrupted. Patients were not to worry if the plant was unobtainable locally out of season. The lady from Orléans for whom Geoffroy recommended the waters of Sainte-Reine was told that she could obtain the remedy properly prepared from several Parisian apothecaries.[90] Barille's remedy strongly savoured of the hermetic and the empirical. As Geoffroy's practice was generally free of exotic prescriptions, its promotion may well reflect the state of the market. There were so many lithontriptics available in the eighteenth century, promoted by qualified physicians as well as quacks, that Geoffroy may have felt it necessary to favour one relatively harmless concoction to stop his patients trying others. On the other hand, given the difficulties of curing the disease (which Geoffroy, as we shall see readily granted) perhaps he was willing to promote any nostrum which showed the slightest sign of being beneficial. Certainly, he also encouraged his patients to wear a magic stone:

> Quelques personnes se trouvent fort bien pour la gravelle et les colics nefrétiques d'une pierre nefretique ou pierre de jade que l'on applique a crud sur la peau a l'endroit du rein malade [.] on peut essayer ce remede sans rien risquer.[91]

Geoffroy's course of treatment was intended to cleanse the body completely of the malignant humour which oppressed it and was naturally a long-term process. But the Parisian physician was well aware that many of his patients were in considerable pain, if only periodically. Another part of his therapy, therefore, consisted in assuaging their discomfort in the short term. Quinine was prescribed in cases of intermittent fever and cataplasms for violent headaches. In asthma attacks patients were advised to take a special herbal *tisane*, made *inter alia* from hyssop, agaric and marjoram, which was taken with a spoonful of Narbonne honey.[92] In particular and understandably, Geoffroy sought to alleviate the pain of passing stones. What was needed, Geoffroy believed, was to melt the *glaires* which surrounded the granules and made their excretion difficult, and at the same time to relax the urethra so that the stones might pass more easily. This was to be done in a variety of ways, in part by bleeding and bathing the patient, and administering *lavements*, in part through herbal drinks. The *lavements* in this case might be composed of blackcurrant and whey, the potions of emollient concoctions made of linseed, turpentine and even egg yolk. Commonly the plant, wall-pellitory, was prescribed as a diuretic to relax the urethra.[93]

Geoffroy, then, was a cautious, flexible practitioner who preferred to take the disease by stealth rather than by outright attack. He was also pragmatic, recognizing that his prescriptions could not always be followed to the letter by his patients (however willing). Herbs might not be in season locally; a patient might find a particular part of the treatment onerous or unfulfillable. He was particularly sensitive to the problems of consuming mineral waters on site. In general, this was the preferred course of treatment, but Geoffroy realised that journeys to Forges and other vaunted *stations* were not always possible. To obviate the difficulty Geoffroy suggested several alternatives. Patients could always attend a local spa with the same properties as the one preferred. Many of Geoffroy's Breton patients were allowed to attend Dinan rather than Forges, although the Paris physician was convinced that Dinan water was not as good.[94] Failing that, it was always possible to consume the water at home, or even, *faute de mieux*, concoct·one's own. A lady from Laval in Maine suffering from a weakness of the stomach in 1729 was told that artifical ferruginous water could be made by immersing blacksmith's nails in a bottle of red wine. All that had to be done was cork the bottle and leave the ingredients to infuse, giving the bottle a shake from time to time.[95]

However, Geoffroy was never one to pander to his patients. If he could be accommodating, he was also firm. Patients who questioned his wisdom or who refused essential parts of his treatment were dealt with summarily. Take the case of the 63-year-old, lieutenant-colonel, Monsieur de Guyon of Noyers in northern Burgundy, purportedly suffering fom pickled blood ('une saumure de sang'). On 23 July Geoffroy had sent him a consultation through a third party, the *abbé* Guyon, who lived by the Paris Place Royale, now the Place des Vosges (Geoffroy at this date lived in the Marais). A few days later he received another letter from the patient's sister explaining why Geoffroy's treatment could not be followed. The lieutenant-colonel thought *demi-bains* were of no use, he disliked milk, and anyway he had taken a cold (always assumed by patients a reason to quit a regime). Geoffroy replied on 10 August, sticking by his original consultation. He was willing to compromise on the *demi-bains*, but the milk diet was absolutely essential.[96] Admittedly,

Geoffroy always spiced the pill of his displeasure: he was always polite. When the Countess d'Orville announced that she had abandoned his treatment after a ten-day trial, Geoffroy did not condemn her outright. Although he was certain that the treatment was not the cause of her hot chest, he praised her for discontinuing the *tisane* and *bouillons*. It would give her chest time to re-establish itself. Nevertheless, she should resume the *bouillons* as the sure way to reduce her swollen stomach.[97]

Moreover, if polite, Geoffroy was also frank. Once he had analysed the nature and site of the disease, he expressed his views on the possibility of its cure. Where the malady was inveterate and complex he openly admitted that the case was a difficult one which might not have a happy conclusion. In some cases he would only promise relief. Thus the asthma of one Madame de Noirville was beyond his competence. Now 54, the lady had been suffering the complaint for nearly 30 years and had reached the stage where she was coughing up a bituminous substance on rising. Geoffroy, however, told her not to be disheartened. He could make the malady bearable, and she should not despair, 'car on ne laisse pas de vivre longtemps avec cette indisposition'.[98] Geoffroy was just as honest with his nephritic patients where the stone was too large to rend. A lady diagnosed as having an ulcerous kidney was told that she was beyond cure: 'Nous n'avons trouvé jusqu'à present aucunement lithontriptique ... veritablement capable de briser le pierre' (an indication perhaps of Geoffroy's true opinion about the star-thistle elixir and its many rivals). Once more, though, Geoffroy offered his patient hope. The lady was not in perpetual pain, the spasms could be reduced, and the malady was not life-threatening. Many people died with a stone in the kidney and never knew they had one.[99] Geoffroy, where possible, therefore, attempted to relieve anxiety. But he was no mountebank peddling miracle cures.

Concluding Remarks

Thanks to the survival of Geoffroy's medical correspondence it has been possible to reconstruct the medical practice of an eighteenth-century French physician in far greater detail than hitherto. As it stands, however, it is a reconstruction in isolation and in consequence of limited interest. What the medical historian would really like to know is whether or not Geoffroy's practice was typical. Did physicians replicate his pattern of treatment all over France, or did Geoffroy represent Parisian medicine? Did physicians trained in the capital practise medicine differently from their colleagues (a much larger number) trained at Montpellier? Did partisans of the different medical philosophies definitely champion different cures as the polemics suggest? Unfortunately, at present we cannot even begin to answer these questions. As there are very few detailed studies of medical practice anywhere or at any time in early–modern Europe, we have no way of telling whether there were distinctive national patterns of therapeutics, let alone a difference between Paris and the provinces.[100] Indeed, it may be the case that these questions will never be satisfactorily answered. In a country where patients revealed little about their medical experiences and the correspondence of physicians has not survived in abundance, it will prove difficult to compile a series of similarly detailed profiles of medical practice for comparative purposes. In the course of my research I have unearthed several utilizable sources (especially from the second half of the century), but none that is as rich as the Geoffroy correspondence.[101] The most obvious complementary source is the archive of the Société Royale de Médecine, which has been used for a variety of purposes by medical historians, but never to write a history of late-eigteenth century medical practice.[102]

That Geoffroy's pattern of treatment had its supporters is quite clear from the correspondence itself. A number of patients who consulted the Paris physician were in the hands of medical men who attempted to cure through gentle depletion. Geoffroy often complimented the local physician on his treatment, blaming its inefficacy not on the remedies but on the short time that they were deployed.[103] Equally, however, the correspondence makes clear there were differences. One worried father contacted Geoffroy on behalf of his 22-year-old daughter because he was no longer satisfied with the treatment that she was receiving from the physicians of Caen. The latter, it seems, were dogmatic iatromechanists 'qui ne trouve (sic) pas autre (sic) remedes que de la faiere segner de temps en temps'.[104] It is also quite clear that Geoffroy would have had little sympathy with a court doctor like Helvétius who had given his patient Dargouges the violent emetic kermes, purportedly much in vogue at the time of Geoffroy's death.[105] But the correspondence only gives tantalizing glimpses of alternative therapies. It can be no substitute for a series of consultations as rich as Geoffroy's own.[106]

On the other hand, if Geoffroy's correspondence is of limited value for understanding eighteenth-century medical practice, it offers an extremely interesting insight into patient–practitioner relations. There may be no reason to accept that his practice was representative, but there is equally no reason to suspect that his patients were not. What then can we learn from the correspondence?

Obviously, Geoffroy's patients were not always patients in the modern sense of the term. They could disobey his orders; they had their own likes and dislikes; and some were almost certainly shopping around. The intermediary physicians, too, often lamented their patients' wilfulness. The lightly apoplectic Comtesse de Souteron, for instance, who had endured a variety of anti-apoplectic liqueurs (including *eau de Carmes*, a secret specific prepared by the Order), *lavements*, and vesicatories, had refused the application of poultices. 'On est à observer', wrote her physician, 'que l'on jamais pu obtenir de la malade de lui faire des embrocations et des liniments sur les parties paralisés par raport a la qu'elle abhorre a la mort toutes les odeurs qui luy causent des vapeurs extraordinaires.'[107] Nevertheless, what is striking is that so many (even among his most socially prominent patients) definitely did place themselves (body and soul) under his sway. Geoffroy commanded great power and respect. The devotion of a Madame de la Buretiere may have been extreme, but her obedience and deference was not atypical. Such patients, too, were obviously embarrassed by the cavalier, undeferential behaviour of their friends and relations. The Marquis de Bichanteau, corresponding with Geoffroy about his sister's suppressed periods, was suitably mortified by her failure to match his own assiduity. His sister, he told his physician, was not a great one for taking remedies. Four years ago, Geoffroy had prescribed rhubarb for her stomach-aches, but she gave up the treatment after a single month. Still troubled by colic, she compounded the problem by drinking coffee twice a day, claiming that it did her no harm because she had imbibed the stimulant since she was six.[108] Significantly, patients who wrote to Geoffroy directly expressed their esteem in the language of the humble client suing his patron. Geoffroy and by extension all Paris physicians were at the pinnacle of society when the daughter of a *marquise* could end her *mémoire* with the injuction: 'Soyez persuadé de la consideration très particuliere dans laquelle je suis, votre tres humble et tres obeissante servante.' This was the way a prince was addressed, not a lackey.[109]

Geoffroy's power is all the more worthy of note because it was novel. All the evidence we have of seventeenth-century patient–practitioner relations suggests that the nobility at least (and they set the tone) treated their physicians as servants. Madame de Sévigné (died 1696) was the classic example. She changed her doctors repeatedly, patronized without distinction the qualified and the quack, disobeyed both, and totally disregarded their *amour-propre*, even playing a nasty practical joke on one of her medical minions. There is no doubt that she aped the behaviour of her princely betters. Until the end of the century being a court physician was a lucrative but hazardous and ignominious occupation. Henri IV used to employ his chief physician, Du Laurens, to read him bedtime stories in the early hours of the morning.[110] Patients who were deferential to their physicians were the butt of contemporary satire, held up to ridicule for their unnatural and foolish behaviour in plays such as Molière's *Le Malade imaginaire* (1673).[111]

Arguably, Geoffroy and his colleagues were the first generation of society physicians to experience the luxury of practitioner-power (albeit incomplete). Why at the turn of the eighteenth century the nobility should have become more deferential and obedient patients is not yet totally clear. An important preparatory role was played by the aristocratic penchant for taking the waters, which was less than a century old and only properly established in the reign of Louis XIV. As I have argued elsewhere, periodic trips to a spa introduced the court and high society generally to a very different form of patient–practitioner relations. At the spa the physician was king. Imprisoned deep in the French countryside, patients were subjected to a strict regime which depleted both body and soul. Taking the waters was a purgatorial and humiliating experience (especially for a Madame de Sévigné).[112] The catalyst, however, was probably the appointment of Gui-Crescent Fagon as Louis XIV's chief physician in 1693. For over 20 years Fagon was a medical 'tyrant' (to quote Saint-Simon). Unlike his predecessors he had total medical power at court. Not only did he alone have access to the king's body, but he also had the final say in treating other members of the royal family. Courtiers, too, were frequently ordered to put themselves under his care, regardless of their traditional allegiance. Significantly, Fagon could always get his way with the king, who showed the same obedience to his doctor as he himself expected from his subjects. As a result, the stock and the power of the *médecins de cour* rose, as must have ultimately the status and authority of physicians everywhere.[113]

However, this development should not be seen simply as a medical *putsch*, the brainchild of a single, strategically-placed individual. Rather, it should be viewed as part of a much more important phenomenon, the emergence of the bureaucratic and absolute sovereign state, a development in which France led the way. The absolute sovereign state gave a new status to professional men. Administrators and lawyers were no longer the servants and clients of great aristocrats, but sometimes their patrons and masters;

in early seventeenth-century France *intendants* ran the households of the great; at the end of the century a new type of *intendant* ran the state. It was only a matter of time before other professionals benefited from the changing system of values which emphasized the importance of brain above brawn. A move to practitioner–power was guaranteed. The absolute state not only elevated the status of professionals, it also taught and demanded absolute obedience. A *frondeur* nobleman could never be a patient patient. Every neutered courtier at Versailles, on the other hand, was a passive patient in the making. The new ethic of self-control, the so-called 'civilizing process', that provided both the conditions in which the absolute state could be established and its essential cement was the inevitable progenitor of a new form of patient–practitioner relations. A Fagon might have existed before the age of Louis XIV, but patients in a modern sense certainly could not.[114]

This is not to say that the rise of the absolute sovereign state is a sufficient explanation for the development of present-day patient–practitioner relations. What it rather explains is the early appearance in France of a form of practitioner power.[115] Geoffroy's clients, it must be stressed, even the obedient and deferential, were still only quasi-modern patients. Geoffroy's correspondence suggests an élite which was health conscious but not health obsessed. Just as Geoffroy himself did not always promise to cure his patients, this was significantly not their demand. They and their intermediaries sought relief, *soulagement*. Significantly, too, the majority approached him only when their chronic afflictions became unbearable; in normal circumstances they muddled through. Clearly such patients did not believe health was a right and a necessity. It was only once the élite had begun to think in these terms that the physician could become the demi-god of today. And this could only happen in a post-Enlightenment world. The life of the here-and-now had to become of all-consuming importance for the status of the physician to be fully developed. The early-eighteenth century, it must be remembered, was still a pre-Enlightenment age. The Counter-Reformation was still in the ascendant. Indeed, in its Jansenist and most austere form it was affecting some sections of the lay and clerical élite more deeply than ever before. This was still an age when death, if seldom openly courted, was seldom shunned. Moral and spiritual health was more important than physical well-being and the two were not yet confused.[116] Practitioner-power did not mean practitioner dependence. This was to grow as the eighteenth century progressed, although ironically in the short term the development would have a detrimental effect on 'professional' practitioner power. Qualified practitioners were too few, too unsuccessful and too mutually hostile to provide the kind of medical service consumers increasingly demanded. As a result France on the eve of the Revolution was inundated with quacks.[117]

But if the practitioner power of the early-eighteenth century was not born from patient-need, its significance should not be devalued. It was definitely one of the factors helping to create the so-called society of notables which predated and in some ways caused the French Revolution. The elevation of professional status in the course of the seventeenth century did not mean the devaluation of traditional aristocratic mores. Purged of their *frondeur* associations, the élite values of the late-medieval world still survived and flourished in a modified form at court and in the army. Louis XIV was proud to be a member of the *noblesse de race*. In fact, France at the turn of the eighteenth century had two rival and counter- balancing hierarchies of status, each with its apex at Versailles and each headed by the monarch. In the course of the eighteenth century, however, the most affluent and prestigious components of these two hierarchies began to fuse and a new super élite was created based on a common culture. This common culture was primarily founded on shared patterns of investment and consumption. Members of the new élite increased their predominantly landed wealth in the same proto-capitalist ways; they had the same avant-garde tastes in literature, art and furniture; hand-in-hand they patronized the newly-formed masonic societies and filled the provincial academies.[118] In another, albeit minor, aspect this common culture manifested itself in a shared medical experience. Practitioner power ensured that patients, whatever their sex or social and professional background would be treated in the same basic manner. Geoffroy's medical practice was not determined by the provenance of his patients. Titled aristocrats, *parlementaires,* provincial noblemen, great merchants: all were treated as individual representatives of a common humanity, never as social types. Practitioner power, then, was implicitly socially corrosive. It played a part in breaking down the differences between robe and sword, *haute bourgeoisie* and old nobility. It was also, of course, potentially socially radical. Geoffroy's patients primarily came from the groups that would form the new super élite, but his essential pattern of treatment would have been no different if his patients had been paupers. Practitioner power had subversive, egalitarian implications. It is not surprising, then, that the *philosophes* reversed the traditional hierarchy of knowledge and made medicine the key Enlightenment science.[119]

Notes

1. This paper could not have been written without the kind help of Mlle Molitor and the staff of the Bibliothèque de la Faculté de Médecine, Paris.

2. The history of diagnostics before the modern day is traced in Roy S. Porter and William F. Bynum (eds), *Medicine and the Five Senses* (Cambridge: Cambridge University Press, 1993).

3. Physicians would also feel the patient's belly for signs of an enlarged spleen or liver. Urinoscopy was still promoted in the sixteenth century. At Padua the chair in practical medicine established in the mid-century was called *De urinibus et pulsibus*. In the mid-eighteenth century the Montpellier-educated Paris physician and vitalist, Théophile de Bordeu (1722–76), would turn taking a patient's pulse into an art form.

4. On the hierarchy of the sciences, see Laurence W. B. Brockliss, *French Higher Education in the Seventeenth and Eighteenth Centuries: A Cultural History* (Oxford: Clarendon Press, 1987), 1–2.

5. Diaries and account books reveal that physicians in early–modern France would visit their patients several times a day and sometimes every couple of hours. For example, Bibliothèque Municipale, Avignon, MS 5178, *cahiers de visites* of Pellisier, Saint-Rémy en Provence, 1762–5.

6. Among many French e.g., J. de Sainte-Beuve, *Résolutions de plusieurs cas de conscience touchant la morale et la discipline de l'Eglise* 3 vols (Paris, 1689–1704).

7. Nancy G. Siraisi, *Medieval and Early Renaissance Medicine. An Introduction to Knowledge and Practice* (Chicago: University of Chicago Press, 1990), 115–6.

8. See Bibliothèque Nationale, Paris, MS Français 18767, ff., 165–9, 179–80. It is likely that French physicians did give written consultations before this date. At the turn of the seventeenth century several physicians illustrated their published works with specimen case histories in the form of anonymous medical consultations.

9. On the development of literacy, see Robert A. Houston, *Literacy in Early-Modern Europe. Culture and Education 1500–1800* (London: Longman, 1988), especially chs 6 and 7. An interesting attempt to extend the possibility of consulting by letter to the semi-literate was initiated by the French physician, Théophraste Renaudot, in the 1630s. Renaudot had a booklet published depicting parts of the human body. Patients were asked to indicate on the diagrams the location of their aches and pains, then choose from a list of symptoms: see his *La Présence des absens* (Paris, 1642). Discussed in Howard M. Solomon, *Public Welfare, Science and Propaganda in Seventeenth Century France. The Innovation of Théophraste Renaudot* (Princeton, NJ: Princeton University Press, 1972), 175–6 and

appendix C.

10. See Andrew Wear, 'Medical Practice in Late Seventeenth- and Early Eighteenth-Century England: Continuity and Union', in Roger French and Andrew Wear (eds), *The Medical Revolution of the Seventeenth Century* (Cambridge: Cambridge University Press, 1989), 294–320. Changes in medical philosophy are described in Brockliss, *French Higher Education*, ch. 8.

11. *Mémoires de Saint-Simon* Gonzague Truc (ed.), 7 vols (Paris: Gallimard, 1948–61), ii, 53.

12. Biblothèque Municipale Nîmes, MS 414, no. 24, Boissier de Sauvages to Baux, 13 June, 1731. In the first edn of his famous nosology, Boissier de Sauvages (1706–67) produced only an outline sketch of his ideas.

13. Tobias Smollet, *Travels through France and Italy* Frank Feselstein (ed.) (Oxford: Oxford University Press, 1979), 89–104.

14. Paul-Joseph Barthez, *Consultations de Médecine. Ouvrage posthume de P. J. Barthez* (ed.) J. Lordat, 2 vols (Paris, 1810).

15. Bibliothèque de la Faculté de Médecine (hereafter BFMP), Paris, MS 5241–5.

16. The phenomenon in England has already been explored but only to a degree: see Guenther Risse, 'Doctor William Cullen, Physician, Edinburgh. A Consultation Practice in the Eighteenth Century', *Bulletin of the History of Medicine,* 48 (1974), 338–51; and A. F. Oakley, 'Letters to a Seventeenth-Century Yorkshire Physician', *History of Medicine,* 2 (1970), 24–8; also comments in Dorothy and Roy S. Porter, *Patient's Progress. Doctors and Doctoring in Eighteenth-Century England* (Cambridge: Polity Press, 1989), 76–8. Andrew Wear of the Wellcome Institute, London, is working on Hans Sloane's consultation correspondence.

17. See especially Roy S. Porter (ed), *Patients and Practitioners. Lay Perceptions of Medicine in Pre-Industrial Society* (Cambridge: Cambridge University Press, 1985); Roy Porter, *Health for Sale. Quackery in England 1660–1850* (Manchester: Manchester University Press, 1989); Porter and Porter, *Patient's Progress;* Irvine Loudon, *Medical Care and the General Practitioner 1750–1850* (Oxford: Oxford University Press, 1986); Lucinda McCray Beier, *Sufferers and Healers: The Experience of Illness in Seventeenth-Century England* (London: Routledge & Kegan Paul, 1987).

18. For an example of what can be done from printed medical texts, see Laurence W. B. Brockliss, 'The Medico-Religious Universe of an Early Eighteenth-Century Parisian Doctor: The Case of Philippe Hecquet', in French & Wear, *Medical Revolution,* 191–221.

19. Hence the importance of the letters of Mme de Sévigné, one of the very few French women of the classical period to be obsessed by her health: see *Madame de Sévigné, Molière et les médecins de son temps* (Marseilles: Centre méridional de Rencontres sur le XVIIe siècle,

1973); and Laurence W. B. Brockliss, 'The Literary Image of the *Médecins du Roi* in the Literature of the Grand Siècle', in Vivian Nutton (ed.), *Medicine at the Courts of Europe 1500–1837* (London: Routledge, 1990), 129–33.

20. A controversy begun with the seminal article of N. Jewson, 'Medical Knowledge and the Patronage System in Eighteenth Century England', *Sociology,* 8 (1974), 369–85.

21. The basic source for Geoffroy's life is the *éloge* read by Fontenelle on 4 April, 1731: see *Histoire de l'Académie Royale des Sciences* (1733), 93–100. Additional details are provided in the notices on the Geoffroy family in *Dictionnaire de Biographie française* 15, cols 1132–3, 1134–5, 1143–4. Unless otherwise stated information provided in the section below comes from these sources.

22. Fontenelle says 1693. Pharmacy, like surgery and physic, was largely a corporate profession in early–modern France. The right to practise in a particular town came from being received as a master apothecary by the local corporation. Training in one town and settling in another was commonplace.

23. This was an institution set up in 1635, independent of the faculty, to provide practical tuition in botany and anatomy (and later pharmacy and surgery). Its crowning glory was its botanical garden, a facility that the Paris faculty did not possess.

24. Henry Guerlac, *Newton on the Continent* (London: Cornell University Press, 1981), 100. Geoffroy was a frequent correspondent of Sloane's for the rest of his life: see the catalogue of Sloane MSS in the British Library, *sub nomine.*

25. Copies of the dissertations can be found in the British Library, Department of Printed Books, 1182 e 3 (nos 23, 24 and 30). Paris MD's were automatically members of the Paris College of Physicians. For the requirements that had to be fulfilled to become a Paris MD, see Brockliss, *French Higher Education,* 74–5.

26. *Dictionary of Scientific Biography, sub* Geoffroy; Hélène Metzger, *Les Doctrines chimiques en France du début du XVIIe siècle à la fin du XVIIIe siècle* reprint edn (Paris: Blanchard, 1969 [1923]), ch. vi., *passim*; Guerlac, *Newton,* 77–6, 101, 139–40.

27. Established by Francis I in the 1530s. By the eighteenth century there were four medical chairs attached to the Collège Royal.

28. *Tractatus de materia medica sive de Medicamentarum simplicium historia* 3 vols (Paris, 1741). A 7-volume French translation appeared in 1743. The treatise is complete for the mineral reign but only reaches 'Meliolotus' in the section on plants. This section was completed anonymously in 1750 and another on animals was produced by Nobleville and Salorne in 1756–7.

29. Bibliothèque de la Faculté de Médecine, Paris, MS 18, 'Commentaires de la Faculté', *sub anno*. The professors were elected at the beginning of the academic year.

30. British Library (hereafter BL), Sloane MSS, 4044, ff. 51–2: Geoffroy to Sloane, 31 May, 1715. In this and other quotations cited below the original orthography is followed.

31 BL, 1182 e 3 (no. 45). This dissertation is discussed with reference to the contemporary embryological debate in Laurence W. B. Brockliss, 'The Embryological Revolution in the France of Louis XIV: the Dominance of Ideology', in Gordon R. Dunstan (ed.), *The Human Embryo. Aristotle and the Arabic and European Traditions* (Exeter: University of Exeter Press, 1990), 158–96.

32. The case which dragged on until the middle of the century is briefly discussed in Paul Delaunay, *Le Monde médical parisien au dix-huitième siècle* 2nd edn (Paris: Rousset, 1906 [1905]), ch. 5. The case is only mentioned in passing in Toby Gelfand, *Professionalizing Modern Medicine. Paris Surgeons and Medical Science and Institutions in the 18th Century* (London: Greenwood, 1980), 85.

33. *Catalogus librorum viri C. D. Stephani-Francisci Geoffroy* (apud Gabrielem Martin: Paris, 1731): there are copies in both the Bodleian and British Libraries.

34. David Sturdy, 'Pierre-Jean-Baptiste Chomel (1671–1740): A Case Study in Problems Relating to the Social Status of Scientists in the Early Modern Period', *The British Journal for the History of Science*, 19: 3(1986), 318–19; J. P. Nicéron, *Mémoires pour servir à l'histoire des hommes illustres dans la république des lettres, avec un catalogue raisonné de leurs ouvrages* 43 vols (Paris, 1729–45), xli, 98–9 (Hecquet, notice). I am engaged in a study of medical libraries in eighteenth-century France.

35. BFMP, MS 5241, ff. 35–6. This fact is not too surprising. It has been argued for England that it was only in the eighteenth century that physicians began to attend children as part of a more positive attitude towards child-rearing: see Porter and Porter, *Patient's Progress*, 103–5.

36. BFMP, MS 5242, fo. 150 (case no. 47 in this MS).

37. BFMP, MS 5242, ff. 167–8 (case no. 61). *Mémoires* on behalf of both Mme and Mlle Danse. For an account of this merchant family, see Pierre Goubert, *Familles marchandes sous l'Ancien Régime. Les Danse et les Motte de Beauvais* (Paris: Ecole Pratique des Hautes Etudes, VIe Section, 1959).

38. BFMP, MS 5242, fo. 95 (no. 33): letter to Geoffroy 26 October, 1723.

39. BFMP, MS 5241, ff. 43–8: letters to and from Geoffroy 10 June and 3 July, 1729. From the tone of the letter the marquis had corresponded with (or perhaps even seen) Geoffroy on several occasions.

40. BFMP, MS 5242, fo. 1 (case no. 1), no date. The letter does not reveal whether the lady, who had taken three weeks getting to France via London, was visiting the country for her health or pleasure.

41. Admittedly, Geoffroy must have owed his teaching post at the Jardin du Roi to the king's chief physician, so it is a little peculiar that he did not inherit any of Fagon's court clients when the latter retired in 1715.

42. See BFMP, MS 18, fo. 189r, faculty minutes. The Bull *Unigenitus* of 1713 was the most sweeping of several papal condemnations of Jansenism. The standard history of the movement is still Augustin Gazier, *Histoire générale du mouvement janséniste* 2 vols (Paris: Champion, 1922–4). For the history of the Bull *Unigenitus* in the University of Paris, see Charles M. G. Brechillet Jourdain, *Histoire de l'Université de Paris aux XVIIe et XVIIIe siècles*, 2 pts in 1 vol. (Paris, 1862–6), pt i, 300–72, *passim*.

43. BFMP, MS 5241, ff. 22–6. For the cult of the deacon Pâris, see B. Robert Kreiser, *Miracles, Convulsions and Ecclesiastical Politics in Early Eighteenth Century Paris* (Princeton, NJ: Princeton University Press, 1978); Cathérine-Laurence Maire (ed.), *Les Convulsionnaires de Saint-Médard. Miracles, convulsions et prophéties à Paris au XVIIIe siècle* (Paris: Gallimard, 1985).

44. BFMP, MS 5241, fo. 116.

45. Unfortunately, the letters provide little information about Geoffroy's charges.

46. For example, BFMP, MS 5241, ff. 94–6: letter 8 January, 1719; MS 5242, fo. 112, no date (no. 37). Hébert, it seems, had got to know Geoffroy while staying in Paris.

47. According to a royal edict of 1707 only graduate physicians could treat internal diseases in France. The most recent account of the hierarchic structure of the ancien-régime medical profession is Matthew Ramsey, *Professional and Popular Medicine in France, 1770–1830. The Social World of Medical Practice* (Cambridge: Cambridge University Press, 1989), ch. 1.

48. For example, BFMP, MS 5242, ff. 55–8, letter 18 March, 1726 in the hand of Mme de la Buretiere of Châteaudun (no. 18). The lady had become Geoffroy's patient in September 1724.

49. BFMP, MS 5242, fo. 217v: in response to a letter of 10 September, 1724 (no. 78).

50. Generally, it is impossible from the letters to tell whether patients were advised by their medical practitioners to seek Geoffroy's advice or whether patients forced their practitioners' hand. Not surprisingly, the practitioners hint that the initiative came from themselves.

51. BFMP, MS 5242, ff. 127–8, no. 40: letter 12 April, 1730.

52. Patients often added their own postscript to letters if they felt that there was relevant information that the doctor had forgotten.

53. BFMP, MS 5242, fo. 134, no. 42: undated letter with no address, 1729.

54. BFMP, MS 5242, fo. 97: letter 11 November, 1723. Morfontaine was probably not the name of the *curé* but of his village. For recent

studies of community feeling (both rural and urban) in eighteenth-century France, see: Yves Castan, *Honnêteté et relations sociales en Languedoc, 1715–1780* (Paris: Plon, 1974); and David Garrioch, *Neighbourhood and Community in Paris 1740–1790* (Cambridge: Cambridge University Press, 1986).

55. BFMP, MS 5242, ff. 83–5, no. 29: undated letter (late February, 1728). Poitevin taught at the Collège de Beauvais *c.* 1710–*c.* 1735; his course of philosophy survives in MS for the years 1730–2. See Brockliss, *French Higher Education*, 223n, 352, 355, 357, 380n, 465. The Ettmuller referred to here was presumably the Leipzig professor, Michael (1644–83), rather than his son. Some of M. Ettmuller's works were published in French in the early eighteenth century.

56. The collection of letters is loosely classified (there is no index) according to separate diseases. MS 5242, nos 47–66, deals with asthmatic cases. Geoffroy differentiated between humoral and convulsive asthma; in the second case there was no pituitous expectoration: see the case of a Bernardine nun, December 1724 (ff. 173–4).

57. In the early months of 1730, Geoffroy was preoccupied with faculty business, overwhelmed with patients and himself laid low with a fluxion of the chest. As a result he did not reply to a letter from Mme Pecquet de Sainte-Victoire written 7 January until 17 April: see BFMP, MS 5241, fo. 124.

58. BFMP, MS 5242, ff. 40–1 (no.14). The intermediary is one De la Goudonniere, who wrote to Geoffroy on other occasions and was probably a physician at Falaise.

59. BFMP, MS 5242, ff. 211–12 (no. 77).

60. BFMP, MS 5242, ff. 51–2 (no. 18): the account is concocted from the physician's *mémoire* and the patient's additional comments.

61. This may have been either a qualified master surgeon or an unlicensed specialist. Eye diseases in the eighteenth century still tended to be the province of the wandering empiric.

62. In the seventeenth and eighteenth centuries this was one of the most popular French spas: see Laurence W. B. Brockliss, 'The Development of the Spa in Seventeenth-Century France', in Roy S. Porter (ed.), *The Medical History of Waters and Spas*, suppl. no. 10 of *Medical History* (London: Wellcome Institute for the History of Medicine, 1990), 23–47.

63. Taton presumably knew that Geoffroy had taken a scientific interest in Saint-Amand water. In 1699 Geoffroy had sent the Royal Society a report on the spa. See BL, Sloane MSS, 4037, fo. 222: Geoffroy to Sloane, 7 March, 1699.

64. Madame de la Buretiere's physician talked in his initial letter of consulting one or two *médecins* of quality.

65. Etampes is about 25 miles from Fontainebleau. Dargouges was almost certainly a Paris *robin*. Fleury was probably the name of his

country estate.

66. BFMP, MS 5241, ff. 27–30: letter 21 May, 1730. This was J. Cl. Adrien Helvétius (1685–1755), doctor of the Paris faculty. His father, Adrien Helvétius, had popularized the use of ipecacuanha in France.

67. BFMP, 5241, fo. 116. Geoffroy in his reply assured the countess that the mucous could not have formed as the result of his remedies. Rather it was the result of 'un peu de rhume que vous sera survenu dans un tems froid'.

68. BFMP, 5241, fo. 64: letter 2 September, 1717. Forges was another leading French spa. Voltaire took the waters there in 1724 and was equally suspicious of its virtues. 'There is more vitriol in a bottle of Forges water than in a bottle of ink, and frankly I do not believe that ink is very good for the health.' Cited in Theodore Besterman, *Voltaire* (London: Longmans, Green & Co., 1969), 103.

69. BFMP, 5242, fo. 48: letter 3 January, 1725. The letter is in the third person but not written by a physician. At the end, Mme La Buretiere apologizes for not writing herself, for she is in no fit state to do so.

70. Before taking the whey, Madame de la Buretiere had paid a visit to Geoffroy in Paris, thus cementing the relationship by a personal meeting.

71. *Ibid.*, ff. 55–8. This letter was written by Mme de la Buretiere. Either Geoffroy did not reply, or the reply is lost.

72. For details of early-eighteenth century medical theory, see Brockliss, *French Higher Education*, ch. 8, and Brockliss, 'Philippe Hecquet', 196–201.

73. Especially the dissertation entitled: 'An medicus Philosophicus Mechanico-chymicus'. Cf. also Geoffroy's comments on Hecquet's triturationism in a letter to Sloane, 31 August, 1712: see BL, Sloane MSS, 4043, ff. 85–6.

74. Hecquet was one of the greatest sinners in this respect. Geoffroy himself did not publish in the vernacular but his spermatozoist thesis was translated and extended by a colleague, Nicolas Andry (1652–1742).

75. BFMP, MS 5242, fo.41: letter 2 December, 1729.

76. BFMP, MS 5242, fos. 144–7: consultation, 22 August, 1728. Geoffroy does not seem to have shared the view of eighteenth-century Englishmen that gout was a preservative; while in its throes, sufferers supposedly could not catch any other disease: see Porter and Porter, *In Sickness and in Health*, 147–9.

77. These were two stones attached like eyes to the crayfish's body: see Robert James, *A Medicinal Dictionary* 3 vols (London, 1743–5), *sub nomine*.

78. Mineral water was bottled for transportation from the third quarter of the seventeenth century, although the trade was only fully organized in the early eighteenth century: see L. W. B. Brockliss,

'The development of the spa', 40; Pascale Cosme-Muller, 'Entre science et commerce: les eaux-minérales en France à la fin de l'ancien-régime', in Jean-Pierre Goubert (ed.), *La Médicalisation de la société française 1770–1830* 9 of *Historical Reflections/ Réflexions historiques* (Waterloo, Ontario, 1982), 257–69.

79. Brockliss, 'Philippe Hecquet', 203–4.
80. Porter, *Health for Sale*, ch. 6.
81. BFMP, MS 5242, fo. 85 (no. 30): letter 10 December, 1729.
82. BFMP, MS 5242, fo. 44: letter, undated (August 1727) (no. 15).
83. BFMP, MS 5242, fo. 174: no date (December 1724) (no. 62).
84. BFMP, MS 5242, ff. 11–14: consultation 17 March, 1729.
85. BFMP, MS 5242, fo. 38: consultation 14 April, 1730.
86. See *ibid.*, fo. 39. The lady in question was advised to go to Forges; the waters were very good for melancholic diseases. Balaruc is near Montpellier.
87. BFMP, MS 5242, ff. 125–6: consultation no date (September 1727). While there the countess was to drink Vichy water and bathe in Bourbon water. Mme de Sévigné had done the same in 1687.
88. BFMP, MS 5242, fo. 182r: consultation 29 June, 1730 (no. 66). Sainte-Reine is near Dijon.
89. BFMP, MS 5241, ff. 54–6: consultation 30 October, 1729.
90. BFMP, MS 5242, fo. 184r.
91. BFMP, MS 5242, fo. 193: consultation 11 April, 1729. Nephrisis was particularly prevalent in Paris at the turn of the eighteenth century: see Martin Lister, *A Journey to Paris in the Year 1698* (London, 1699), 232–3. Lister describes the activities of one of the most famous cutters of the stone at this date, Jacques Baulant (known as *Frère* or *Père* Jacques: he was not a cleric). If they could, patients understandably preferred to deal with the disease with lithontriptics.
92. For example, BFMP, MS 5242, ff. 139–41, consultation for Madame de Cerny [?], no date.
93. For example, BFMP, MS 5242. ff. 195–6: consultation 17 September, 1728 for a lady of 50 attacked with nephritic pains since she was 12 (no. 72).
94. See remarks in BFMP, MS 5242, fo. 39: consultation 14 April, 1730 (case 13).
95. BFMP, MS 5241, ff. 81–3: consultation 29 July, 1729. Artificial mineral waters were only made on a commercial scale from the end of the eighteenth century: see N. G. Coley, 'The Preparation and Uses of Artificial Mineral Waters (*c.* 1680–1825)', *Ambix,* 31 (1984), 33–48.
96. BFMP, MS 5241, ff. 99–101.
97. BFMP, MS 5241, fo. 116.
98. BFMP, MS 5242, ff. 153–5: consultation 14 September, 1730. Geoffroy himself had a chest complaint that may well have carried

him off a few months after this letter.

99. BFMP, MS 5242, fo. 221v (no. 79). The patient was advised to take a specific daily infusion of *pareira brava*, white nettle flowers and St John's Wort, plus the usual emulsions at times of *accès*. Earlier in his life Geoffroy had not dismissed the possibility of finding an efficacious lithontriptic. See letter to Sloane, 30 September, 1710: BL, Sloane MSS, 4042, fo. 181.

100. Even for England the information is sparse. Despite the increasing volume of literature on eighteenth-century English medicine, there is a notable absence of hard information about individual medical practice. There were definite national differences. The English took up cold water treatment and sea-bathing a century before the French. Cf. the remarks in E. Julia-Fontenelle, *Manuel Portatif des eaux minérales le plus employées en boisson* (Paris, 1825), 170–84.

101. The correspondence of many physicians survives but often the letters are only tangentially about their medical practice. Physicians were collectors, local historians, archaeologists, etc., who were in the van of the Enlightened community of the provinces. At present I am working on one such figure, Esprit Calvet of Avignon (1728–1810).

102. The Annales school used the archive to map the prevalence of particular diseases in the late-eighteenth century. The best study of the *Société* is Caroline Hannaway, 'Medicine, Public Welfare and the State in Eighteenth Century France: the Société Royale de Médecine de Paris (1776–1793)', Ph.D. dissertation, Johns Hopkins University, 1974.

103. For example, BFMP, MS 5242, ff. 167–8, case of Mlle Danse of Beauvais who had a breast ulcer.

104. BFMP, MS 5242, fo. 112v: the girl, a nun-nurse, was suffering from headaches and haemorrhaging from the ear; she had been bled five times; the author of the *mémoire* was the apothecary Hébert.

105. BFMP, MS 5241, ff. 27–30. Geoffroy is extremely complimentary about the drug considering that he never advocated its use; perhaps he was humouring his patient. According to Hecquet kermes was used by the young, inexperienced practitioner on the make: see Philippe Hecquet, *Le Brigandage de la Medecine dans la maniére* (sic) *de traiter les petites veroles et les plus graves malades par l'Emetique, la saigneé du pied et le kermes mineral* (Utrecht, 1732–3), especially pt i.

106. These, of course, must be MS consultations for the reasons stated in the first section of this paper. Since writing this paper I have had the good fortune to discover a collection of consultations written by Geoffroy's contemporary, the Montpellier physician, iatrochemist and court doctor, Pierre Chirac (d. 1732). Chirac is generally associated with the introduction of kermes (amorphous trisulphide of antimony) into the French pharmacopoeia, but a study of his consultations suggest that he usually advocated the same mildly depletive remedies as Geoffroy. In a similar vein, his patients were

placed on a light diet and subjected to a ritualistic round of *bouillons*, tisanes, *lavements*, and baths. Unfortunately, only the consultations have survived, not the incoming letters: see Library of the College of Physicians, Philadelphia, MS 10a 183, Chirac, 'Consultations' (from the papers of Cuthbert Constable). Constable, an East Yorkshire Catholic, seems to have studied under Chirac and taken copies of a representative sample (?) of his consultations in the 1700s.

107. BFMP, MS 5242, ff. 123–4: *mémoire* 9 September, 1727.

108. BFMP, MS 5241, ff. 43–9: *mémoire* 10 June, 1729. Coffee was always one of the drinks Geoffroy banned.

109. BFMP, MS 5241, ff. 49–51: *mémoire* for the Marquise de Pontfarey, Laval, 1 July, 1729.

110. Brockliss, 'The Literary Image of the *Médecins du Roi*', 124, 129–33.

111. Molière's views on physicians are discussed at length in *Madame de Sévigné, Molière et les médecins de son temps, op. cit.* note 19 above. For another example of patient–power towards the end of the century, see Elborg Forster, 'From the Patient's Point of View: Illness and Health in the Letters of Liselotte von der Pfalz (1652–1722)', *Bulletin of the History of Medicine*, 60, 3 (1986), 297–320.

112. Brockliss, 'The Development of the Spa', 43–5. See also Pierre Thomas Du Fossé, *Mémoires pour servir à l'histoire de Port-Royal* (Utrecht, 1739), 490–1. The noble Du Fossé, visiting Bourbon in 1696, specifically called the experience 'humiliant'.

113. On Fagon, see Brockliss, 'The Literary Image of the *Médecins du Roi*', 134–7. There are also two outdated studies: A. Corlieu, 'Guy-Crescent Fagon (1638–1718)', *France médical*, 48 new series (1901), 169–74, 189–92; A. J. Grozieux de Laguérenne, *Guy-Crescent Fagon, archiâtre de Louis XIV, surintendant du Jardin royal des plantes (1638–1714)* (Paris, 1930).

114. The most important studies of this revolution in noble behaviour are by Norbert Elias: see his *The Civilizing Process* 2 vols (Oxford: Blackwell, 1977–82) and *The Court Society* (Oxford: Blackwell, 1983). Elias ignores the important ingredient of stoicism in the creation of the new ethic: see Gerhard Oestreich, *Neostoicism and the Early-Modern State* B. Oestreich and H. G. Koenigsberger (eds), trans. D. McLintock (Cambridge: Cambridge University Press, 1982).

115. Modern research by Porter *et al.* suggests that in eighteenth-century England, in contrast, practitioner–power of any kind was unknown. Significantly for the argument here, the eighteenth-century English, proud of their 'liberties', were notoriously ungovernable. Supposedly, French émigrés in the 1790's were amazed to find that the English would rather be robbed than suffer the presence of a police force: see Alexis de Tocqueville, *L'Ancien Régime et la Révolution* (ed.) J. P. Mayer (Paris: Gallimard, 1967), 143.

116. On the development of secularism in eighteenth-century France, see

especially John McManners, *Death and the Enlightenment. Changing Attitudes to Death in Eighteenth-Century France* (Oxford: Oxford University Press, 1985); Michel Vovelle, *Piété baroque et déchristianisation en Provence au XVIIIe siècle* (Paris: Plon, 1973). Some of Geoffroy's patients did express a fear of dying.

117. This point will be argued in the book that I am writing with Colin Jones on early–modern French medicine (to be published by Oxford University Press). The power of quacks proved very difficult to erode before the late nineteenth century even when the medical profession was reorganized: see Ramsey, *Professional and Popular Medicine*, especially chs 3–7.

118. On the development of this new élite, see especially Franklin L. Ford, *Robe and Sword: The Regrouping of the French Aristocracy after Louis XIV* pbk edn (New York: Harper & Row, 1965 [1962]); Guy Chaussinand-Nogaret, *La Noblesse au XVIIIe siècle. De la féodalité aux lumières* (Paris: Hachette, 1976); Daniel Roche, *Le Siècle des lumières en province: académies et académiciens provinciaux 1680–1789* 2 vols (Paris: Mouton, 1978).

119. Looking beyond the Revolution the early development of a form of practitioner–power in France may be the starting point for understanding the detached attitude of the medical professors and researchers of the Paris school towards their patients. As will be seen in a later chapter Anglo-American visitors to early nineteenth-century Paris found the reification of the patient perplexing and distasteful. Of course, Geoffroy's patients were still definitely individuals; his was not a 'clinical' practice.

3

Private Practice and Public Research: The Patients of R. T. H. Laennec

Jacalyn Duffin

'Que de gens bien mis,
que de gens crottés ...'
From a contemporary drinking song

In the last 15 years, historians have begun to study medical history 'from below', by examining the experience of the long-ignored patient. The medical past, they remind us, consists not only of doctors and diseases but also of patients and illness. The interaction between patient and doctor is more than a means of medical livelihood; it is often fundamental to therapy and it can be vital for research.[1]

René Théophile Hyacinthe Laennec (1781–1826) was the inventor of the stethoscope and the first to develop auscultation as a means of physical diagnosis. This achievement made him one of the founders of a new type of nosology based on the objective detection of internal organic changes, rather than on the observation of subjective disease symptoms. Several biographies, most more or less hagiographic, have been made of the personal and social circumstances of his discovery, and his life has been the subject of articles, displays, conferences and two feature length films.[2]

On the other hand, Laennec's patients, who were the basis of his practice and research, have been mentioned in only a few anecdotal accounts; there has been no attempt to assemble these people into a practice profile. Using biographies, letters and the extant manuscript case records, this paper will explore Laennec's practice through his patients, both private and public, their origins, political and intellectual sympathies, their reasons for consulting Laennec, and their opinion of his treatment. It will also examine their impact on his work.

Laennec's Career and Fortunes

Laennec was born in Brittany on 17 February, 1781. His mother died when he was five years old. Although their father was still living, he and his brother eventually went to live with their uncle, Guillaume Laennec, a surgeon in Nantes, under whose tutelage Laennec began his medical instruction. In 1801, he went to Paris to study with J. N. Corvisart des Marets (1755–1821), clinician at the Charité Hospital and Napoleon's personal physician. He completed his degree in 1804.

Despite great success as a student, Laennec was not wealthy (see Table 1). His father had sued him for support in the lean years shortly after his graduation and this, together with the costs of maintaining an unmarried sister and a tubercular brother, placed him in relative poverty. In 1816, he was appointed to the Necker Hospital, through the influence of his friend, Becquey, under-secretary in the Ministry of the Interior, and his precarious financial condition then began to improve (see Table 2).

Shortly after the Necker appointment, Laennec discovered that heart sounds could be transmitted through a rolled-up notebook. He investigated the relationship between chest sounds and pathological change by listening to the (often tubercular) patients in his hospital wards and by performing autopsies when they died. In less than three years he published the first edition of his treatise, *De l'auscultation médiate* in 1819.[3]

Laennec suffered from chronic ill health and after the publication of his book, he retired to his home in Brittany for two years. Upon his return to Paris in 1822, he received many honours, including an appointment at the Charité Hospital and to the Chair of Medicine at the Collège de France. He continued to see private patients, but devoted most of his energy to the hospital. Due to the changes in Laennec's circumstances, all the styles of nineteenth-century French practice, identified by Jacques Léonard, from the country doctor to the 'grand patron', can be found in the career of this single physician.[4]

Laennec described his routine in a letter written to a medical friend in 1817.[5] Rising at 7.30 or 8.00, he gave consultations while he dressed. Mornings were spent in hospital visits and with students; afternoons and evenings until 10 p.m., in rounds, with a one hour break for dinner; the hour before bed at 11 p.m. was devoted to correspondence. He continued to work on auscultation for a second edition, published only weeks before his death of tuberculosis, on 13 August, 1826, at the age of 45.[6]

Laennec's political and personal sentiments greatly influenced his practice. He has been portrayed as an innovator with conservative inclinations.[7] The study of Latin and Greek had been abolished during the Revolution, but, at the risk of appearing reactionary, Laennec did not hide his love of classical scholarship. In his thesis, he proposed a new interpretation of Hippocrates, designed to be both philologically correct and conceptually compatible with the new style of anatomo-clinical medicine.[8] He prepared to compete for the chair of Hippocratic medicine and was greatly disappointed when it was abolished in 1811. Although post-Revolutionary atheism officially ended with the Concordat of 1801, its influence continued to be felt in the hiring practice of academic institutions for several more years. During this time, Laennec became a devout Catholic and in 1802 joined the Congregation, a Catholic society founded in secrecy by the Jesuit priest, Delpuits.[9] After the Restoration of the monarchy in 1815, many academic physicians remained politically liberal, but Laennec was openly sympathetic to the crown. His position at the Collège de France and his university appointment were both the result of direct intervention by the royal family during the conservative 'crackdown', following the failure of the Carbonari movement in 1822. The liberal-leaning and less religious members of the medical faculty were aware of and resented Laennec's acceptance of royalist favours.

Some of Laennec's private patients came from the clergy and the aristocracy, but his hospital patients came from the working classes. Sources for this essay include the two editions of his treatise on auscultation (in which he often discussed individual cases by name) and his manuscripts, comprising letters, preparatory notes for his lectures at the Collège de France, a few private consultations, and 770 case records of the public hospital patients examined at the Necker, Charité, and Hôtel-Dieu Hospitals.[10] In addition, several of Laennec's patients wrote about encounters with their doctor. Most of these documents pertain to the period after the invention of the stethoscope.

Private Patients

The private patients of Laennec often shared his geographic origins, political sympathies, religious preferences and artistic tastes, and they included several well-known individuals and aristocrats. Now, in the aftermath of the febrile celebration of the bicentenary of the French Revolution, it is a little difficult if not cavalier to explore the history of the Bourbon Restoration, especially that of its supporters. Recent work on this period has concentrated on the opponents to the Restoration, defined as they chose to define themselves, as the

'Generation of 1820'.[11] Historians have tended to justify the actions of the opponents, finding intelligence, tolerance, and merit in their achievements and opinions. Only a few historians have been inclined to defend the Restoration, but not without complications. De Grandmaison, who admired the Congregation, addressed the problem of favouritism in the Villèle ministry, while minimizing the contribution and political influence of the Congregation in the persons of Mathieu de Montmorency and *grand maître* Frayssinous.[12] Similarly, Rouxeau, who idolized Laennec, tried to defend the political interference on Laennec's behalf by citing the outstanding intellectual merit and 'courage' of the man who benefited from it.[13] Nora Hudson observed that 'it is not uncommon to regard the ultra-royalists of the Restoration as having more affinity with prejudice than with doctrine.'[14] Similarly, Alan Spitzer remarked that reconstructing the original appeal held in the conservatism of Cousin and Chateaubriand 'puts a considerable strain on our historical empathy'.[15]

Thus, Laennec must be identified with the 'wrong' side of the 'Generation of 1820'; yet, most historians have been unable to reject his merit even if they choose to devalue his fellow physician-royalists. This has fostered some awkward prose. For example, Ackerknecht and Spitzer describe the royalist physicians as 'nonentities', who capitalized on their connections to take the place of 'virtually all the outstanding members' of the faculty who were perceived to be 'politically unreliable'.[16]

Clergy

Shortly after his religious conversion, Laennec befriended the young Breton priest, Hyacinthe-Louis Comte de Quélen, who, in 1807, became a member of the house of Napoleon's uncle, Cardinal Fesch. Quélen recommended Laennec's services to the Cardinal, who appointed him his *premier médecin,* in the spring of 1809. Rouxeau claimed that Laennec had to overcome his 'natural repugnance' to such situations in order to accept the position,[17] but it is certain that he did not have much repugnance for the 3,000 francs a year, which came with the post and constituted at least a third of his income. There were expenses: Laennec was obliged to borrow 700 francs for such essentials as the 'costume de cour', 'chapeau à claque' and sword, official attire for the household of the Cardinal. Nevertheless, he felt that the new title would convey public confidence; judging by his subsequent rise in fortune, this seems to have been true (Table 1). The retainer compares favourably with the average annual income for rural practitioners of approximately 900 francs estimated by Jacques Léonard and his colleagues.[18]

Attendance on Fesch is said to have been difficult: he was preoccupied by the vagaries of his political fortune and insisted on daily medical visits, but he does seem to have liked his doctor.[19] At first, Laennec served for three years, until the Cardinal fell into disgrace in March 1812; he then returned for a few months before Fesch left Paris for Rome in 1815.

This connection with high-placed clergy made Laennec one of the doctors of choice for ailing men of the cloth. A file entitled, 'Consultations of the Cardinals', contains the autopsy reports of Cardinal Eriskin (1809) and of Cardinal Vincenti (1811).[20] A 17 page report describes the sickness and death of Cardinal 'X', probably a Monseigneur Ruffo who fell ill of angina while visiting France and died on, as Laennec called it, 'The Ides of March', 1810.[21]

Laennec also attended Félicité de Lamennais (1782–1854), a fellow Breton from Saint-Malo. This liberal priest-philosopher attempted to reconcile Church and throne and, when this failed, to cultivate a bond between the Church and the people independent of the state. In 1814, he sent his friend, the abbé Tesseyre, to pay Laennec's medical bill.[22] Lamennais may have chosen Laennec because of his openly avowed religious and royalist leanings.[23] Four years later, however, he found him overly stern and expensive and turned to other doctors.[24] He wrote the following to the Comte de Senfft:

> There is no doctor in Paris more capable nor more knowledgeable than Laennec; the problem is that he is too much so. Because of this, after what I have seen, his practice is too much dependent on certain systematic ideas, which he has formulated. For this reason, I prefer Fiseau.

Notwithstanding the advice, Senfft did consult Laennec. Lamennais politely replied:

> M. Laennec is not only an excellent doctor, he is also a man of strong principles and remarkable spirit. Therefore, I am not surprised that you are pleased to have found him.[25]

What exactly Lamennais meant by 'systematic ideas' is not clear. It may have been Laennec's use of the stethoscope, which some contemporaries found excessive to the exclusion of other modalities of diagnosis. Alternatively, it may have been his practice of using high-dose antimony emetics, or it might have been Laennec's obvious royalism at a time when Lamennais was disillusioned with the crown.

Certainly patients chose their doctors, but it seems evident, in this case, that the doctor chose or, at least, maintained an interest in his patient. When Lamennais published the second volume of his *Essai sur l'indifférence en matières de la religion* (1820), Laennec wrote him a congratulatory letter concerning the section on insanity, in which he offered certain of his own observations about the relationship between emotional ills and political unrest. The comments could be summed up as, 'a healthy mind results from healthy, strong society'. Lamennais published the letter in the preface of the second and subsequent editions.[26] The doctor became a participant in the life work of the patient, but the reverse is also true. For his own Collège de France lectures on mental illness *(vésanie)*, Laennec made remarks that bear a decidedly Mennaisian stamp: he called for more order and authority; and he thought that political and moral chaos were both product and cause of insanity.[27]

For at least ten years, Laennec was consultant physician to a strict religious community of women in Paris and he published his experiences with tuberculosis there.[28] His observations led him to the conclusion that tuberculosis resulted from psychological stress and privation, an opinion apparently endorsed by his own experiences with the same disease.[29] He remained a devout Catholic, but, possibly due to the growing rift between Church and throne, his popularity with the clergy appears to have declined after his connection with Fesch had dissolved and a new bond with nobility emerged.

Soldiers

In February 1814, the military hospitals of Paris were filled with injured soldiers, and public hospitals were needed for their care. Typhus was rampant; a third of the more than 700 doctors, students and nurses who tended these patients, succumbed to the disease. Private citizens fled the city and Laennec's finances took a proportionate drop. He volunteered at the Salpêtrière Hospital where his charges included many soldiers of Breton origin. Although these soldiers were hospital patients, Laennec made them his private concern. The Breton language, or Celtic, was still spoken and the soldiers did not always understand French. Far from their home, these young war-wounded pined away in the stench and confusion of the enormous city hospital. Since Laennec noticed that the men improved emotionally and physically when they were grouped together in one ward, he planned a small research project on what might anachronistically be called, the 'psychosomatic' aspects of care. He sought and obtained permission to create a special ward of

Breton soldiers and found three Breton doctors to assist him. He made it a practice to speak in their native tongue.

The Bishop of Quimper wrote to thank Laennec for his work. In his reply, Laennec outlined the programme he had implemented and its positive results:

> What I have done is very little.... In this calamitous community, the Bretons had more to complain about than the others. Isolated ... almost all overcome with homesickness, they fell into profound discouragement and many refused any sort of help. All my colleagues found them even more difficult to understand than the Germans and the Russians because they made no use of sign language. Those that I could assemble in my ward were a little less unfortunate. I had the consolation of losing only one sixth, a terrifying mortality in normal times, but low in this moment. I lost approximately one third of my French patients and this was the average mortality in most of the military hospitals of Paris.[30]

This original research project, undertaken in the heat of crisis, emphasized two aspects of new medical practice: psychosomatic medicine and statistics, priority for the latter traditionally being given to P. C. A. Louis.[31]

Private Citizens

No narrative of Laennec's clients would be complete without reference to the patient at the centre of his account of the discovery of auscultation. One morning in October 1816, he was called to see a young female, whose name and age he did not reveal. He suspected a cardiac lesion and he decided to attempt to listen to her chest; however, the girl was well developed, if not quite plump, and the concerned parents hovered nearby. How was he to enhance the transmission of sound and yet minimize what would appear to be an invasion of the girl's modesty? He seized one of his notebooks, rolled it into a tight cylinder, applied one end to her chest, the other to his ear and was astonished at the clarity of the heart sounds. As this was prior to auscultatory interpretation, the exercise could provide no further information in this particular case. The outcome was not recorded and no manuscript pertaining to this – the most important of all his private consultations – has been found.[32]

Better-known patients, though certainly of less research significance, were the Breton writer, statesman and politician, René de Chateaubriand (1768–1848) and his spouse, Céleste Buisson de la Vigne (1774–1847). Chateaubriand hid during the Revolution and the Terror, but was honoured by Napoleon, who granted him state appointments and sent him as ambassador to Rome in 1804. Together with Cardinal Fesch, he had been assigned the difficult task of encouraging the Pope to appear for the coronation of Napoleon. Chateaubriand eventually broke with 'the tyrant' Bonaparte and supported the return of the aristocracy, of which, conveniently, he was a member.

Chateaubriand may have been an aristocrat, but he was never financially secure. He married for money, then ignored his wife for the first decade of their marriage. Nevertheless, his devoted spouse and a network of mistresses and patrons supported and encouraged him in his opinions and his art. He was narcissistic and given to fits of anger or depression and he indulged in ill health for many years. At the end of his life, he was virtually immobilized by gout. Possibly through the 'Brittany connection' or perhaps through devotees of the Congregation, he first encountered Laennec sometime before 1812. In that year, he was afflicted with palpitations and, since some of the physicians he consulted suspected an aneurysm, he feared the worst. His wife wrote this account, testimony of their love-hate relationship:

> The palpitations of Monsieur increased to the point that he was certain he suffered from a fatal disease. As he did not lose any weight and his colour was good, I was fairly certain he had a nervous condition. This didn't prevent me from being anxious all the same and I implored him to see Laennec, the only doctor in whom I had any confidence ... I let him leave, but my anxiety was so great, that he had gone no more than a quarter of a league, than I left myself and arrived only moments after he did. I hid until the end of the consultation. Laennec arrived: after a long narrative, in which he [Chateaubriand] did not minimize his woes, the doctor told him that he had nothing wrong; Monsieur de Chateaubriand gave him a complete list of his ailments; Laennec was firm and would prescribe nothing, except, perhaps, that he take his hat and go for a stroll. 'But what if I placed a few leeches?' said my husband. 'If that would make you happy, you can go ahead,' said Laennec 'but I advise you to do nothing.' I can't describe how I suffered until he left. I watched for the doctor in the passage way and asked him what was the matter with my husband: 'Nothing at all,' he replied and bidding me goodnight, he disappeared. Five minutes later, I heard the patient, charmed and cured, come down the stairs singing and laughing that certain persons had wanted to bury him alive; and when he came home around 11 o'clock, he was delighted to find me there so he could tell me that Laennec had found his state so alarming that he didn't even want to use leeches:

125

> he had only a small rheumatic pain ... his imagination, working on
> a pain to which he wouldn't have paid the least attention at another
> time, had created for him a real disease.[33]

These memoirs, written at Chateaubriand's urging, were cribbed
without acknowledgement, for the *Mémoires d'outre-tombe*, but the
passage on the consultation with Laennec was omitted.
Chateaubriand later gave an enthusiastic notice of his doctor's book
on auscultation, the work of a 'knowledgeable Breton compatriot'.[34]

Madame de Chateaubriand and Laennec saw each other often.
She suffered from a bronchitic condition, possibly bronchiectasis,
and her capricious health forced her 'from time to time to heave
great sighs in the direction of the little doctor'. She called Laennec a
petit secco, a little dry stick, but when he left Paris in 1819, she
vowed she would have no medicine other than common sense and
asses' milk. Twelve years after Laennec's death she was still praising
his skills and mourning her loss.[35]

The interest seems to have been mutual. The name of Madame de
Chateaubriand figures in Laennec's lecture notes and in his personal
letters.[36] The nature of her illness fascinated him. Apparently, in 1818,
she had had all the signs of pulmonary consumption and one colleague was convinced she would die. Laennec reminded himself of
this on several occasions, as an example of the unreliability of clinical
signs and as a reason for hope in phthisis, which, at the time, could be
defined by its gloomy prognosis. On his own death-bed, he cheered
himself with this memory:

> Calculated properly, I can only compare my case to that of
> Madame de Chateaubriand eight years ago. Cayol was certain she
> would die of phthisis in two or three months, notwithstanding the
> stethoscopic signs. I stuck to my position and at the end of ten
> months, the huge quantity of sputum decreased by half, the fever
> fell and I left for my vacation with peace of mind.[37]

Laennec may also have attended Madame Juliette Récamier
(1777–1849), beautiful muse of Paris, wife (in name only) to an
elderly banker and mistress of Chateaubriand. Inspiration to several
prominent statesmen and artists, she has been praised for her
intelligence and generosity in prose and immortalized for her
beauty, in the masterpieces of Jacques-Louis David and François
Gérard. Madame Récamier met Chateaubriand during the last
illness of their mutual friend, Germaine Necker, Madame de Staël
(1766–1817). Both women had been exiled from Paris for their
anti-Bonapartist activities and their political influence. For the

purposes of this essay, the interest of their encounter 'au chevet de' Madame de Staël lies in the fact that Laennec had been summoned there too.

Madame de Staël's narratives of the events surrounding the Revolution and the birth of the empire were decidedly unpopular with Napoleon. In exile in Switzerland, she had maintained a liberal, artistic forum. In an account of her last illness, her doctor, Antoine Portal (1742–1832), described a visit by Laennec, which took place in June 1817, less than one year after his discovery. The patient had suffered from pleural effusion since the preceding February:

> She complained of a squeezing pain in the upper part of the chest over which a newly graduated doctor placed a large blister. Another well-known doctor [Laennec], using a horn of paper, which he placed with one end on a part of the thorax and the other in his ear, believed he diagnosed a hydrothorax and could even hear a sort of undulation. This method of investigating the interior of the chest didn't convince me and I did not share his opinion, in spite of the regard I might have had for him. [38]

The Duc de Broglie, son-in-law of Madame De Staël, also witnessed Laennec's visit and observed that the consultant 'stood himself in great need of medical care'.[39] Madame de Staël died one month later on 14 July, 1817 and, to Laennec's discredit, her autopsy did not reveal a pleural effusion.

Among other well-known people attended by Laennec was Victor Cousin (1792–1867), philosopher and professor at the Sorbonne.[40] Cousin has been called the 'chien de garde' and apologist for the Restoration; however, since his course at the Sorbonne was abruptly 'terminated' in 1820, he became popular with those opposed to ultra-royalism.[41] In his own lectures, Laennec applied Cousin's word 'eclectic' to what he considered to be the ideal medical philosophy: one that eschewed exclusive theories and embraced useful notions from the past, including the concept of a 'vital force'. Laennec's vitalism was perceived, by some, as a throwback to outdated notions from Antiquity and, by others, as a direct product of his Catholic faith, but Laennec related it to Cousin's new 'system' of philosophy for the nineteenth century. 'Eclecticism' later became the name for the school of medical thought led by Gabriel Andral, following Laennec's death.[42]

Cousin introduced Laennec to the musicologist, C.-C. Fauriel (1772–1844), who shared his interest in folk culture, poetry and music. During their 'exciting encounters', Laennec played the flute and Fauriel sang Breton songs. The scene was gently described by C.

A. Sainte-Beuve (1804–1869), literary journalist and critic, who was also a doctor and a former student of Laennec.[43] Other artists seem to have figured in the private practice, including Alexandre Dubois (later known as Dubois-Drahonnet), who was a popular but struggling painter, unable to pay his bills. In return for medical services rendered, he painted the only known full-sized life portrait of his doctor in 1812.[44]

Laennec left no case records of Cousin, Fauriel or the Chateaubriands, but his papers contain the histories of a few other private patients. These documents mostly concern bourgeois patients who could afford individual attention, and only a few pertain to the poor, who, for reasons of fear, shame, or pride, avoided the hospital. There are the cases of an 18-year-old 'nymphomaniac', a congenitally retarded girl, an old soldier with cancer, and a law student with mumps involving the testis.[45] There is also a long narrative of the last illness of Athanase Vorogidès, a doctor born in Constantinople who had studied medicine in Vienna and Bucharest.[46]

Some consultations were conducted through the post.[47] Charles Saunier of Côte d'Or near Dijon, probably a wine dealer, wrote at least twice seeking Laennec's help. The first letter came from a Parisian hotel. Saunier may have come to the city to visit a relative, since Perrine Saunier, a 25-year-old seamstress, was in Laennec's hospital at the time.[48] Charles Saunier consulted Laennec in person on 7 June, 1825 for headache and a chest complaint; however, during the course of the interview, Laennec elicited the history of a dog bite some eight years before. Fears about the possibility of rabies were aroused, either because of the doctor's queries, or because the man had been preoccupied with the idea for many years. In his letter, he asked eight questions about rabies. Laennec must have replied, for he was thanked in the second letter and sent 40 francs. Despite the reassurances, Saunier was still afraid of hydrophobia and expounded on his symptoms for three pages. Laennec annotated both letters and kept them with his lecture notes for the Collège de France. On the first he wrote 'melancolia. fear of hydrophobia' and placed it with the lecture on rabies, presumably in order to remind himself to answer Saunier's eight questions, which typified the ignorance of common knowledge.[49] He labelled the second letter, 'rare example of unreasonable anxiety (fear of rabies) which has none of the features of vesania' and he filed it with his lectures on mental illness.[50]

Aristocrats

The royalty who resurfaced at the departure of Napoleon were called 'émigrés'. Their return to power and the lap of luxury, after having fled their country during its troubles, gave them a selfish reputation.[51] Laennec attended many members of this class and, since they were not always rich, his devotion may have stemmed from respect for their position. He was circumspect about their names and what little documentation survives is obscured by deliberate omissions. Hence, there are records for 'Mlle xxx', the 'Duchesse de C...', 'Monsieur le comte H...'. There are at least three (probably) different people designated simply by the title 'N...' . From personal correspondence an additional list of Laennec's regal clientele can be assembled: the Duchesse d'Estissac, the Marquise de Chavagne, the Marquis de Talaru, the daughters of the Comtes de Kersant and de Senfft, Madame de Levis, Madame de Mercy, and Madame de Lorient.[52]

The best known of these patients was the Princess of the Two Sicilies, Marie-Caroline-Ferdinande-Louise, the Duchesse de Berry (1798–1870). This enterprising young woman was the widow of the Duc de Berry, second nephew of King Louis XVIII. Seven months after her husband's assassination in 1820, she gave birth to a son, called the 'miracle child'. Her father-in-law, the Comte d'Artois, became Charles X in 1824 and the Duchesse de Berry enjoyed considerable influence at court; her son was viewed as a direct heir to the Bourbon line and some hoped Charles X would abdicate in his favour. In 1830, the Duchesse led a failed attempt to replace the 'usurper' Louis Philippe with her son, 'Henri V'. Among her strongest supporters was René de Chateaubriand.[53]

Laennec's appointment as physician to the Duchesse de Berry was arranged by his former professor, the court doctor J. N. Hallé (1754–1822). His presentation took place on 1 January, 1822. Henceforth, for a salary of 4,000 francs a year, he was to attend his royal patient daily at her chateau.[54] Once again, as in the days he served Cardinal Fesch, Laennec was required to dress in courtly attire complete with a sword. Apparently, the Duchesse found his method of percussion somewhat brutal, but she liked her new doctor and gave him an Italian cello. There is a legend that the 'miracle child', then 16 months old, enjoyed riding on Laennec's gold-headed cane.[55] How much Laennec had to do with the Duchesse is not clear. His name does not appear in her biographies, although ample anecdotal space is given to her 'accoucheur', Dr Deneux.[56]

Hallé died in February 1822, leaving vacancies in the Medical Faculty and at the Collège de France. Laennec's colleagues elected the physiologist, François Chaussier (1746–1828) to the latter.[57] The King, however, ignored the election results and granted the position to Laennec on 31 July, 1822. This event occurred in the middle of a conservative backlash against anti-royalist activities: between February and October of the same year, ten men were executed for their association with the Carbonari movement. Undoubtedly, Laennec owed this appointment to the prevailing sentiment and his association with the Duchesse de Berry. The following year, he became a professor in the medical faculty in succession to those purged for their perceived political orientations. His honours included the Légion d'Honneur and election to the Académie de Médecine.[58] Royalist connections were thought to have been decisive in his triumphs of 1822–23.[59]

Public Patients

Although Laennec's famous clients have attracted the greater attention, his research owed at least as much if not more to the anonymous hospital patients. The hospitals in which Laennec worked, had embraced changes endorsed by the Revolution. Patients were to be used as subjects for teaching and research; if they died, their bodies were autopsied.[60] After his discovery of auscultation, Laennec kept records of many (exactly what proportion has not been determined) of his public hospital cases. Large gaps in the sequence of dates imply that only a fraction of these records have survived. Nevertheless, there are 770 case histories of patients he attended during the last ten years of his life, 1816–1826.[61] Approximately 50 of these cases, often with the names of the patients, were published in each of the two editions of his treatise on auscultation.

The manuscript records are rarely in Laennec's own hand, although he occasionally dictated or annotated them. He usually assigned the writing to students, requiring them to provide a detailed history and, where indicated, an autopsy report. As many as three or four different accounts of the same case can be found, presumably because Laennec assigned interesting patients to several different students.[62] Some documents, written in Latin, appear to be daily entries, while longer accounts, in French, are case summaries.[63] A detailed history of medical and social circumstances surrounding the illness was provided and reference was often made to the patient's temperament. The clinical and autopsy diagnoses graced the cover of every case as a title.

Not all were chest patients, but Laennec used these records to test the reliability of his stethoscopic signs and to correlate the sounds he heard in the living patient's chest with lesions he observed in the corpse. The evolution of the stethoscopic nomenclature and signs can be traced through these documents. For example, Grmek has identified the heuristic value of the exaggerated vocal fremitus heard over lung cavities in the case of the woman, Goigy (also interpreted as Grigy or Guigy), 'mother and wife of soldiers'. She seems to have been the first patient in whom Laennec appreciated pectoriloquy, likely because she was talking instead of breathing deeply while her doctor tried to listen.[64]

The records suggest possibilities for the demographic history of Paris, but several factors would tend to skew the selection: wards were for women or men only; Laennec may have been more inclined to preserve the records of those who had died, in preference to those who had been discharged; he began to be known as a lung specialist and other cases may have been sent elsewhere; and finally, the patients would probably have come from the sixth and seventh arrondissements where his hospitals were located.

Nevertheless, some comparisons can be made between this group of people and the demographic analyses of contemporary Paris. For 662 of the 770 patients an occupation was given. Table 3 shows the distribution of 646 of these patients grouped according to occupation. There were 189 different occupations, some so precise they defied the usual classification. The pattern corresponds to other demographic studies of early nineteenth-century France.[65] Almost one quarter of the male patient population worked in the construction industry, the most common occupations being mason and stone cutter (involving 41 individuals). The most common employment among women was dressmaker (34), followed closely by maid (30), and lingerie maker (27). The sewing of clothing concerned a total of 75 of the 662 patients.

Early nineteenth-century Paris is vividly evoked with special mention of activities such as pin-maker, ribbon-maker, flounce-maker, shepherd, spaghetti-maker, junkman, bottle-seller, mule-keeper, fan-painter, chimney-sweep, midwife, lamplighter, writer, male nurse and rope dancer, each represented by one patient. There were six water carriers, two teachers, two female gardeners, and three each of lemonade salesmen, butchers, lapidaries and weavers. There were jewellers, coachmen, milliners, printers, bakers, pastry chefs, students in law and medicine, theatre workers and dancers, but no musicians, aristocrats, politicians or doctors.

Of the 662 patients with occupations, 234 were women, only ten of whom were listed as 'housewife'. Those with no occupation given were not always women, but for these individuals many other details are often lacking, including the name and sex. One important group of workers was the day labourer, as often female as male. At least half of the domestics were male and some of the heavier jobs, such as porter, were occupied by females. Perhaps because they could work at home, married women tended to be 'lingères' leaving the outside domestic jobs to single women. Some of the workers were quite young: a girl of 12 years, who died, was identified only as a 'mattress maker'; a 16-year-old carver recovered from his disease, but a 17-year-old milliner and an 18-year-old mason both died.[66] Others were quite old: an 80-year-old woman, who died of pneumonia after five weeks in the hospital was found at autopsy to have been suffering from widespread cancer; on admission, she had been described as a labourer.[67]

From 1816 to 1826, there was a trend to more faithful recording of employment. This may reflect an increasing consciousness of occupational disease. In fact, sometimes the mine or the factory is specified, as in the cases of four workers from the white lead factory at Clichy, north of Paris.[68] Three of these men were diagnosed as having lead poisoning; one died. Other workers (masons, copper smelters and lapidaries) were also thought to have 'coliques métalliques', although their symptoms were mild.[69] This diagnostic zeal suggests the post-Revolutionary doctor was so attuned to the possibility of labour-related illness that, when confronted with any patient at risk, he could diagnose little else. It also contrasts with the apparent lack of sensitivity to work-related illness observed at the end of the eighteenth century, suggesting that the Revolution may have sensitized the medical gaze with respect to the labourer.[70]

It is difficult to select a representative sampling of the public patients. Medically speaking, many examples can be found of ante-mortem diagnosis confirmed by autopsy. However, the following five cases, not necessarily demonstrative of stethoscopic success, do represent typical hospital experiences and offer the life-histories of people who were not usually able to leave their own record.

1. Wife Dumont, a 61-year-old woman of good constitution and sanguinous temperament, ... suffered confluent smallpox at the age of 7 which left only a few permanent scars on her face. Her periods appeared at 19 years, she married at 20 and had 11 children, six of

whom are still alive. Her periods stopped without complication when she was 50. All her life she worked very hard. Often she sought oblivion in wine. Ten years ago, she noticed that carrying a heavy load or becoming very angry made her heart beat harder than usual. Eight years ago, she was treated with violet and honey tea for catarrh, but she did not stop working. She notices that her cough improves in summer and worsens in winter. Lately, her palpitations have been more frequent accompanied by a choking sensation and violaceous changes to her nose and lips especially when in the cold. Exposed to all the atmospheric vicissitudes of this season, her respiration became laboured, her cough much worse and, abandoning her usual occupation, she presented herself to the Necker Hospital on 12 October, 1816.

In this early record from the month in which Laennec claimed to have made his discovery, no occupation was given, nor was there any mention of the stethoscope.

On physical examination, a well-nourished woman with yellowish skin and smallpox scars. The nose was very large and dark purple in colour especially at the tip. There was a scar on her right leg from an old injury and there were several varicosities. Respiration was short and noisy sometimes interrupted by choking and coughing spells productive of frothy sputum. Percussion of the thorax was mediocre, posteriorly and in the region of the heart. The pulsations of the heart were tumultuous and easily felt over the base of the sternum. The pulse was rapid by intervals, but equal in both arms. The jugular veins were distended and in the one on the right, there was a marked trembling. The tongue was moist but the patient complained of severe thirst and bitterness. The abdomen was distended and tender to deep palpation. There was constipation, the urine was scant and dark, but intellectual functions were intact. The breathing worsened and delirium caused the patient to try to leave her bed several times. She died at 5.30 in the evening.[71]

Even without auscultation, the clinical presentation is entirely consistent with the post-mortem findings of enlarged heart and tricuspid valve abnormalities. The lungs and liver were engorged with blood. There were signs of previous pleurisy and the cervix uteri was obliterated by a polyp.

2. Entitled 'Boulimia'. Herbé, a 22-year-old soldier in the colonial regiment, with pale skin and red hair was admitted to the hospital in December 1819 for aching pains in his legs and emaciation, despite a voracious appetite which he had some difficulty to satisfy. His illness went back two years and appeared to begin with a venereal condition which he had contracted in Martinique and for

which he had been given a lengthy treatment, this winter, consisting of, so he said, 64 bottles of Van Swieten liquid and many frictions [mercury]. Since his therapy he had no symptoms of syphilis, did not masturbate, and did not have any commerce with women. His principal symptoms on admission were an extreme thinness so that his arms and legs resembled those of a six-year-old child ... *he did not cough at all*.... Towards the end of December he noticed an increase in his urinary volume, out of proportion with the amount of liquid he drank. We verified this phenomenon and thought he had diabetes, but it disappeared in a few days without treatment.... On Christmas day he had two nervous attacks, or convulsions ... but he improved and ... still with his great appetite, left hospital at the beginning of January.

He was re-admitted on 6 February, 1819, with a productive cough ... there was marked pectoriloquy under the right clavicle.... On 1 March, he was found in a state of prostration, with extreme agitation and great difficulty in breathing. Breath sounds on the right were well heard, but there were no sounds on the left even though the chest was resonant to percussion. The heart beat was rapid. The cough had ceased. He was prescribed four leeches to the left chest ... but he died in the evening.[72]

The autopsy revealed extensive bilateral pulmonary tuberculosis with cavities in both lungs. No mention was made of pneumothorax, although the clinical findings might have suggested it.

3. Marie-Louise Usé, a 22-year-old gardener, hysterical ['hystérique'] since the age of ten and subject to frequent vomiting, sustained a contusion to her epigastrium on 15 April, 1822 and was admitted to the hospital with all the symptoms of intense peritonitis on 9 May.... The stomach was tender ... there was constipation. She had a smooth red tongue, severe headache and intense almost continual vomiting which aggravated her pains.

She received baths, leeches to the groin, and mercury frictions, all to no avail. She developed dysuria. [The record is heavily corrected and annotated in Laennec's own hand. He was conducting research on antimony tartrate, an emetic with drastic side effects.]

On 2 July, she was treated with orange leaf tea to which had been added tartar emetic. Her vomiting was no worse than before ... at the end of three days of therapy she felt well and wished to discontinue treatment ... her fever returned on the 22 July, the emetic was started on the 24th and by the 27th, she was cured.... At home she remembered the in-hospital therapy and took a strong dose [of tartar emetic] when needed and was cured the same day.[73]

Laennec appeared to correct the student's notes for emphasis as much as for accuracy.

The following case was labelled 'Quartan fever?', but seems to have been recognized as malingering.

> 4. Joseph Fleuret, a 47-year-old locksmith was admitted with a five-week history of quartan fever. Each attack began at 3 a.m. The patient had had the disease before. The skin was yellowish, the spleen perhaps a little enlarged. All other functions ... [were]... in good condition and [he had] a very big appetite.
>
> Today, 10 May, the day the attack should have occurred. The patient maintained that he did have a brief chill at 3 a.m. and even more abundant sweating than usual. At 6 a.m., there was no evidence of fever and the skin was only slightly moist as is normal after sleep. We have doubts about this fever.
>
> The 11th. Displeased about the doubts raised concerning the existence of his fever and finding that he isn't getting enough to eat, the patient insists on leaving the hospital. Agreed.[74]

This case was labelled 'Nostalgia'.

> 5. A young girl, 18 years of age, with fair complexion and chestnut hair, was admitted to hospital with no particular localizing signs. She was weak and unhappy with facial pallor and dark circles around her eyes. She had no difficulty breathing and did not cough. She was so depressed that it was thought she was suffering from nostalgia.[75] In fact, she had been in Paris only for a short time and longed to return to her native village near Amiens. The pulse was regular, but weak and rapid. The chest resounded a little less than normal on the left, but respiration was clear on both sides.... She continued like this for a few days; then, the depression and sadness deepened. Fever appeared, which became continuous and increasing; the abdomen was slightly tender; she developed the Hippocratic facies ['grippé ... tiré']. Her mental faculties were altered and she drifted into stupor ... leeches were applied, but her condition worsened and she died almost three weeks after admission.

On autopsy, tubercles were found in the right lung and the peritoneum. The cerebral convolutions were flattened and there was increased serosity in the pia mater and ventricles.[76]

Conclusion

Laennec's career was intimately associated with his patients in an iterative process that led to a gradual increase in his fortunes: the more patients he treated, the more his attentions were sought; the greater his social position, the greater his institutional stability. Both practice and research were shaped by social class, academic position, and personal convictions. The private patients provided the major part of his livelihood, but the hospital practice provided the patients and cadavers necessary for his research. Far from being mutually exclusive, however, the activities of practice and research were intertwined. Laennec willingly brought his research into the private setting; moreover, he often relied on ideas learned from his patients when it came to the interpretation of his findings.[77]

In Laennec's early years, the lack of a hospital or a faculty appointment hampered his ability to establish a large practice. The private patients seem have chosen their doctor for his Breton origins and his political or religious leanings, which stood in opposition to most of his colleagues in the Napoleonic period. Following the discovery of auscultation and Laennec's elevation to a position of prominence, his ability to attract such persons was greatly enhanced. The ambivalence of Lamennais and the fidelity of Madame de Chateaubriand make it clear that 'doctor-shopping' took place in post-Revolutionary Paris and that the choice was influenced by a physician's politics, religion and position, as much as by his personality, comportment, and medical accomplishments.[78]

Laennec's later practice was sharply divided along class lines, because of the social circumstances of the hospital patients. Private patients generally came from the upper and middle classes and were seen at his residence or in their own homes. These people provided his main source of income; the stipends offered by Cardinal Fesch and the Duchesse de Berry were his greatest financial support. There is insufficient information to claim that the attentions he gave the rich were substantially different from those he gave to the poor; however, in his concern for the anonymity of aristocrats, he appears to have approached them with greater solicitude.

At the end of the eighteenth century, the hospital was a place where the poor went to die. One hundred years later, as precise diagnosis and the promise of cure became increasingly allied to the technology of institutional facilities, rich and poor patients came to share the similar hospital experience.[79] Laennec's stethoscope, as the first in a long line of modern diagnostic instruments, has become a symbol of the medical technology that transformed the nature of hospitalization; his hospital records, therefore, offer a unique glimpse of hospital life at the dawn of diagnostic technology.

Laennec's records demonstrate that the post-Revolutionary hospital, in which the stethoscope was first used, was much like its eighteenth-century predecessor. The presence of teaching and research notwithstanding, it catered to the working-class sick, seldom the destitute, never the rich. It appears the hospital patients tried to carry on with their occupations, even when they were severely ill. Their case histories also tend to support the observation that the working-class patient tried self-help and non-expert treatment before turning to an institution.[80] As a result, Laennec's hospital may have held only a minority of the urban sick; however, poor patients could not gain access to him in any other setting.

Evidence from late eighteenth-century Britain and early nineteenth-century America suggests that experimental and student procedures were withheld from affluent patients until they had been tried on the poor.[81] In contrast, Laennec claimed to have made his first rudimentary stethoscope in a private home and did not hesitate to experiment with it on private patients. Auscultation was painless, harmless, and, as it was modestly performed through the patient's clothing, it was singularly non-invasive. For these reasons, it carried little risk, but scornful colleagues did ridicule the posture adopted for listening to chest sounds. An image-conscious practitioner might be expected to avoid situations that could provoke laughter or draw undue attention to the errors of inexperience from influential observers. Nevertheless, within a year of his discovery, Laennec boldly used his stethoscope to examine Madame de Staël.

Being auscultated by Laennec possibly held a special cachet and may have become a not-to-be-missed experience for a certain class of people in the tubercular Paris of the mid-1820s. Unlike the hospital patients, some of the wealthy seem to have had infinite time and capacity for being sick. It is not known how often the doctor was asked to listen to the chests of those who, like Saunier, had consulted him for non-thoracic reasons. Perhaps Laennec catered to these demands, but he did not shrink from calmly disagreeing with a vigorous Chateaubriand intent on being ill.

Laennec's patients, both public and private, influenced his research. Numerous patients and cadavers were needed to define the chest sounds and relate them to organic changes. His consummate skill as a pathologist is often cited as the major reason for the successful development of auscultation; the skill was essential, but the hospital position was equally important, if not the *sine qua non* of auscultation. Only in a ward of chest patients, could he have gathered the clinical and pathological experience necessary to establish the meaning of the lung and heart sounds with such speed and accuracy.

Patients contributed to Laennec's investigations not only as 'biological material', but also on an intellectual level. Sometimes, this was fortuitous: for example, the situation of the Breton soldiers suggested an experiment to assess the relationship between psychological and physical well-being. On other occasions, Laennec seems to have deliberately sought his patients' participation. Thus, he could 'choose' his private patients as they chose him; he was interested in their politics, religion, philosophy and art. Their adventures and misadventures were important to his perception of himself, as a doctor, as an educated participant in society, and as a patient. With them, he agreed that the return of the monarchy was not simply a return to the 'Ancien Régime', but the creation of a sane and natural order through adaptation of the best elements of the old monarchy to the new structures of the Revolution.[82] Thus, he and Lamennais shared ideas on the relationship between moral order, social order and mental illness. Similarly, he invoked the philosophy of Cousin, when he integrated the 'vital force' into his lectures on human physiology and turned his stethoscope into a tool for its investigation.[83] As a patient himself, Laennec was sustained in his own last hours by recalling the recovery of Madame de Chateaubriand.

Finally, there is an ironic difference in Laennec's relationship with his private and public patients. Fesch, Lamennais, the Chateaubriands and the Duchesse de Berry all survived their doctor, most by more than 20 years. Just as Laennec relied on their financial support, his intellectual and physical health depended on their continued existence – in short, their well-being contributed to all aspects of his own. On the other hand, it was research on public patients that allowed Laennec to perfect his new method of auscultation. Despite any concern he may have felt for the sufferings of the poor, the success of his hospital research was absolutely dependent on their dying. Unlike the well-known and more affluent patients, most members of this group died long before their doctor; yet, it was his involvement with the lives and deaths of these humble people that brought the doctor his lasting fame.

Table 1: Laennec's Finances until Necker Appointment in 1816

	Medical Earnings	Other Income	Expenses
1804	150F		*(tuition)* 900F *(thesis)* 500F *(shirts)* 120F
1805	400F	1,200F *(pension)* 1,000F *(journal editing)* 75 louis *(treatise on parasites)*	
1806	?	600F/yr *(pension)*	
1807	2,400F	1,200F *(journal editing)*	*(rent)* 270F/yr *(furniture)* 508F
1808	3,400–3,600F		
1809	? + 3,000F Fesch		*(father's debt)* 30,000F
1810	? + 3,000F Fesch		*(father)* 600F/yr
1811	8-9,000F [3,000F Fesch]		
1812	?		*(sister)* 1,200F/yr
1813	10,000F		
1814	5,400F		
1815	5,400F		*(father)* 1,200F/yr
1816	5,400F		

Table 2: Laennec's Finances after 1816

	Income	Known Expenses
1816	? *(Necker Hospital)*	*(cabriolet)* 3,000F
	? *(private practice)*	
1819	7,000F *(Treatise on auscultation)*	*(scientific expenses)* 1,000F
1822	4,000F *(Duchesse de Berry)* 5,000F *(Collège de France)* 20,000F *(consultations)*	*(rent)* 1,700F/yr
1823	10,000F *(Faculty salary) (+ ? Charité Hospital)* 5,000F *(Collège de France)* 4,000F *(Duchesse de Berry)* 20,000F *(consultations)* 10,000F *(for a single consultation in Bordeaux)* *(was to be 50,000F if patient was saved)*	*(rent)* 1,700F/yr
1824	5,000F *(Collège de France)* 4,000F *(Duchesse de Berry)* 10,000F *(Faculty)* 20,000F *(consultations)*	*(rent)* 3,000F/yr *(lump sum invested)* 12,500F 3,750F/yr
1825	5,000F *(Collège de France)* 4,000F *(Duchesse de Berry)* 10,000F *(Faculty)* 20,000F *(consultations)*	*(rent)* 3,000F/yr *(invested)* 3,750F
1826	5,000F *(Faculty)* *(leaves Duchesse de Berry and* *Collège de France 1819–26)*	*(rent)* 3,000F/yr *(invested)* 3,750F *(to drain marsh)* 16,000F

Laennec's will and estate

1824	'séparation des biens' settled 15,000F on wife; 40,000F on himself; pension to father 1,000F/yr; reduced to 600F/yr in a codicil, 1826
1826	3,000F/yr awarded by Crown to his widow (until 1830)
1827	5,000F award to the *Treatise on Auscultation*

Table 3: Occupations* of 646 of Laennec's Hospital Patients

Building and Quarries

mason	34
joiner	22
painter/plasterer	14
carpenter	10
stone cutter	7
digger	5
welder	4
roofer	3
Total	**99**

Commerce, Arts, Public Servants

merchant	34
office	19
military	12
postman	5
student	4
artist	3
teacher	2
Total	**79**

Alimentation

chef	20
baker & pastry	19
water, juice seller	10
butcher	5
wine/beer	5
kitchen maid	3
refiner	1
Total	**63**

Equipment and Maintenance

metal worker	37
carriageworks etc.	26
fine craftsman	18
porcelain/cutlery	7
saddler	7
jeweller	5
cooper	3
sweep	1
Total	**104**

Textiles and Fashion

dresses/lingerie	75
shoes	30
tailor	13
laundry	10
hats	11
weaving/spinning	6
bedding	3
hairdresser	2
dyer	2
Total	**152**

Unskilled labour

labourer	female	34
	male	30
domestics	female	37
	male	16
housewife		10
concièrge, huissier		4
coalporter		3
Total		**134**

Agriculture

gardener	10
farmer	5
Total	**15**

* categories after Louis Henry, *Techniques d'analyse en démographie historique,* (Paris: Institut National d'Etudes Démographiques, 1980).

Notes

1. Roy Porter, 'The Patient's View: Doing Medical History from Below', *Theory and Society* 14 (1985): 175–98; Arthur Imhof, 'The Hospital in the Eighteenth Century; For Whom?' and Charles Rosenberg, 'And Heal the Sick: Hospital and Patient in the Nineteenth Century', both reprinted from the *Journal of Social History* 4 (summer 1977) in Patricia Branca, (ed.), *The Medicine Show: Patients, Physicians and the Perplexities of the Health Revolution in Modern Society* (New York: Science History Publications, 1977), 141–63 and 121–40, respectively; Roy Porter, (ed.), *Patients and Practitioners. Lay Perceptions of Medicine in Pre-Industrial Society* (Cambridge: Cambridge University Press, 1985); Edward Shorter, *Bedside Manners: The Troubled History of Doctors and Patients* (New York: Simon and Schuster, 1985).

2. The best biography is Alfred Rouxeau, *Laennec avant 1806* vol. 1 (Paris: Baillière, 1912) and *Laennec après 1806*, vol. 2 (Paris: Baillière, 1920), re-issued in facsimile as *Laennec*, 2 vols (Quimper, France: Les éditions de Cornouaille, 1978). See also: Henri Duclos, *Laennec* (Paris: Flammarion, 1932); Roger Kervan, *Laennec, médecin breton* (Paris: Hachette, 1955); Paul Kligfield, 'Laennec the Discoverer of Mediate Auscultation', *American Journal of Medicine*, 70 (1981): 275–8; Henri Saintignon, *Laennec: sa vie, son oeuvre* (Paris; Baillière, 1904); Gerald B. Webb, 'René Théophile Hyacinthe Laennec', *Annals of Medical History* 9 (1927): 27–59; Gerald B. Webb, *René Théophile Hyacinthe Laennec, a Memoir* (New York: Paul B. Hoeber, 1928). Proceedings of a bicentennial conference on Laennec filled the entire issue of *Revue du Palais de la Découverte*, no. spéciale 22 (1981). The two feature length films are Maurice Cloche and Association Internationale Cinématographique, 'Laennec', 1949 and Yvan Kovacs and Antenne II, 'La passion de Théophile', February, 1981.

3. R. T. H. Laennec, *De l'auscultation médiate ou traité du diagnostic des maladies des poumons et du coeur fondé principalement sur ce nouveau moyen d'exploration*, 2 vols (Paris: Brosson et Chaudé, 1819).

4. Jacques Léonard, *La France médicale. Médecins et malades au XIXe siècle* (Paris: Gallimard, 1978), 97–100.

5. Letter to Courbon-Pérusel, 22 April, 1817, cited in Rouxeau, *Laennec*, vol. 2, 189.

6. R. T. H. Laennec, *Traité de l'auscultation médiate et des maladies des poumons et du coeur*, 2nd edn 2 vols (Paris: Chaudé, 1826).

7. Pierre Huard, 'Les facettes multiple de René Théophile Hyacinthe Laennec (1781–1826)', *Bulletin de l'Académie de Médecine* 165 (1981) no. 2: 249–54.

8. R. T. H. Laennec, *Propositions sur la doctrine d'Hippocrate relativement à la médecine pratique* (Paris: Didot, 1804). Jacalyn

Duffin, 'L'Hippocrate de Laennec repris: la fièvre à l'ombre de l'anatomie pathologique', in Paul Potter, Gilles Maloney, and Jacques Desautels, (eds), *La maladie et les malades dans la collection hippocratique*. Actes du VIe Colloque International Hippocratique (Québec: Sphinx, 1990), 433–61.

9. Charles Alexander Geoffroy de Grandmaison, *La Congrégation 1801–1830* (Paris: Plon, 1889), 35, 162; see also G. Berthier de Sauvigny, 'Le congrégationiste, le chrétien', *Revue du Palais de la Découverte*, no. spéciale 22 (1981): 225–328. On being told he was meeting devout medical students the Pope exclaimed, 'medicus pius, res miranda!', cited in Saintignon, *Laennec*, 50. Grandmaison did not mention that Laennec was present at the papal audience, but gave a detailed description of the presentation ceremony in the Chapelle des Allemands of the church of Saint Sulpice, 50–7.

10. Essential for any exploration of Laennec's manuscripts is the catalogue by Lydie Boulle, Mirko Grmek, Catherine Lupovici and Janine Samion-Contet, *Laennec: catalogue des manuscrits scientifiques* (Paris: Masson, 1982). The personal letters, which were the basis of Rouxeau's biography, are not included in the catalogue; however, they have been transcribed in five theses of medicine directed by Dean of Medicine Kerneis, Nantes. See F. Vial, 'La correspondence de Laennec à travers les fonds Rouxeau', *Revue du Palais de la Découverte* no. spéciale 22 (1981): 214–24.

11. Robert Warren Brown, 'The Generation of 1820 during the Bourbon Restoration in France. A Biographical and Intellectual Portrait of the First Wave, 1814–1824', Ph.D. Dissertation, Duke University, 1979; Alan B. Spitzer, *The French Generation of 1820* (Princeton: Princeton University Press, 1987); Alan B. Spitzer, *Old Hatreds and Young Hopes: The French Carbonari against the Bourbon Restoration* (Cambridge Mass.: Harvard University Press, 1971).

12. Grandmaison, *La Congrégation*, 317–18. See also G. Bertier de Sauvigny, *The Bourbon Restoration* (Philadelphia: Pennsylvania University Press, 1966).

13. Rouxeau, *Laennec*, 2: 288.

14. Nora E. Hudson, *Ultra-Royalism and the French Restoration* (Cambridge University Press: 1936), 181–2.

15. Spitzer, *Generation of 1820*, 96.

16. Spitzer, *Generation of 1820*, 248. Erwin H. Ackerknecht, *Medicine at the Paris Hospital, 1794–1848* (Baltimore: Johns Hopkins, 1967), 101.

17. Rouxeau, *Laennec*, 2: 123.

18. Jacques Léonard, Roger Darquenne and Louis Bergeron, 'Médecins et notables sous le consulat et l'Empire', *Annales ESC* 32 (1977): 858–65, especially 860–1.

19. Fesch gave Laennec a bust of himself and a crucifix. Délégation à l'Action Artistique, La Société Française d'Histoire de la Médecine, L'Académie Nationale de Médecine et la Délégation aux

Célébrations Nationales, *Laennec: l'inventeur de l'auscultation. Catalogue de l'exposition,* 1981 (Paris: Firmin-Didot, 1981), 52.

20. Nantes, MS. Classeur 1, lot f, ff. 181–9.

21. Nantes, MS. Classeur 7, lot e–1(I), ff. 1–17; see also Rouxeau, vol. 2, 101–5.

22. Alfred Roussel, *Lamennais d'après des documents inédits,* 2 vols (Rennes: Caillière, 1893), 1: 48.

23. Nora E. Hudson, *Ultra-Royalism,* 126–7.

24. Letters to 'Jean' (his brother) 28 January, to 28 March, 1818, F. de Lamennais, *Correspondence générale,* edited by Louis le Guillou, 9 vols (Paris: Colin, 1971), 1: 386, 390, 397, 409.

25. Letters to the Comte de Senfft, 27 November, 1823, Lamennais, *Correspondence,* 2: 428–9, 431–2.

26. F. de Lamennais, *Essai sur l'indifférence en matière de religion,* 8th edn (Paris: Belin-Mandar et Devaux, 1829), 2: 90–3.

27. 'Vésanies', 8th lesson, *Collège de France, 1823–24,* MS. Cl. 2a(B), ff. 172r–174v.

28. Laennec, *Traité,* 2nd edn, 1826, 1: 647. Laennec did not identify the community, but said it had not received official sanction and was barely tolerated by Church authorities, because of the austerity of its practices.

29. Jacalyn M. Duffin, 'Sick Doctors: Bayle and Laennec on Their Own Phthisis', *Journal of the History of Medicine and Allied Sciences* 43 (1988): 165–82.

30. 2 June, 1814, cited in Rouxeau, *Laennec,* 2: 120–1.

31. L. L. Rostan claimed credit for this experiment. Jacalyn Duffin, 'Vitalism and Organicism in the Philosophy of R. T. H. Laennec', *Bulletin of the History of Medicine* 62 (1988): 525–45, especially 540. In other manifestations of his view of psychosomatic medicine, especially his reticence to report a gloomy prognosis, Laennec appears to have been like his contemporaries. Jacques Léonard observed that nineteenth-century French physicians preferred to hide the truth of terminal illness from their patients, believing in the beneficial effect of an optimistic outlook on physical condition. Léonard, *La France médicale,* 127–9.

32. Laennec, *Traité,* 2nd edn, 1826, 1: 7–8. A more detailed, possibly embellished, account of this case, involving children tapping on a log in the courtyard of the Louvre, was told by Laennec's former student and Breton compatriot, Alexandre Kergaradec le Jumeau, 'Discours de Laennec sur l'inauguration de la statue à Quimper le 15 août 1868', *Bulletin de l'Académie Impériale de Médecine,* 33 (1868): 807–16.

33. Céleste Buisson de la Vigne, Vicomtesse de Chateaubriand, *Mémoires et lettres de Madame de Chateaubriand,* edited by Joseph le Gras (Paris: Jonquières, 1929), 42.

34. Cited in Henri Duclos, *Laennec,* 237–8 and in Gilbert Chinard,

'Laennec and Chateaubriand', *Bulletin of the History of Medicine*, 7 (1939): 95–6.

35. Buisson de la Vigne, *Mémoires*, 218, 225, 260.

36. Laennec wrote, 'Catarrhe muqueux chronique ... Mme de Chateaubriand a eu', 29th lesson, Collège de France, second year, 1823/4, Nantes, MS. Classeur 2 lot a(B), fo. 256v.

37. Laennec, letter (his last) to his cousin Mériadec Laennec, 4 August, 1826, cited in Rouxeau, *Laennec*, 2: 421.

38. Cited in Rouxeau, *Laennec*, 2: 190–1, 198.

39. Achille Charles Léonce Victor, le Duc de Broglie, *Personal Recollections*, translated and edited by Raphael Ledos de Beaufort, 2 vols (London, Ward and Downey, 1887), 1: 366. Since Madame de Staël had previously suffered from scarlet fever, her early death of dropsy and breathlessness may have been due to rheumatic heart disease. Jean Christopher Herold, *Mistress to an Age. A Life of Madame de Staël* (Indianapolis: Bobbs Merrill, 1958), 107, 417.

40. Charles Dédéyan, 'Laennec et les écrivains de son temps', *Revue du Palais de la Découverte*, no. spéciale 22 (1981): 245–59.

41. Alan B. Spitzer, 'Victor Cousin and the French Generation of 1820', in *From Parnassus. Essays in Honor of Jacques Barzun*, edited by Dora Weiner and William R. Keylor (New York: Harper Row, 1976), 177–94; Spitzer, *Generation of 1820*, 72–96; Hester Eisenstein, 'Victor Cousin and the War on the University of France', Ph.D. Dissertation in Philosophy, Yale University, 1968, 21–52, especially 30–1.

42. Laennec, 2nd lesson, Collège de France, first year, probably given on 4 or 5 December, 1822/3, Paris, MS. 2186(IV), fo. 13v; Gabriel Andral, *Clinique médicale*, 4 vols (Paris: Gabon, 1823–7), 1: 30. See also Ackerknecht, *Medicine at the Paris Hospital*, 101; Jean-François Braunstein, *Broussais et le matérialisme: médecine et philosophie au XIXe siècle* (Paris: Méridiens Klincksieck, 1986).

43. 'Another man who got along very well with Fauriel was, if you can believe it, the great doctor Laennec! ... The Breton songs soon became the favourite pastime ... of these two spirits from such different walks of life. Fauriel knew the words, but Laennec knew all the tunes, tunes learned in his childhood never to be forgotten. He brought his flute (and you have to have seen Laennec to really imagine him cast as Lycidas) and while his friend recalled the words, he tried to jot them down.... A touching scene the mere idea of which brings a smile, so worthy of these souls, of these hearts truly antique and pure.' C. A. Sainte-Beuve, *Portraits contemporains*, 3 vols (Paris: Didier, 1847), 2: 565–6.

44. The result so pleased the subject that the portrait was shipped to Brittany, preventing the dismayed artist from entering it in the Paris salon. Later, Dubois was commissioned by the family to add a stethoscope to his work. The copy, which hangs in a stairwell of the

old medical faculty in Paris, was reproduced in Rouxeau, *Laennec.*

45. Nantes, MS., Classeur 1, lot f(VI) (A), ff. 110–12 and 114–23v; lot k(XI), ff. 249–56; lot n(XIV), ff. 262–3.

46. This account is written by Laennec's cousin, Mériadec Laennec, Nantes, MS., Classeur 1, lot j(X), ff. 238–46.

47. Several of these have been published. See for example, Jean–Pierre Kerneis, 'Postface pour des documents inédits,' *Revue du Palais de la Découverte* no. spéciale 22 (1981): 329–43; Valléry-Radot, 'Trois lettres inédites de Laennec', *Histoire de la médecine* 2 (1952): 31–7; M. Laignel-Lavastine, 'Une ordonnance de Laennec', *Bulletin de la Société Française d'Histoire de la Médecine* 13 (1914): 17–21. See also Jean des Cilleuls, 'Une consultation donnée par Laennec en 1805', *Histoire de la médecine,* 6 (no. 7) (1956): 15–18.

48. Nantes, MS., Classeur, II, ff. 506–7.

49. Nantes, MS., Classeur 2, lot a(A), fo. 66r–v.

50. Nantes, MS., Classeur 2, lot a(B), ff. 175r–176r.

51. Margery Weiner, *The French Exiles, 1789–1815* (London: John Murray, 1960).

52. Nantes, MS., Classeur 1, lot f(VI) (B), fo. 169; Nantes, MS., Classeur 1, lot f(VI) (B), ff. 178–80; Laennec, *Traité,* 2nd edn 1826, 2: 90–1; Nantes, MS. Classeur II, ff. 496r and 511r; Classeur III, lot 3, fo. 176r; Nantes, MS. Classeur 1, lot t(XX) 396–415. This is further complicated by the reserve of Laennec's biographer, Alfred Rouxeau, who suppressed the names of aristocrats indebted to Laennec.

53. Vincent W. Beach, *Charles X of France. His Life and Times* (Boulder, Colorado: Pruett, 1971), 410–13.

54. This handsome amount guaranteed·Laennec a comfortable existence. The manner of interaction and payment seems to represent a return to an earlier style characteristic of practices in both France and England. See Guy Chaussinand-Nogaret, 'Nobles médecins et médecins au cour au XVIIe siècle', *Annales ESC* 32 (1977): 851–7; N. D. Jewson, 'Medical Knowledge and the Patronage System in 18th century England', *Sociology* 8 (1974): 369–85. I have been unable to find comparable monetary figures for the French Restoration; however, according to the accounts of Antoine Portal, médecin du Roi, amounts paid to medical persons in the court of Charles X ranged from 3,000 F to 30,000F, Louis-Désiré Véron, *Mémoires d'un bourgeois de Paris* [1855], *textes choisis par Pierre Josserand,* 2 vols (Paris: Guy le Prat, 1945), 1: 106.

55. Rouxeau, *Laennec,* 2: 279–82.

56. Baronness Orczy, *The Turbulent Duchess* (New York: Putnam, 1936), 52–3; Vincent Cronin, *The Romantic Way* (Boston: Houghton Mifflin, 1966), 23–78.

57. Rouxeau, *Laennec,* 2: 285.

58. 22 August, 1822 and election 24 January, 1823 (ratified 6 April,

1823), respectively, Rouxeau, *Laennec,* 2: 286, 296.

59. Laennec may have replaced the republican sympathizer, Antoine Dubois, who had allied himself with Deneux at the Restoration and would be purged from the Faculty on 23 November, 1822. Véron, *Mémoires,* 1: 101–2, 109–11; Ackerknecht, *Medicine at the Paris Hospital,* 40; Paul Delaunay, *D'une révolution à l'autre, 1789–1848. L'évolution des théories et de la pratique médicales* (Paris: Editions Hippocrate, 1949), 18; Spitzer, *Old Hatreds,* 139–41, 259.

60. Russell Maulitz, *Morbid Appearances: The Anatomy of Pathology in the Early Nineteenth Century* (Cambridge: Cambridge University Press, 1987), 142–3.

61. The hospital cases occupy three files kept at at the Musée Laennec, in Nantes, MS. Classeurs I, II and III.

62. For example there are four separate accounts of the last illness of 70-year-old Adrien Fouleux, Classeur I, lot e, fo. 4r, Classeur III, fo. 280r–v, 327–9, and 334–7. As Boulle *et al.,* have observed, these different records often appear in different handwriting, e.g. 'Legrand', *Laennec. Catalogue,* 63.

63. Accompanying each report are the dates of entry and of discharge or death; the hospital, ward and bed number; the patient's name and, if a married woman, the maiden name as well; the age, occupation, and origin, if not Parisian. Problems arise in determining the exact numbers of different individuals because the students occasionally made mistakes. Hence, some patients appear to have been more than one person.

64. Classeur I, lot b, ff. 29–32v. See also M. D. Grmek, 'L'invention de l'auscultation médiate, retouches à un cliché historique', *Revue du Palais de la Découverte,* no. spéciale 22 (1981): 107–16.

65. The categories and grouping of these occupations are based on those given in the demographic studies by Louis Henry, *Manuel de démographie historique* (Paris and Geneva: Droz, 1967), 46–8 and *Techniques d'analyse en démographie historique* (Paris: Institut National d'Etudes Démographiques, 1980), 22–4.

66. Classeur II, ff. 35r–36v; Classeur II, fo. 241r; Classeur I, lot c, fo. 27.

67. Jobet, Classeur I, lot c, fo. 23.

68. Gournay, Classeur III, lot 1, ff. 1–6; Dupont, Classeur II, fo. 256r–v; Lebel, Classeur II, fo. 526r; Maillet or Mailler, Classeur III, lot 10, ff. 474r–480v.

69. Vaché or Vacher, Classeur I lot a[I], fo. 19v and Classeur II, fo. 501; Duflau, Classeur II, fo. 400r; Dehor, Classeur I, lot a [I] fo. 19r; Derval, Classeur III, lot 2, fo. 101.

70. Arlette Farge, 'Work-related diseases of artisans in eighteenth-century France', translated by Elborg Forster, in *Medicine and Society in France, Selections from the Annales, Economies, Sociétés, Civilisations,* edited by Robert Forster and Orest Ranum (Baltimore and London: Johns Hopkins University Press, 1980), 89–103.

71. Dumont, 1816, Classeur I, lot b, ff. 15r–16v.
72. Herbé, 1819, Classeur I, lot b, ff. 159r–160v.
73. Usé, 1822, Classeur I, lot c, ff. 78r–79r.
74. Fleuret, 1824, Classeur II, fo. 250r.
75. Nostalgia was a specific diagnostic category; see Duffin, 'Sick Doctors'.
76. Anonymous, 1819, Classeur I, lot b, ff. 167–169v.
77. The interaction between Laennec and his patients was not unlike the relationship between medical knowledge and the consultation in late eighteenth-century Britain described by Jewson, 'Medical Knowledge'.
78. This is not to suggest that all patients came to their practitioners in this manner. Roy Porter has emphasized how little is known of patient loyalties in medical history, 'Introduction', *Patients and Practitioners*, 17.
79. Rosenberg, 'And Heal the Sick', 134.
80. Ginnie Smith, 'Prescribing the Rules of Health: Self-Help and Advice in the Late Eighteenth Century', in Roy Porter, (ed.), *Patients and Practitioners*, 249–82. This pattern had been observed in a comparison of late eighteenth-century hospitals in Copenhagen and Berlin. Using the conceptual device of a 'morbidity onion', Arthur Imhof proposed that an increase in the intermediary (non-institutional) levels of care might explain why people admitted to hospital appear to have been much sicker than those in either contemporary cities or later hospitals. Imhof, 'The Hospital', 145.
81. Rosenberg, 'And Heal the Sick', 132. When William Withering first used digitalis, he tested it on charity patients. See 1785 facsimile in J. K. Aronson, *An Account of the Foxglove and its Medicinal Uses, 1785–1985* (London: Oxford University Press, 1985), 2.
82. Nora E. Hudson, *Ultra-Royalism*, 181–2.
83. Jacalyn Duffin, 'Puerile Respiration: Laennec's Stethoscope and the Physiology of Breathing', *Transactions and Studies of the College of Physicians of Philadelphia*, Ser. 5, 13 (1991): 125–45.

4

The Development of Medical Specialization in Nineteenth-Century Paris

George Weisz

We are only beginning to understand how specialization came to dominate our contemporary western medical systems. Both psychiatry and obstetrics have come in the last decades to symbolize the professional power of medicine and have thus generated an extensive historical literature. But few other specialties have been closely examined in anything like their full social and scientific complexity. Even less is known about the larger processes which led to the appearance and spread of specialties. All of these lacunae are magnified in the case of France which has yet to find its historian of specialization.

Some of our ignorance simply reflects the enormity of the task. How can one examine fully the 20 or so specialties that were established in most western nations by 1914 (not to mention those which appeared later)? One alternative is to survey a broad area from a narrow perspective. In two very astute books, Rosemary Stevens has focused on the professional and institutional ramifications of specialization in England and the United States in the twentieth century.[1] Her analysis is illuminating on many levels but is necessarily superficial in its treatment of specific specialties. More seriously, it neglects or takes for granted the very nature of specialization itself. The closest Stevens comes to accounting for the emergence and spread of specialization are some brief passages about it being an inevitable consequence of advances in twentieth century science and technology.[2] Nearly two decades of activity in the sociology of science has – whatever one thinks of the varieties of social constructivism – made it impossible to accept such formulations uncritically.

Most work in this area has adopted a different approach and concentrates on the history of a single specialty in a particular national context. The more sophisticated (or sociologically inclined) use the case study to elaborate or critique a theoretical model of the specialization process. The classic work in this vein by George Rosen was written nearly 50 years ago and retains much of its pertinence.[3] Rosen's model emphasizes the intellectual focus on particular organs and organ systems that emerged out of the Parisian school of pathological anatomy and that combined with specific instrumental or scientific innovations to produce specialty groups. Critics are perhaps unfair in reducing his views to this intellectual model of specialization. He was well aware of social factors such as urbanization and the self-interested pecuniary motives of individual physicians pursuing specialization.[4] But critics are certainly correct in arguing that his model, based on the case of ophthalmology as it is, applies with difficulty if at all to certain specialties. Sydney Halpern has pointed out that the development of paediatrics grew largely out of socio-political concern with a particular population category, children.[5] Russell Maulitz has described the rise of the rather amorphous domain of internal medicine in the United States 'as a series of historical contingencies' that led to a negotiated consensus about the boundaries of the field.[6] Bonnie Blustein has pointed out that some specialties consisted in fact of general practice for specific populations.[7] And many scholars have discussed the central role of individual entrepreneurship and collective competition in the emergence and development of specific specialty fields.[8] Some take issue with the Rosen model, while others appeal to variants of the 'professionalization' model. Such case studies, whatever their specific orientation and whether they embrace or eschew models and theoretical generalizations, have deepened our understanding of the diversity inherent in the specialization process. It is clear that knowledge, technique and practice on one hand and institutional conditions, collective self-interest and socio-political ramifications on the other, play themselves out differently in the case of each specialty, the same specialties in different nations, and even the same national specialty at different historical moments.

Studies of individual specialties will undoubtedly continue to be our primary strategy for understanding the full complexity of the processes involved. But in concentrating exclusively on the individual 'specialty' at the expense of the larger framework of 'specialization' we risk misinterpreting our data for lack of an adequate context. Relating our findings to theoretical models which are usually formalizations of results from other case studies is a poor substitute for that context. We can achieve it only by examining specialization systemically but empirically in its rich historical detail. This is a tall order to be sure but possible, I believe, if one is prepared to use historical source materials in somewhat unconventional ways and to pose questions that can be answered with the aid of such sources. This may mean forgoing temporarily issues of explanation (and especially those relating to the motivation of specialists) and accepting the more modest task of historical description.

In this essay, I attempt to describe or map the changing contours of medical specialization in the city of Paris during the nineteenth and early twentieth centuries. I utilize several conventional historical sources, medical journals and educational archives, for instance. But I will be relying primarily on lists of one sort or another; lists elaborated by historical actors, and lists that I myself have compiled from a variety of sources. I will be particularly concerned with Parisian medical directories as indicators of the spread of specialties. Such sources can be treated quantitatively so that I present from time to time summary data to illustrate the evolving scope of specialist practice. But I leave detailed quantitative analysis for another paper. Here, I will be more interested in the specialist categories presented in such lists as indicators of how historical actors themselves viewed the evolving domain of specialization.

The Early Ninteenth Century

During the early nineteenth century, the important distinctions in medicine were those among the eighteenth-century professional groupings, physicians, surgeons and pharmacists. On its establishment in 1820, the Academy of Medicine was divided into three sections representing these three professional categories. (These sections were in 1829 replaced with 13 sections representing a mix of professional and disciplinary groupings.) The Parisian hospital system in its various lists of personnel also utilized these three categories exclusively for identification purposes until mid-century.

More generally, the government published an annual volume, the *Almanach officiel,* listing the various state and semi-public institutions and their personnel. Included during the early decades of the nineteenth century, were annual listings of the medical practitioners of Paris officially recognized by public authorities. In the volume of 1805, practitioners were classed under four rubrics: 83 individuals were listed as *médecins,* 106 as *chirurgiens,* 2 as *médecins-oculistes,* and 2 as *oculiste, citoyens* (which presumably meant that they did not have medical diplomas). Even this minimal recognition of specialties disappeared in later editions where the categories utilized were aimed at distinguishing between the types of medical degree practitioners possessed. In this period of rapid transition and conflict, it seemed important to distinguish among degrees from various institutions of the *ancien régime* and post-revolutionary period. The 451 physicians in the *Almanach* of 1812 were thus divided into 3 diploma categories as were the 83 surgeons.[9] Pretty much the same number of practitioners in 1820 (490 physicians and 81 surgeons) were divided into the same six categories, with the addition of a seventh for foreign physicians.

If the headings used in such official listings of practitioners reflected the views of authorities, practitioners had an opportunity to introduce specialist identifications among the other sorts of information placed next to their name. The historian cannot know what such tags meant in practice, whether an individual was claiming special competence or, less likely, actually limiting his practice to specific types of patients and conditions. (This uncertainty applies to all the specialist directories which we shall be examining.) But what is clear is that Parisian doctors in the early nineteenth century rarely described themselves in terms that indicated specialization of knowledge or practice. In the *Almanach* of 1805, for instance, there were in addition to the four practitioners in the two oculist categories, three individuals among those in the listing of surgeons who identified themselves as *accoucheurs,* specialists in birthing, three others who identified themselves as specialists in the treatment of hernias and one calling himself a dentist. Specialty tags seem to have lost favour in subsequent years. Only three individuals in the *Almanach* of 1812, two oculists and one herniary specialist, utilized them. It may be significant that all three had pre-revolutionary diplomas. By 1820, specialties were slightly more in vogue. In that year, 11 practitioners identified themselves as specialists. No less than five were *oculistes* of one sort or another, two others were *accoucheurs.* A *dentiste* and a *herniare* were also to be found.

That diseases of the eyes and birthing were among the few specialties that enjoyed any recognition at all in the early nineteenth century is confirmed by one of the first privately published medical directories, the *Almanach général des médecins pour la Ville de Paris* published in 1830.[10] The purpose of this commercial venture was to satisfy the seemingly endless need for information about medical institutions and practitioners. The listings of Parisian medical practitioners in this directory are far more detailed than those in the *Almanach officiel.* Each might contain the year of the diploma, as well as information which indicated specialized interests, notably the title of the doctoral thesis and of published writings. In a few cases, the individual actually described himself as a specialist.[11] In a sample of the first 436 listings, the vast majority (86%) were described as '*médecin*' including a few whose institutional title was hospital surgeon. Only 31 individuals identified themselves as surgeons which was one of the two constituent elements of early nineteenth-century medicine.[12] The next largest category was *accoucheur* (sometimes alone, sometimes connected by a hyphen to *médecin* or *chirurgien*) with 20 listings. There were five *oculistes*, three *dentistes* and one specialist in hernias. There were also a number of individuals whose main identification was *médecin* but who indicated near the end of their listing some form of specialization. Thus Chamat (p. 201) identified as *médecin* included the phrase 'occupies himself especially with scrofulous illnesses' while Chambeyron (p. 201) also listed as *médecin* added the phrase 'legal medicine of the insane'. But such clarifications were few in number and are difficult to categorize.

All in all, the choice of specialties remained very limited. And there was clearly a reluctance to describe oneself as anything other than a *médecin*. This was even the case for several individuals who were actually developing specialties, like the psychiatrist Esquirol (who identified himself simply as a *médecin*). Specialties were still linked in the minds of many to charlatanism and patent medicines,[13] and it may be that the doctrine of the unity of medicine which had led to the formal unification of medicine and surgery at the end of the eighteenth century continued to influence the way in which medical practitioners presented themselves.[14] The only major exception to this general reluctance to identify with specialties was obstetrics.

As we saw, the number of individuals identified as *accoucheurs* was not much less than the number identified as surgeons. Although obstetrics lacked the professional associations and journals that sociologists would identify with an emerging specialty, it had a specialized clientèle, parturient women, that was the object of state attention for populationist reasons. It had its own hospitals like the Paris Maternité because this class of patients had been segregated from other hospital inmates since the eighteenth century. Its initial *raison d'être* seems to have been to decrease mortality in childbirth through the provision of obstetrical training, initially aimed at midwives and later at doctors.[15] By 1830, the three national medical faculties all contained chairs of *accouchement*. The faculty of Paris in fact had two such chairs, a clinical chair and a theoretical chair which combined *accouchement* with diseases of women and children.[16] The reorganization of the Academy of Medicine in 1829 separated this specialty from its parent surgery by establishing a separate section of obstetrics,[17] giving it further official recognition. Although recognition was slower to come in the Parisian hospital system where obstetrical wards were annexed to medical or surgical services, the Parisian hospital administration began – sometime before 1850 – to refer to physicians at the Maternité hospital as *médecins-accoucheurs*.

Obstetrics can thus be seen as the first of the nineteenth-century medical specialties in France. It had developed in the eighteenth century out of political perceptions of social need and the tendency in Paris to segregate different types of poor patients in distinct hospital institutions. Its emergence seems to have owed little to the professionalizing activities of the specialists themselves. It had achieved considerable professional recognition by 1830. In contrast, the specialty of *oculiste* seems a throwback to earlier patterns of medical practice. Ocular surgery had become accepted by the Parisian surgical corporation in the late eighteenth century.[18] But its major asset in the early nineteenth century was royal favour. The Royal Medical Service included two *oculistes* (Demours and Guillié), while another, de Wenzel, was a Baron (a title conferred by a foreign monarch). Since the reign of the Bourbons came to an end in 1830, this proved a fragile basis for a specialty, especially one regularly identified by doctors with charlatanism.

It is worth mentioning that there was a varied array of specialist hospital institutions in Paris during the early nineteenth century. Children, women, the elderly, the insane, sufferers of chronic or venereal diseases were only some of the categories of patients segregated for reasons of administrative rationality, humanitarianism and morality. Such institutions were beginning to play a major role in the development of specialist medical knowledge through the research and teaching opportunities which they offered.[19] But while work in such hospitals undoubtedly made certain doctors experts in particular fields, it did not produce, early in the century, firm specialist identity. Obstetrics in this respect was quite unique.

Specialist Journals in the 1830s and 1840s

Specialization during the 1830s had its proponents. In 1838, Félix Ratier published a defence of specialization.[20] One year later, two journals devoted to medical specialization came into existence. Appearing in June was *L'Esculape, Journal des Spécialités Médico-Chirurgicales*. It was edited by a Dr S. Furnari who was described in medical directories as a specialist in diseases of the eyes. The journal was to appear three times a week and remained in publication for three years. A second journal, the *Revue des Spécialités et Innovations Médicales et Chirurgicales* appeared in November and was published, irregularly until the 1860s. It was edited by Vincent Duval, a specialist in orthopaedics, who described himself as Director of Orthopaedic Treatments of the Parisian Hospital system since 1831. While his institutional status in the 1830s is somewhat unclear,[21] well-known hospital physicians and surgeons were certainly among his contributors.[22] He claimed to have been encouraged to create such a revue of specialties by his teacher Broussais.[23]

Since both journals were interested in the entire range of specialties, they were not very different from many general medical journals published at the same time. Nevertheless, both were clearly sensitive about medical hostility to specialization. Each journal opened with an editorial essay defending the legitimacy of competent medical specialization based on a general medical education common to all doctors. In doing so, each journal also quoted well known figures who had made comments favourable to specialization; both journals cited at length the same lines from Bichat's *Recherches sur la vie et la mort* in their opening comments and mentioned the many famous figures who had in fact specialized in a particular area of medicine.[24]

During its first year of publication, *L'Esculape* had on its masthead a listing of the medical specialties which it included within its domain. The listing disappeared in the two subsequent years, suggesting that the editor was not entirely happy with his efforts to map medical specialties. Nevertheless, the categories used outline one possible system of classification for medical specialties. The masthead can be usefully compared with some of the editor's remarks in his opening article. His competitor, Duval, wrote a review in 1841 of the specialties to which his journal had made a contribution.[25] While not a complete inventory of specialties, the seven categories of specialties he discussed shed further light on the understanding of specialization at the end of the 1830s.

L'Esculape's masthead begins with '*Accouchemens*' or birthing. Every French listing of medical specialties I have ever seen begins with this category. The consistent priority of this specialty is, as they say, 'overdetermined'. The word begins with a letter that is at the top of alphabetical lists. It concerns birth, in many ways the primal human (and medical) act. It describes the oldest of the recognized specialties in France. Despite this alphabetical start, the list is not in fact alphabetical and as a whole obeys no obvious logic. 'Accouchement' is followed as it usually is in such listings by 'Maladies des femmes et des enfants'. The linkage sanctioned by a chair at the Paris Faculty of Medicine combining the three subjects is based on the obvious connection between birth and the women and children who are the objects and consequences of obstetrical intervention. From then on, specialties appear in an almost arbitrary order.

Specialties on the banner of *L'Esculape*, 1839

Accouchemens	Chirurgie herniaire
Maladies des femmes et des enfants	Maladies des oreilles
Orthopédie	Hygiène et chirurgie militaire
Maladies des voies urinaires	Hygiène publique et privée
Chirurgie dentaire	Maladies vénériennes
Maladies des yeux	Maladies de la peau
Médecine légale	Eaux minérales
Maladies du système nerveux	

Subjects reviewed in *Revue des Spécialités et des Innovations Médicales et Chirurgicales*, 1841

Epidémies	Ophthalmologie
Hernies	Maladies cérébrales
Orthopédie	Obstétrique
Syphilis	

Most are based on anatomical structures. Others are based on classes of patients (women and children) forms of treatment (mineral waters, hernial surgery) types of disease (venereal) and social functions (legal medicine, military hygiene and surgery, public and private hygiene). Among the organically based specialties, was '*maladies des yeux*', a term that had replaced the traditional somewhat unsavoury '*oculiste*'. The field was just then in the public eye due to a new surgical technique to cure strabism which had been discussed at some length in the Academy of Medicine. Orthopaedics was associated primarily with the sectioning of muscles and tendons in order to cure deformities. '*Maladies des voies urinaires*' (called more generally '*maladies des organes génito-urinaires*' in the editor's introduction) was most closely associated with operations for the stone, particularly lithotrity. The anatomical turn in mental medicine was evident in the fact that this was called '*maladies du système nerveux*' in the masthead. (The competing *Revue des Spécialités et Innovations Médicales et Chirurgicales* went even farther in the direction of localization referring to it as '*médecine cérébrale*'.) It was well on its way to becoming a recognized specialty thanks to the activities of Esquirol and his circle and to the Asylum Law of 1838.[26]

Perhaps the most surprising categories are those which are not ordinarily thought of as medical specialties. Legal and forensic medicine, associated by the editor in his introduction with *'toxicologie'* had assumed increasing importance in the legal process and had its emblematic figure in Orfila, as well as a place in the curriculum of the Paris Faculty of Medicine. (In addition to a chair of legal medicine at the Paris Faculty, there was a chair held by Orfila in medical chemistry.)[27] Military hygiene and surgery were also institutionalized in military hospitals and the curriculum of the Val-de-Grace hospital which trained military doctors. Public hygiene came closest to the usual model of an emerging specialty with a group of individuals around a journal, the *Annales d'hygiène publique* (founded in 1829),[28] a chair of hygiene at the Paris Faculty of Medicine, as well as a section in the newly reorganized Academy of Medicine (1829) which it shared with legal medicine. Duval in the *Revue des Spécialités et Innovations Médicales et Chirurgicales* discussed a variant of public health which he called *'épidémies'* and which he associated with Nicolas Chervin and anticontagionism.[29]

There is a strong tendency on *L'Esculape's* masthead (although not in the text of articles) to avoid the technical greek and latinate terms for specialties. This was to be characteristic of specialist classifications well into the twentieth century. It is also worth noting the importance of orthopaedics in the early process of specialization; the editor of one of the journals was an orthopaedist, and the specialty was one of those that appeared both on the masthead of *L'Esculape* and in Duval's discussion of recent developments in medical specialties.

Medical Dictionaries

It would seem from the defensiveness of specialist journals that specialization faced considerable opposition from the medical profession. One way of gauging élite opinion on the matter is through an examination of medical encyclopaedias or dictionaries. The first half of the nineteenth century was something of a golden age for such dictionaries. Medical knowledge was advancing quickly, yet with considerable scope for conflicts of fundamental doctrine and perspective. The result seems to have been an endless fascination for encyclopaedic works which managed to summarize, classify, condense and interpret existing medical knowledge. Some of these works were prepared by members of the Parisian medical élite which dominated the Faculty of Medicine and the hospital system.

I have come across three such dictionaries of the early nineteenth century (among six that I found in the Osler Library) with something to say about medical specialization. None of them recognizes 'specialization' itself as a category deserving of mention. Very few specialization categories, in fact, are mentioned at all. The ones receiving treatment come as no surprise in view of our preceding discussion.

Obstetrics, for instance, is characteristically covered in a variety of ways. The earliest publication in our sample, the *Dictionnaire des Sciences Médicales* which began appearing in 1812, has an entry for '*Accoucheur*', a specialized attendant who, since the teaching of medicine has become more 'philosophical', is a doctor 'who has acquired profound theoretical knowledge in the different branches of the healing art, who has practised with success surgery and medicine, and who has dedicated himself to the treatment of maladies of women and of newborns'.[30]

That some ambivalence surrounded even this specialty is suggested by another work of this type, the *Dictionnaire de Médecine et de Chirurgie Pratique* which began to appear in 1829. There is no entry on specialized birthing practitioners but only on '*Accouchement*', birthing itself. The essay written by Ant. Dugès, Professor at the Medical Faculty of Montpellier, and taking up 40 pages, starts by denying the existence of obstetrics as a separate branch of knowledge.

> Despite the fact that some consider the science and art of *accouchement* to be a special branch of medicine, and this has even been given its own name (*obstétrique*), one should not however believe that this branch really has an independent existence. Obstetrics is composed of knowledge borrowed from all the other branches of the healing art; It has nothing of its own but the totality, the chain of these borrowings....What has made it constitute itself as an entity, in spite of the heterogeneity of its elements, is less a rational link between them than the practice adopted for some time now by certain surgeons of devoting themselves exclusively to the practice of *accouchements*, and by others of abandoning them completely. The profession of *accoucheur* or that of midwife, created in time immemorial, has become an **art** and has presupposed or brought with it a **science** which includes the necessary principles of its practice.[31] [his emphasis]

Dugès, appointed in 1824 as the first incumbent of the chair of obstetrics at Montpellier, felt strongly enough about the intellectual status of obstetrics to have moved three years later to a chair of surgical pathology.

Other specialties fared far worse in the three early encyclopaedias. The *Dictionnaire de Médecine*, whose 15th volume appeared in 1826 published an entry on oculists by Raige Delorme; this was the occasion for a critique of specialization which 'gives rise to more abuses than it provides advantages for science'.[32] The criticism of this occupation got progressively stronger as the essay advanced. Only an entry on dentists in another volume of this work written by Marjolin[33] had anything remotely positive to say about a specialist group.

The situation, however, began to change somewhat in the second edition of the *Dictionnaire de Médecine* which began appearing in 1832. By 1840 and 1841 when the volumes 21-23 which took the encyclopaedia from 'Nev' to 'Pér' appeared, a change in editorial policy had taken place. One finds entries for *'Obstétrique'* (now one of the three fundamental divisions 'of the art of medicine which the specialization of studies and the necessities of practice have established most naturally'[34]); *'Odontechnie'* (the art of dentistry which, it was argued, had long suffered from the lack of medical knowledge that characterized its practitioners[35]); *'Ophthalmologie'* in which the author Velpeau criticized professional specialization on the grounds that eye diseases could not be separated from the other body systems;[36] *'Orthopédie'* and *'Pédiatrie'*, the practitioners of which remained largely unmentioned. The overall tone was not necessarily supportive of specialization. But the existence of such articles provided some recognition that the fields involved were distinct domains of knowledge which was a necessary prerequisite for the specialization of practice.

In fact, the recognition of distinctive areas of knowledge went back even farther than 1840. All of the encylopaedias I have discussed were created by boards of editors dividing up the domain of medical knowledge. Even the earliest ones recognized some specialties as constituting discrete areas of knowledge, for editing purposes at least.

Medical knowledge was characteristically divided into three categories, following the pattern of organization of chairs in the medical faculties. A list would usually begin with the basic sciences on which medicine depended; it would go on to the basic medical divisions, medicine and surgery which could themselves be broken down into such categories as pathology and therapeutics. Often pharmacology in one form or another was also included. Finally, there were specialized applications of medicine like *'accouchement'* or *'hygiène'*. There was plenty of room for variation and ambiguity in such lists but this pattern reappeared quite frequently.

For reasons of space, I will limit myself to the third category of specialized applications of medicine. I emphasize that these represented not professional specialties but domains of editorial expertise. Nevertheless, I would suggest that such recognition was crucial for emerging specialization.

As early as 1812, five categories of specialist knowledge were thought to require special editors.[37] The second edition of the *Dictionnaire de Médecine* which began appearing in 1832 had no less than nine such categories, not including medical philosophy and medical history. But one cannot infer from this that specialization was achieving greater recognition within French medicine (though I believe on the basis of other evidence that it was). Wide variations of editorial practice in such matters can be inferred from the fact that the *Nouveau Dictionnaire de Médecine et de Chirurgie Pratique*[38] appeared in 1864 with only three such specialized editorial categories. (There was also little treatment of specialties in the contents.)

Three fields were singled out with special editors in all five of the dictionaries we have mentioned (although formulations and combinations of elements were variable). Not surprisingly, *'accouchement'* appeared on all five editorial lists in one form or another; so did *'hygiène'* and *'médecine légale'*. All three, of course, were also on the masthead of *L'Esculape* in 1839, and all were the subjects of chairs at the Paris Faculty of Medicine. *'Maladies syphilitiques'* and *'maladies cutanées'* (or *'de la peau'*) appeared on four lists, each as a separate category, while *'maladies mentales'* was on three. (These three domains were also singled out in *L'Esculape*.) There are two surprising omissions. Diseases of the eyes and orthopaedics, so prominent in the specialty journals, were totally absent from the editorial lists, suggesting that these were subsumed under other categories, notably surgery. (The surgeon, Velpeau, wrote several articles on *ophthalmologie*.) It may also be that there was some suspicion of specialists in these fields which were most closely associated with an entrepreneurial approach identified with charlatanism.

Editorial categories and the men who filled them give some indication of the role of specialized hospitals in generating specialized expertise. They suggest that the role of such hospitals was significant but that other paths to expertise existed. The most widely recognized clinically based editorial category was *'accouchement'*. In our four dictionaries which began publishing from 1812 to 1832, a total of seven men had responsibility for this field. Of the four who worked on the earliest one which began to appear in 1812, two were identified as faculty professors, another was adjunct surgeon at the

Salpêtrière hospital for women and another (Gardien) is listed simply as a doctor of medicine. The four men responsible for obstetrics in the three later works were all identified as faculty professors.

In the field of mental medicine, the single editor in the Dictionary of 1826 was listed only as a doctor of medicine (Georget). In the work which began to appear three years later, one editor (Foville) was listed as a doctor at the Rouen asylum, a second, Magendie, was a well-known physiologist at the Collège de France, and a third, Londe, was listed only as a doctor of medicine.[39] In the second edition of this Dictionary, published in 1832, Georget, still listed as a doctor of medicine, was joined by Ferrus a physician in the psychiatric wing of the Bicêtre Hospital.[40]

Among the other specialty areas, an editor in venereology, Cullerier, was at the Hôpital des Vénériens, but two other editors listed no institutional affiliation. Of the four editors in dermatology, two were closely affiliated with a specialized hospital, the Saint-Louis (devoted to skin problems) and a third was at Saint-Antoine, a general hospital;[41] a fourth (Casenave) had no affiliation. Two of the three editors in paediatrics were at the Hôpital des Enfants Malades while the third worked at the central bureau of admissions of the Parisian hospitals (where all doctors started their hospital careers).

So while working in a specialized hospital was not absolutely necessary for consideration as an expert in a field, it certainly helped in certain cases. It is also likely that some of those without an institutional affiliation had in fact trained with someone at such a hospital at an earlier stage of their careers.[42]

Practitioners in 1852

In 1852, Henri Meding published a volume entitled *Paris Médical: Vade-Mecum des Médecins Étrangers dans Paris*. It was full of information that might be of use to a physician; the topology of Paris, hospital institutions, recent publications and medical journals. At the back was a listing of 1,460 Parisian medical practitioners. The listing is fairly comprehensive since administrative statistics showed 1,442 doctors and 175 *officiers de santé* in Paris in 1845–47.[43] But information was sparse, with most individuals having little more than an address. Consequently, it would be dangerous to make too much of its contents. But the directory does nevertheless provide some indication of the general scope of specialization.[44]

The majority of listings were lacking altogether in self-descriptions. Forty-nine individuals were identified as surgeons, which no one would have considered a specialty designation at mid-century. One hundred and twelve others, or 8% of the listings, included something like a specialty designation, although once again we do not know exactly what this meant in practice. Lack of uniformity in the form and categories used suggests that practitioners rather than the editors provided the description which was in the nature of advertising to peers.

Comparing the listings of 1852 with those of 1830, suggests that specialization had made substantial progress but that most specialties remained small and fragmented. The two largest specialties in the earlier listing continued their predominance. Once again, *accoucheurs* made up by far the largest category of specialists, with 23 listings. However, their numbers seem to have declined substantially since 1830.[45] It is not clear whether this decline reflected the new speciality opportunities which were now available or some constraints on obstetrical practice. Well behind were two other categories. Eleven individuals were specialists of the eyes, with *maladies des yeux* having definitively replaced the term *oculiste*. A new category that since 1830 had made its appearance among the largest specialties was *maladies mentales,* a heterogenous category, it is true, made up of six individuals who actually used the term and six who described themselves as alienists at particular asylums.[46]

Nine individuals had some connection with mineral waters, six of them describing themselves as inspectors of mineral waters. They may well have been concerned only with calling attention to their possession of an administrative post rather than to specialist status. But it would be difficult to deny inspectors some form of specialist status if one attributes it to alienists.

Eight individuals identified themselves as homeopaths; one cannot know in any specific case whether this was meant as something like a specialty designation or more probably as a public repudiation of all orthodox medicine. Less problematic were the seven specialists in children's diseases and five in women's diseases, with three individuals in both groups. However, there was, surprisingly, no overlapping between obstetrics and women's diseases despite the fact that the term *'obstétrique'* ordinarily covered diseases of women as well as birthing. This suggests that some separation between the two fields was beginning to take place. (The same applies to paediatrics and obstetrics.) Among the many specialities represented by five or less individuals, ones that seem surprisingly small are orthopaedics (in view of its prominence in the specialist medical journals), venereology and dermatology (in view of their specialty hospitals and the prominence of their practitioners on the editorial boards of medical dictionaries). Even more glaring considering their intellectual prominence are the very few references to public health and legal medicine. This may reflect the prejudices of the editors (ones apparently shared by all the later directories we will be discussing) or may simply mean that these were not perceived as specialties which defined individuals but rather as particular sorts of medical activities that were typically combined with clinical practice. It is also possible that the kind of advertising represented by such self-identification in a professional directory was irrelevant to individuals in these fields, since they were not in search of referrals or clients but rather of posts allocated by local authorities.

Looking at some of the other information which individuals included about themselves, we get some sense of the role of specialization within the medical élite and vice versa. Of the 112 listed specialists (excluding surgeons), ten individuals had posts at middle and senior levels in the Faculty of Medicine and ten others had posts in the Parisian hospitals. To this one should probably add the six individuals with asylum posts which were clearly less prestigious than those in hospitals but which provided a relatively desirable administrative cachet. All together, about one quarter of those identifying themselves as specialists can be considered members of the Parisian medical élite. Most of the posts were concentrated in a small number of specialties, particularly obstetrics and paediatrics.

The Development of Intellectual Specialization

During the 1860s and 1870s, specialization gradually spread as a result of two processes: the creation of specialized medical journals and the introduction of specialties into the medical school curriculum. The two processes were in fact interconnected. Most of the early journals were founded and supported by élite physicians at the faculty and in hospitals (or other state institutions such as those for the blind or the deaf). They were predominantly in those fields on the verge of full acceptance into the medical curriculum.

Many of the medical journals created during this period survived for only a year or two. Since I am interested in journals as an indicator of professional activity and medical acceptance, I will in what follows only be concerned with those journals that survived for at least a decade.[47]

Before 1865, specialist periodicals tended to be in more marginal fields. Public health with its places in the Faculty and the Academy of Medicine was the earliest and probably most prestigious of the nascent specialist domains to have its journal, the *Annales d'hygiène publique* (1829–1922). The field got a second publication, *Santé publique*, in 1869 (lasting until 1887).

Some of the fields which spawned publications would eventually achieve recognition as specialties. Thus the *Annales de maladies de la peau* lasted from 1843 to 1852.[48] Enjoying greater longevity was the *Annales médico-psychologiques* from 1843 to 1948. (This was joined for a decade by a second publication, the *Journal de médecine mentale* published from 1861–70.) The few fields spawning new publications in the 1850s and 1860s tended to be fairly marginal if not controversial. No less than four new journals of hydrology appeared between 1854 and 1858, and all continued to publish for an extended period. Homeopathy, after several false starts got the *Bibliothèque homéopathique* (1832–42) and the *Journal de la Société Gallicane de médecine homéopathique* (1850–90). Dentistry, which remained unregulated and whose place in medicine was problematic, got *Art dentaire* in 1857. Two journals were devoted to animal magnetism.[49]

Although there was not a great deal of new publishing activity in the 1860s, specialties got a boost from the expansion of teaching at the Paris Faculty of Medicine. There continued to be considerable opposition within the Faculty to the introduction of specialty teaching to the curriculum; a commission convened at the end of the 1850s rejected the idea of creating new specialty chairs not, it would seem, because professors rejected specialist teaching but because they did not wish to reduce the prerogatives of the existing clinical chairs.[50] The conflict was eventually resolved by a compromise. During the early 1860s, a newly appointed reformist dean, Pierre Rayer, introduced six new *cours complémentaires* in the clinical specialties. These were taught by junior level personnel, the *agrégés*, rather than by professors and were not part of the core curriculum. But even this second class position represented an advance for the specialties involved; mental and nervous diseases, skin diseases, venereal diseases, diseases of children, diseases of the eyes and diseases of the urinary tract.[51]

The reformers' motives seem to have had less to do with emerging specialist practice in France than with the development of specialist medical education in Germany. In this as in many other respects, German initiatives were a model to be emulated. This imperative to equal Germany in the educational and scientific spheres gained in intensity after the French defeat at the hands of Germany in 1870.[52] The system of *cours complémentaires* was not perceived to be working very well. More importantly, perhaps, the creation of chairs in clinical specialties was seen as a key aspect of that restructuring of medical education and higher education in general that was gaining support among the nation's political and intellectual élites. Such specialty chairs were thought particularly vital to maintaining France's position within international medical science and to attract the foreign doctors who had once come to France to complete their post-graduate education but were now travelling to Germany.[53] Debate of this issue began within the educational administration and the Faculty in 1875. Although there was some disagreement about the subjects which deserved representation and about whether professors in newly created specialist positions should be equal in title and prerogatives to those in existing chairs, there was little opposition to the principle of expanding the role of specialties.[54] In 1877, a clinical chair in mental maladies was established, the first of seven chairs in the various clinical specialties that were introduced before 1890. These seem to have been essentially the products of the imperatives of international educational and scientific competition rather than the result of pressure from indigenous specialty groupings which developed more slowly than their counterparts in the United States. Some Faculty reports on these matters explicitly distinguished between professional specialization which was of little interest and scientific specialization which was vitally important in the competition against foreign science.[55]

> If we ask for specialized chairs, it is in order to have professors devoting themselves entirely and without second thoughts to the study of certain specialized parts of science; it is in order that French science be capable in this area of wrestling with [lutter avec] foreign science;[56]

Only intellectual criteria, moreover, were used in debating which specialties should be the subjects of chairs. Those established before the turn of the century were:

1. '*clinique de maladies mentales*' (established in 1877 and separated from '*maladies nerveuses*' with which they were often associated). The Faculty elected to the chair Benjamin Ball who had little psychiatric experience, in preference to the alienist, Magnan. The argument used by Charcot to defend Ball emphasized the latter's general mastery of pathology in comparison to the narrow expertise of his opponent. But it is rather unlikely that such arguments expressed bias against specialization *per se*.[57] It is more probable that the terms of the debate reflected competition between neurologist-pathologists who were firmly ensconced in the hospital system and alienists who were segregated in their own system of asylums and who, by and

large, lacked the legitimacy conferred by the paradigmatic methods of anatomo-pathology.[58]

2. *'clinique des maladies des enfants'* (1878)

3. *'clinique ophthalmologique'* (1878). This was the only specialized chair using a greek-derived name until the twentieth century. It was also the most scientifically prestigious of the new specialties. Academic reports and debates referred specifically to the discoveries which the ophthalmoscope had made possible.[59]

4. *'clinique des maladies cutanées et syphilitiques'* (1879) which combined two specialties often but not always practised together. All the sources we have so far used to map specialties before 1870, in fact, treated them as two separate fields; individuals identifying themselves as specialists in 1852 chose one or another designation, never both. Nevertheless, the earliest journals in the field combined the two specialties,[60] suggesting intellectual if not practical links.[61] The LeFort report voted by the Faculty in 1878 (as well as the Broca report three years before) recommended that only derma-tology be raised to the status of a clinical chair on the grounds that venereology was both distinct and of little scientific interest.[62] It is not clear whether it was the Faculty assembly or the Ministry which decided to combine the two subjects. But the Ministry appointed to the chair, without consulting the Faculty (as was the usual practice) the venereologist Alfred Fournier, suggesting that political or at least public health considerations were involved. Ironically, Fournier showed little interest in dermatology.[63]

5. *'clinique des maladies du système nerveux'* (1882) created for Charcot and bringing to the Faculty the nervous diseases excluded from the chair of mental medicine in 1877.

6. *'clinique d'accouchement'* (1890). This was the second obstet-rical chair at the Faculty. A third one was established in 1908.

7. *'clinique des maladies des voies urinaires'* (1890). This field had been explicitly excluded from the status of a chair in the 1870s on the grounds that it was not sufficiently advanced scientifically. During the next decade it apparently gained some scientific credibility.

All seven fields were fairly venerable, having been on *L'Esculape's* banner of 1839 listing the medical specialties. Six of the specialties can be traced back to the specialized hospitals of the early nineteenth century which treated particular sorts of clients. (The exception is the latest of the chairs devoted to urinary diseases.) And all had been the subjects of *cours complémentaires* since the 1860s. Five more clinical specialty chairs were created in the decade before 1912.

In the middle of all this institutional activity, specialty medical journals began to appear, the earliest in the field of dermatology-venereology in 1868. During the decade between 1871 and 1880, there appeared no less than five long-running journals of ophthalmology. Obstetrics-gynaecology saw four journals appearing during the decade. Although most of the new journals represented the best-established specialties that were already being taught as Faculty courses and that would be the first to attain chairs, there were a few more recent and less prestigious specialties among the journals. Otorhinolaryngology saw its first journal appear in 1875; because it was not being talked about as the subject of a chair, this journal was one of the few which engaged in polemics about the importance of the specialty and its right to a chair at the Faculty. For the most part the journals of the 1870s were content to improve the status of the specialty and the career prospects of editors and writers by producing specialized medical knowledge.

After 1880, the publication of new specialized journals intensified, bringing the benefits of publication to other specialties, paediatrics in 1883, orthopaedics in 1887 and electricity-radiology in 1893. By 1905, about 125 specialist journals (excluding 11 journals of surgery) that I have been able to identify were in publication.[64] Most fields had several journals and a few, notably obstetrics–gynaecology, had over a dozen. By this time, moreover, the more established fields were represented by Parisian and occasionally national specialist societies, though these never seem to have achieved the importance of parallel societies in the United States. They were part of international networks of specialty societies that convened from time to time at international congresses.

By the beginning of the 1880s, specialization in medicine was becoming widely accepted, but not all reservations had been overcome. An indication of this ambivalence is provided by the 10th volume of the *Dictionnaire Encyclopédique des Sciences Médicales* (edited by A. Dechambre) which appeared in 1881 with an entry (the first to my knowledge) on *'Spécialités médicales'*. The author, A. Chereau, emphasized that, unlike the specialists of old who lacked science,

> Most of our specialists of today are graduated men, who have demonstrated knowledge, and who, while cutting up the art, do not bring the profession into disrepute. So-called special works do not impede in any way so-called general works, and analysis cannot do harm to synthesis. After all, it is specialists who have produced most of the useful inventions and, from this point of view alone, they fully deserve that we offer them a friendly and brotherly hand.[65]

The apologetic tone of this article suggests that in certain circles at least, doubts about specialization persisted. Although intellectual and academic specialization had gained acceptance, specialization of practice was only beginning to be fully embraced by the medical profession.

Specialization of Practice

There were several elements involved in the institutionalization of specialty practice. Formal regulation and certification did not develop anywhere to any significant extent until after the First World War.[66] As in other countries, medical associations in France expressed fear that general practitioners would be relegated to an inferior status if specialty certification were introduced. More pertinent and specific to France was the weight of administrative centralization which, together with the lack of powerful corporate bodies or professional associations, made it impossible to negotiate specialist certification until after the Second World War.[67] Centralization also made it difficult to introduce post-graduate specialist training within the faculties. Although some formal graduate programmes were functioning by the 1930s, the low status certificates they awarded – in public health, forensic and colonial medicine – seem to have been geared mainly to doctors looking for state jobs of one sort or another. Clinical specialties were poorly represented.[68] But some specialty teaching went on in the medical faculties. The practical ward training of the required clinical rotations *(stages)* oriented many practitioners towards specialist practice even if, in theory, they were supposed to constitute the general education of physicians. And informal post-graduate courses for specialists *(cours de perfectionnement)* also seem to have been offered by some faculties.[69] Above all, specialized practice was gradually being structured for the medical elite by changes in the Parisian hospital system.

Specialization among members of the Parisian medical elite depended on its acceptance within the hospital system where elite clinical careers were pursued. Formally, however, hospitals evolved at a somewhat slower pace in this respect than did the medical faculty. The existence of specialized hospitals helped some fields, though not others, in the sense that it was possible to pursue clinical practice and research while training students in the field. Likewise it was possible for clinicians to make agreements with the central admitting bureau of the hospital system to direct certain types of patients to their wards, creating wards that were *de facto* specialized. But these did not provide formal recognition to the specialty and did not give ambitious young clinicians any particular incentive to become specialists. The naming of several individuals in the late 1820s and 1830s to provide specialist treatment (Civiale and Leroy d'Étiolles for surgery of the urinary tract, Jules Sichet for ophthalmology, Vincent Duval for orthopaedic treatment) took place outside the regular system of recruitment for hospital posts.[70]

Slowly, the educational and intellectual developments we have so far described transformed the Parisian hospital system which had for most of the century recognized only three categories of practitioners in its midst: physicians, surgeons and pharmacists. (The title *accoucheur* was sometimes used but it had no particular administrative meaning.) The Parisian hospital administration, the Assistance Publique, began from the 1870s to create specialized wards and many hospital physicians and surgeons were known as specialists.[71] But these medical practitioners continued to be referred to in its lists of personnel as simply physicians, surgeons and occasionally *accoucheurs*, implying that they fulfilled a specialized institutional as opposed to medical function. Furthermore, the competitive examinations for an appointment to the hospital system continued to be based on general medical or surgical, but not specialist, knowledge. When added to the fact that the *agrégation* for entry into the junior ranks of the faculty was also based on general medical knowledge,[72] it becomes apparent that aspiring members of the medical élite could not devote themselves fully to specialties until they were firmly installed in élite medical institutions. Even then, appointments to specialist wards were usually based on factors like seniority, making the match between specialist and ward something of a hit-or-miss affair.

Specialists campaigned in a variety of ways for recognition. In 1878, the municipal council of Paris voted a motion introduced by one of its members, the psychiatrist Bourneville, to create a small corps of obstetricians in the hospitals. Despite some controversy caused by the opposition of hospital surgeons, this was implemented in 1881. Gynaecological surgery, however, remained firmly in the hands of surgeons which marked the character of French obstetrics in a variety of important ways.[73] Several years later, a competition *(concours)* was introduced for hospital alienists.[74] In 1887, the venereologist, Alfred Fournier, took advantage of depopulationist fears to submit to the Academy of Medicine a report on prophylactic measures to be taken against venereal disease. Among the many wide-ranging measures which he proposed was that the personnel of hospital venereal services, from the lowest to the highest levels, be selected by *concours*, testing knowledge of venereal disease and therapeutics. The Academy voted in favour of this recommendation which was, however, overshadowed by far more controversial aspects of his proposal, notably the shape of an eventual law to control and regulate prostitution.[75]

The Academy's vote produced no results. But in 1897, the medical politician, Paul Strauss, launched a campaign within the Municipal Council of Paris to bring more specialization to the hospital system. The administrative council of the Parisian hospital system took up the question and established a commission led by Paul Brouardel, dean of the Paris Faculty of Medicine, to examine the issue.[76] The commission surveyed five specialties and decided to create a corps of specialists chosen by *concours* in ophthalmology. The regulations to this effect appeared in 1899. The commission decided to reserve judgement on a definitive organization of otorhinolaryngology (ORL), deciding more modestly to recognize officially two special services at Lariboisière and Saint-Antoine hospitals that had been split off from the regular medical services. Hospital physicians and surgeons were asked to apply for positions in these wards and commit themselves to specialize in this field.[77] Three years later, it was decided to create a corps of hospital specialists in ORL nominated by *concours*.[78] In the cases of gynae-cology and neurology, the commission decided that existing resources were adequate. Concerning dermatology–venereology, it was decided that a new specialist hospital and more outpatient clinics were required; but the commission stopped short of creating a separate specialist corps which would have been opposed by hospital physicians.

Shortly thereafter, Alfred Fournier tried to precipitate matters by presenting another paper to the Academy of Medicine on the prevention of syphilis in which he proposed a variety of measures including the creation of a specialized category of hospital venereol-ogists recruited through *concours;* these were to be *'gens de métier'* rather than venereologists by improvisation. Referring to the administrative recognition of hospital obstetricians and alienists, he asked rhetorically whether venerology did not deserve the same treatment; 'does it not have this right by virtue of the infinite number of its patients, by virtue of the importance of the illnesses which it treats, and by virtue of the social consequences of these illnesses'.[79] There was some opposition to the proposal on the grounds that specialization was bad for the profession. 'Each branch which is removed is a part of its patrimony which slips away from it'.[80] But it was supported in the Academy by other specialists like the ophthalmologist, Panas.[81] A committee was formed to review Fournier's proposal but I have been unable to find any trace of its report during the next five years, suggesting that the committee had been paralysed by opponents of specialization.

Venereology, unlike ophthalmology and otorhinolaryngology, seems to have failed to make much headway within the hospital system, because the need did not seem pressing to administrators and possibly because it had little scientific status.[82] But there also seems to have been a reluctance to fragment the hospital corps, unless it seemed absolutely necessary. In 1901, a corps of dentists was established in the Parisian hospitals; these were required to have both medical doctorates and dental diplomas. But no new specialist categories would be introduced during the next two decades.

In 1920, the number of specialties recognized by the hospital administration had not grown at all. This seems to have had little impact on the actual spread of specialization in hospital institutions; a list of Parisian hospital physicians and surgeons published in the *Guide Rosenwald* of that year listed the vast majority as specializing in a particular domain of medicine. But the problems of matching specialists to wards persisted well into the twentieth century.[83]

Directories in the 1880s and 1890s

For the Parisian medical élite, hospitals and medical education determined the shape of specialization. For those outside the élite, however, there were few institutional constraints. Anyone could pretty much call himself anything. All the various processes we have described provided a stimulus for medical practitioners to identify themselves as specialists. One can see the timing very clearly in the major medical directory of the period the *Annuaire Roubaud*[84] which began to appear in 1848. It was rather slow in the early years to include specialist designations, for reasons that are unclear. While Meding's listing of 1852 contained 112 self-identified specialists, and Hubert's *Almanach général de médecine pour la ville de Paris* (1851) listed 61, Roubaud in 1853, had only three, one in *'maladies mentales'*, one in *'maladies des yeux'*, a third in *'lithotripsie'* and *'chirurgie des cavités'*. In 1860 there were 37 self-identified specialists, in 1870, 85, and in 1880, 144. Four years later there were 233. These self-descriptions, at first presented idiosyncratically, gradually took on uniformity, presented in italics and within parentheses. But the editor of the directory felt no need even in the 1880s to organize this information for the benefit of readers into lists of practitioners for each specialty.

The elaboration of such lists was of considerable significance for specialty practice. The heterogeneity characteristic of self-described specialty designations indicates that the creation of chairs and specialty journals had only a gradual effect in codifying specialty categories. Specialist lists are a useful way of gauging the extent of the codification which had taken place; they may have also contributed to the crystallization of specialist categories, particularly those outside the orbit of élite institutions.

The first listing of specialists that I have found occurred in a rather bizarre publication called the *Annuaire des Spécialités médicales et pharmaceutiques* which first appeared in 1880 under the editorship of P. Bouland, yet another orthopaedist. This directory started with an alphabetical listing of practitioners according to name. But unlike the *Annuaire Roubaud* which depended on the information which practitioners themselves provided, the editor seems to have combed existing directories and journals for information about specialists. Among those listed were several figures from outside France including Rudolf Virchow. The alphabetical entries included each individual's major publications rather than any specialty label. This would ordinarily be sufficient to permit identification of specialists by experienced practitioners. But the editor also decided to add a short one-and-a-half page listing of specialist practitioners, without any descriptive information, according to specialties, and including foreigners as well as Frenchmen.

This listing was far shorter and seemingly less important than two other listings which followed, one for medico-surgical materials, ranging from batteries to instruments to manuals, and filling 12 pages in the first volume; and a second listing of pharmaceutical 'specialties' (specific remedies) which the editor took pains to distinguish from secret remedies[85] and filling 19 pages. Despite its brevity, the specialist listing was a major innovation, though Bouland's *Annuaire* survived only until 1886. In 1887, however, there appeared a direct competitor to the *Annuaire Roubaud,* the *Guide Rosenwald* which, like Bouland's *Annuaire,* seems to have made most of its profits from advertisements for pharmaceutical 'specialties'.[86] Like the *Annuaire Roubaud,* this new directory was chiefly comprised of an alphabetical listing of Parisian practitioners which included specialist self-descriptions; it also introduced the innovation of providing lists of practitioners outside Paris according to geographical region. Of more significance for our purposes is that it added in its second issue a separate list of Parisian specialists divided according to specialty. In 1892 – and it is hard to believe

that this was unconnected with the existence of a publishing rival –
the venerable *Annuaire Roubaud* broke with tradition by including a
specialist listing to supplement its alphabetical directory.

Specialty Categories
Annuaire des Specialités médicales – 1880

Accouchements	Maladies du larynx
Maladies des enfants	[Maladies du coeur et des voies
Maladies de la peau	respiratoires – 1882]
Maladies vénériennes	Maladies nerveuses
Maladies des voies urinaires	Maladies mentales
Maladies des femmes	Orthopédie et cinésie
Maladies des yeux	Electrothérapie
Maladies des oreilles	Balnéologie
Hydrothérapie	

Guide Rosenwald – 1888

Accouchements	Nez et des oreilles (maladies du)
Coeur (maladies du)	Odontologie
Electrothérapie	Orthopédie et cinésie
Enfants (maladies des)	Peau (maladies de la)
Estomac (maladies de l')	Reins (maladies des)
Femmes (maladies des)	Vénériennes (maladies)
Hydrothérapie	Voies respiratoires (maladies des)
Larynx (maladies du)	Voies urinaires (maladies des)
Mentales (maladies)	Yeux (maladies des)
Nerveuses (maladies)	

Annuaire Roubaud – 1892

Accouchements,	Maladies des voies respiratoires
maladies des femmes et des enfants,	Maladies de la peau
gynécologie	Maladies syphilitiques
Chirurgiens, orthopédistes	Maladies des voies urinaires
Laryngoscopie et rhinoscopie	Maladies des yeux
Maladies de poitrine	Rhumatisme, goutte

Given the existence of such lists of specialists, it would seem a
simple matter to go on at this point to quantitative analysis. In fact,
matters are far from simple. The difficulty that is easiest to solve
is that each one of our sources is seriously incomplete in one way or
another. These discrepancies testify to the fluidity of specialty identifications during the late nineteenth century and will be
discussed in detail in another paper. The more serious problem is
to decide what counts as a specialty during this period since the
designations which individuals provided were not uniform and
many individuals provided more than one, in a bewildering variety
of permutations and combinations. This is precisely the difficulty

faced by the editors of the directories. They had to determine, in the words of one, generally admitted categories of specialties that 'appeared to us compatible with accepted habits – customs or prejudices, if one prefers – but which has no *raison d'être* but for a convention which modifies itself incessantly'.[87]

Any historian wishing to categorize specialties would be foolish not to look closely at the categorization systems elaborated by his historical subjects (especially if he intends to quantify the data which they provide). But there is a more important reason to analyse the specialty categories embedded in these specialty listings. These provide a unique window into the emerging and fluid world of specialization in medical practice that was just beginning to take concrete shape at the end of the nineteenth century.

Let me begin chronologically with the first listing of the *Annuaire des Spécialités médicales et pharmaceutiques* in 1880 which, like the 1839 masthead of *L'Esculape,* contained 15 specialist categories. Specialties are described in terms of patients (children, women), life-events (birth), organs (skin, urinary tract, eyes, ears, larynx), illness type (venereal, nervous, mental) and techniques (electrotherapy, balneology, hydrotherapy) with one combining organs with techniques (orthopaedics and kinestherapy). It may be significant that these latter technical specialties are the only ones described in technical and even latinate terms, reflecting perhaps the professional insecurity of practitioners. Notable for their absence are the specialties defined by social function that were on the masthead of *L'Esculape* in 1839; public health, military medicine and legal medicine. Medical specialization had become defined as clinical specialization in private or hospital practice. Dental and herniary surgery are also absent (the first temporarily, the second definitively). Among the new specialties appearing on this listing and absent from that of 1839 are maladies of the ears, of the larynx and a number of therapeutic techniques, *'cinésie', 'électrothérapie'* and *'balnéologie'.* Replacing *'eaux minérales',* was the more general *'hydrothérapie'.*

The order of listings is strange and can only be explained as a kind of stream of consciousness. It is certainly not alphabetical although *'accouchement',* here as in all the directories appears first. It is followed by *'enfants',* understandably, since children are the normal outcome of childbirth. One would expect *'femmes',* also closely associated with birth and children, to follow next but instead we get *'peau'* (babies' soft skin perhaps?). Since dermatology was identified with venereology, it is not surprising that *'vénériennes'* follows here. (One notes, however, that they are presented as two separate

174

specialties, despite their characteristic linkage in teaching and the titles of journals.) Likewise the spatial proximity of the site and mode of infection of venereal disease, the genitalia, to the urinary tract explains the next listing *'voies urinaires'*. At this point *'femmes'* appears somewhat abruptly. The reason has to do with the way specialized practices were combined. Many physicians seem to have practised both urinary and gynaecological medicine because both were concerned with female genitalia.[88] It can of course be argued quite correctly that urologists also practised on men. But there was no comparable medical specialty related to the male reproductive organs. In its absence, urology was most closely identified with diseases of women.

We next move on to the organs of the head, *'yeux, oreilles, larynx'*, the order of appearance reflecting perhaps views of their relative importance or seniority. (On *L'Esculape's* masthead in 1839, diseases of the eyes also preceded those of the ears while the throat was not yet deemed worthy of a specialty.) There may also have been a principle of movement from top to bottom at work. This impression is strengthened by the fact that a new specialty was added in 1882, illnesses of the *'coeur et voies respiratoires'* (also absent from the 1839 listing). It was placed after diseases of the larynx. The classification then shifts to two illness types whose relationship to specific organs was somewhat more problematic, *'maladies nerveuses'* and *'mentales'*. This separation of the two categories is unusual in a listing of this sort and undoubtedly follows the pattern recently set by the Paris Faculty of Medicine which had just created separate chairs for each specialty field. The three therapeutic specialties are preceded by *'orthopédie et cinésie'* which combines body parts with types of therapy. The inconsistencies of presentation eventually became evident to the editor who introduced a consistent alphabetical principle of presentation in 1885; this did not, however, change any of the categories.

The second volume of the *Guide Rosenwald* published in 1888 essentially follows the pattern established by the *Annuaire des Spécialités médicales* in its last volumes. It is alphabetical, relatively comprehensive, including even marginal specialties, and tends to separate specialties into discrete units even if they are often joined in practice. It extends to ,19, the 16 specialties which appeared in the last volumes of the *Annuaire*. Of the latter, one marginal category, *'balnéologie'*, has disappeared but three new ones have appeared – *'estomac'*, *'reins'* and *'odontologie'* – all organ based. In addition, the *Guide Rosenwald* explicitly separates diseases of the heart and of the respiratory tract. It adds to a part of the body traditionally thought to merit specialization, the larynx, another category made up of the nose and ears. (Both are missing from the masthead of 1839).[89]

The categorization used four years later by the venerable *Annuaire Roubaud*, then in its 44th year, is somewhat different. There are only ten categories and there is clearly a desire on the part of the editor to rationally lump together specialties that are similar or frequently combined into a small number of rubrics. The listing is also recognizably alphabetical, at least for the first term in each rubric.

The first category lumps together three separate rubrics in both the *Guide Rosenwald* and the *Annuaire des Spécialités médicales* – *'accouchement, maladies des femmes et des enfants'* (note that the latter two are presented as a single specialty as they often were in practice) – and adds a new one *'gynécologie'*. The latter term of course was beginning to be used to identify journals in the field[90] and probably reflects the self-identification of certain specialists with a more professional and scientific vision of their field.

The second category is equally idiosyncratic. Orthopaedists are not linked to a particular therapy (*'cinésie'*) but with a group excluded from the *Annuaire des Spécialités médicales*, surgeons. If putting the two groups together (and the comma suggests that they are recognized to be distinct) seems reasonable, the heading is disconcerting on at least two counts. First, this is the only one which does not represent a category of illness (including birth) or form of therapy but denotes the specialist practitioners themselves (surgeons and orthopaedists). Second, conceiving of surgery as a specialty among others was not common. Medicine throughout the nineteenth century was considered to be comprised of two equal branches, internal medicine and external medicine, i.e. surgery. Specialties developed from one or both of these. The specialist listings in the *Annuaire des Spécialités médicales et pharmaceutiques* were thus titled *'Spécialités Médico-Chirurgicales'*. Roubaud's categorization, though idiosyncratic, suggests that the status of surgery was in the process of change.[91] The fact that most of those he lists as surgeons had posts in surgery at the Paris hospitals suggests an intermediate status somewhere between a constituent element of the surgico-medical profession and the one specialty among many others it was ultimately to become. It was one defined primarily by institutional titles and posts in hospitals and medical schools.

The third category is equally strange, using terms for the examination of the nose and larynx (*'laryngoscopie et rhinoscopie'*). This suggests the centrality of these instruments in the consolidation of the specialty. The ears, however, are no longer singled out for specialized attention. Unusually, the next categories separate specialties that had been linked in the *Annuaire des Spécialités médicales*. Instead of a single category of diseases of the heart and respiratory tract, the *Annuaire Roubaud* like the *Guide Rosenwald* gives two rubrics, illnesses of the *'poitrine'* which undoubtedly include the heart) and those of the *'voies respiratoires'*. Illnesses of the skin are classified exactly as they were in the earlier directory as *'maladies de la peau'*. There also remains a separate category for venereal diseases. Maladies of the urinary tract and of the eyes remain unchanged as distinct categories.

Missing from Roubaud's listing are most of the last six categories in the listings of the *Annuaire des Spécialités médicales*, therapeutic techniques like *'cinésie'*, *'electrothérapie'*, *'balnéologie'* and *'hydrothérapie'* and more surprisingly, illness types such as *'maladies nerveuses'* and *'maladies mentales'*. It adds however a new category missing from the earlier list, *'rhumatisme et goutte'*.

The eleven specialties that are common to all three lists if we do not worry too much about how they are lumped together with others (and assume that the heart is the main concern of specialists of the chest) are:

obstetrics•	skin•
children•	venereal•
women	urinary tract•
orthopaedics	eyes•
larynx	heart
respiratory system	

Of the eleven mentioned, all but three – larynx, respiratory system and heart – are well-established, having appeared on the masthead of *L'Esculape* in 1839. Six of them had already been sanctioned with chairs at the Paris Faculty of Medicine (these are marked by a bullet point). The absence of the by now well-established nervous and mental diseases is surprising. If it is not clear that this absence represents anything more than the idiosyncracies of classification in the *Annuaire Roubaud*, it does suggest a certain remoteness of psychiatry to private medical practice.[92]

Later Directories

By the edition of 1904, the *Annuaire Roubaud* had adopted a very different approach to specialization categories. Instead of ten rubrics, it now listed 22, the same number as the *Guide Rosenwald* of 1905. The *Annuaire Roubaud's* expanded listing was achieved at the expense of alphabetical order, though there are patches which seem to be arranged alphabetically. Much of the increase is due to the addition of new categories. Although the directory achieved some of its expansion by separating previously combined categories, it remained characterized by a penchant for putting together related specialties. The *Guide Rosenwald* in contrast stayed pretty much with its old formula and simply added two new listings.

Overall, the categorization system of the *Guide Rosenwald* remained a good deal simpler than that of the *Annuaire Roubaud* which strived for a precision which made it cumbersome. For instance, whereas the *Guide Rosenwald* has two fairly distinct categories, *'accouchement'* and *'maladies des femmes'*, the *Annuaire Roubaud* has a category *'gynécologie-accouchement'* which partially overlaps a second rubric *'maladies des femmes'*. In complicating its categories in this way, the *Annuaire Roubaud* was most likely seeking to distinguish between two different sorts of medicine for women: one that was closely associated with hospital-based obstetrics; and another based on non-élite private practice and dealing with a wide range of conditions, including many that were psychosomatic. Similarly, whereas the *Guide Rosenwald* combined two previously separated categories into a single one – *'maladies mentales et nerveuses'* – either to reflect the realities of practice or because distinguishing them was highly problematical – the *Annuaire Roubaud* had an identical category plus another category in which *'maladies nerveuses'* was linked to electrotherapy. Once again there seems to be an effort to distinguish hospital, faculty and asylum-based psychiatry and neurology from private medical practice dealing with various forms of neurotic and nervous conditions and popularly associated with electrotherapy. We shall see the full pertinence of these attempts at distinction in a future more quantitative analysis of specialization as it is reflected in these medical directories.

Specialty Categories
Annuaire Roubaud – 1904

Gynécologie-accouchements

Maladies des enfants,

Maladies des femmes

Chirurgiens, orthopédistes

Electrothérapie, maladies nerveuses

Hydrothérapie

Laryngoscopie otologie et rhinoscopie

Maladies mentales et nerveuses

Maladies de l'estomac et de la nutrition

Maladies de poitrine et du coeur

Maladies de la peau et du cuir chevelu

Maladies des voies respiratoires

Radiothérapie - radiographie - radioscopie

Maladies vénériennes et syphilitiques

Maladies des voies urinaires et des reins

Physicothérapie

Maladies des yeux

Maladies de la bouche et des dents

Rhumatisme, goutte

Obésité

Médecin pédicure

Vaccine

Guide Rosenwald – 1905

Accouchements	Orthopédie et cinésie
Coeur (maladies du)	Ozone-oxygène
Electrothérapie	Peau (maladie de la)
Embaumements et autopsie	Pédicure
Enfants (maladies des)	Radiographie - radiologie -
Odontologie	radioscopie
Estomac (maladies de l')	Reins (maladies des)
Femmes (maladies des)	Vénériennes (maladies)
Hydrothérapie	Voies respiratoires (maladies des)
Larynx, nez, oreilles (maladies du)	Voies urinaires (maladies des)
Mentales et nerveuses (maladies)	Yeux (maladies des)

By now there seems to have existed some consensus about specialties since most appeared in both of the publications. A few, however did not. The *Guide Rosenwald*, for instance, did not recognize surgery as a specialty while *Annuaire Roubaud* continued to do so. '*Physiothérapie*', '*rhumatisme-goutte*', and '*obésité*' appeared in the latter but not the former, which did however include '*cinésie*' (possibly the equivalent of '*physiothérapie*') and '*ozone oxygène*'. The *Guide Rosenwald* also treated the kidneys to a separate rubric, whereas *Annuaire Roubaud* attached them to the urinary tract. Various other small differences of formulation are also visible.

To the 11 specialties which appeared on the two early lists we can add the following which appeared on both of our later lists.

electrotherapy	mouth and teeth
hydrotherapy	pedicure
mental and nervous disease	vaccine
stomach	radiography
(Larynx) nose, ears	
(the three organs now irrevocably linked)	

With the exception of mental and nervous diseases represented by chairs at the faculty, these specialties had few academic ties. Several (pedicure, vaccine) were practised by very small numbers of practitioners and some others were recognized in spite of the lack of specialty societies and journals. Clearly, specialized practice had taken on a life of its own and was no longer dependent on institutional visibility.

In subsequent years, specialist practice continued to spread. By 1935, the *Guide Rosenwald* included 36 medical specialties. Nearly 4,000 Parisian doctors, over fifty per cent of all practitioners listed in that year, either identified themselves as specialists and/or were included by the editor in one of the specialty categories. We shall examine the quantitative aspects of this development in another paper.

Conclusion

The preceding discussion suggests that the history of medical specialization in nineteenth-century France can be divided into three
periods. During the first from 1800 to 1860 only small numbers of
doctors called themselves specialists and few specialties had any real
institutional basis. Although specialized hospitals were in existence
making it possible for specialist knowledge to be created, only
obstetrics, ophthalmology and psychiatry had much in the way of
institutional foundations and a critical mass of practitioners. Public
health had the former but not the latter. On the other hand, some
doctors practised as specialists and the pertinence of many specialties
as useful categories of medical knowledge was firmly established by
the 1840s, as we saw in our discussion of medical dictionaries.

A second period lasted from the early 1860s to the early 1880s and
was marked by the introduction of specialization into the curriculum
of the medical faculties and by the development of specialist journals. I
have suggested that it was the imperatives of international educational
and scientific rivalry rather than any pressure from specialist practitioners which explains the former development. In the same way, it
was the opening up of the education system to specialties that
stimulated the development of specialty journals and specialist
knowledge more generally. A third period starting in the early 1880s
was characterized by the very rapid spread of specialist practice in the
absence of any significant control or regulation. This period lasted well
into the twentieth century. It came to an end with the introduction of
regulation and certification after the Second World War.

Aside from these periods, the focus on specialty categories gives a
sense of the somewhat chaotic nature of specialty practice that is
missing from studies centring on associations and journals. If one
starts with our own categories and looks backwards, one will surely
find continuity in the past. But one may miss the flux and fluidity
that characterized specialist practice in real life and that distinguishes
nineteenth-century medicine from that of the twentieth.

Notes

I wish to express my gratitude to the Social Science and Humanities Research
Council of Canada for its financial support of this research. I am also grateful
to Donna Evleth and Don Fyson for providing research assistance.

1. Rosemary Stevens, *Medical Practice in England: The Impact of
   Specialization and State Medicine* (New Haven: Yale University Press,
   1966); and *American Medicine and the Public Interest* (New Haven

and London: Yale University Press, 1971).

2. She writes: 'Specialization was prompted by those who sought excellence in particular areas within expanding fields; it was an inevitable and desirable accompaniment of scientific advance'. Stevens, *Medical Practice in England,* 4.

3. George Rosen, *The Specialization of Medicine* (New York, Froben Press, 1944).

4. See Rosen, *The Specialization,* ch. 5.

5. Sydney A. Halpern, *American Paediatrics: The Social Dynamics of Professionalism* (Berkeley: University of California Press, 1988). The author points out that Rosen himself recognized that paediatrics did not fit into his intellectual model.

6. Russell C. Maulitz, 'Grand Rounds: An Introduction to the History of Internal Medicine', in Russell C. Maulitz and Diana E. Long, (eds), *Grand Rounds: One Hundred Years of Internal Medicine* (Philadelphia: University of Pennsylvania Press, 1988), 4–5.

7. Bonnie Ellen Blustein, 'New York Neurologists and the Specialization of American Medicine', *Bulletin of the History of Medicine,* 53 (1979), 170–83.

8. For instance Lindsay Granshaw, '"Fame and Fortune by Means of Bricks and Mortar": The Medical Profession and Specialist Hospitals in Britain, 1800–1948', in Lindsay Granshaw and Roy Porter, (eds), *The Hospital in History* (London and New York: Routledge, 1989), 199–220; Glenn Gritzer and Arnold Arluke, *The Making of Rehabilitation: A Political Economy of Medical Specialization, 1890–1980* (Berkeley: University of California Press, 1985). Ian R. Dowbiggin, *Inheriting Madness: Professionalization and Psychiatric Knowledge in Nineteenth Century France* (Berkeley: University of California Press, 1991).

9. The sharp decline in the number of surgeons reflects the fact that most graduates of the Paris Faculty of Medicine took general medical degrees rather than surgical degrees which were offered but which held few advantages for surgical practice.

10. L. Hubert, *Almanach général des médecins pour la Ville de Paris* (Paris: Gabon, 1830).

11. The specialty tag usually followed the name and preceded other sorts of information.

12. The possession of a surgical degree often determined if a practitioner labelled himself a surgeon or not. But this was not consistently the case.

13. Matthew Ramsey, *Professional and Popular Medicine in France 1770–1830: The Social World of Medical Practice* (Cambridge: Cambridge University Press, 1988), 23–8 for old regime specialists, 239–43 for 19th-century folk specialists.

14. For instance, Cullerier never described institutionally as chief surgeon of the Hôpital des Vénériennes, nevertheless gave 'médecin' as his

professional identification.

15. On obstetrical training in the 18th century, see Jacques Gélis, *La Sage-femme ou le médecin* (Paris: Fayard, 1988). Also Paul Delaunay, *La Maternité de Paris* (Paris: Pousset, 1909).

16. The *agrégation* in surgery became in 1844 the *agrégation* in surgery and *accouchement*.

17. From 1820–29, *accoucheurs* in the Academy had been located in the surgery section.

18. A chair in ocular surgery was created at the Collège de Chirurgie in 1765. Ramsey, *Professional and Popular Medicine*, 25. A. Corlieu, *Centenaire de la Faculté de Médecine de Paris*, (Paris: 1896), 444.

19. There was an elaborate system of private hospital teaching in Paris in the early 19th century with some devoted to what we would consider specialties. For some of these specialized courses see Jacques Poirier, 'La Faculté de Médecine face à la montée du spécialisme', *Communications*, 54(1992), 210–11. However, hospitals in the absence of intellectual or socio-political pressures were insufficient to develop specialties. Thus geriatrics failed to emerge from the several hospitals devoted to the elderly in the 19th and early 20th centuries.

20. F. S. Ratier, *Lettre aux médecins français sur la nécessité de spécialiser de bonne heure les études des jeunes gens qui doivent devenir médecins* (Paris: Ballière, 1838).

21. According to Corlieu, *Centenaire*, 497, he took over the hospital orthopaedic service only in 1848. This source also identifies him as the first surgeon in Paris to section an Achilles tendon using Stomeyer's procedure.

22. For instance, in the May 1844 issue, Duval's own book on foot and leg deformities was reviewed in the journal by Dr Dalasiauve of the Bicêtre. In the issue of December 1840, a special section on case histories was made up of cases seen in Parisian hospitals.

23. *Revue des Spécialités et Innovations Médicales et Chirurgicales*, 1(1839), 1.

24. S. Furnari, 'Introduction', *L'Esculape, Journal des Spécialités Médico-Chirurgicales*, 1(1839), 1–2; *Revue des Spécialités et Innovations Médicales et Chirurgicales*, 1(1839), 1–5.

25. Vincent Duval, 'Coup d'oeil sur nos travaux', *Revue des Spécialités et Innovations Médicales et Chirurgicales*, 3 (1841), 1–11.

26. On these matters see Jan E. Goldstein, *Console and Classify: The French Psychiatric Profession in the Nineteenth Century* (New York: Cambridge University Press, 1987).

27. There was an unsuccessful effort in 1823 to create a special school of legal medicine and public health to be associated with the Academy of Medicine. (Dupuytren *et al.*, 'Rapport à Son Excellence Monsieur le Ministre de l'Intérieur, sur la proposition de MM. Dariste, Orfila, Pelletier, Caventou et Pelletan, relative à la création d'une École spéciale de médecine légale' in Ministère de l'instruction publique et

des beaux-arts, *Enquêtes et documents relatifs à l'enseignement supérieur,* vol. 37, A. de Beauchamp, (ed.) (Paris: Imprimerie Nationale, 1890), 250–69. In 1860, the *agrégation* in medicine was expanded to include *'médecine et médecine légale'.*

28. On the institutionalization of public hygiene during this period see Ann F. Laberge, 'The Early Nineteenth-Century French Public Health Movement: The Disciplinary Development and Institutionalization of Hygiène Publique', *Bulletin of the History of Medicine,* 56 (1984), 363–79.

29. Duval, 'Coup d'oeil', 3–4.

30. *Dictionnaire des Sciences Médicales,* vol.1 (Paris: Crapart, 1812), 101.

31. Ant. Dugès, 'Accouchement', *Dictionnaire de Médecine et de Chirurgie Pratique,* vol. 1 (Paris: Gabon, 1829), 124.

32. Raige Delorme, 'Oculiste', *Dictionnaire de Médecine,* vol.15 (Paris: Béchet Jeune, 1826), 216–17.

33. Marjolin, 'Dentiste', *Dictionnaire de Médecine,* vol. 6 (1823), 478–9.

34. Raige Delorme, *Dictionnaire de Médecine,* deuxième édn, vol. 21 (Paris: Béchet Jeune, 1840), 189. Its role was still to ensure the complete health of the woman and of the newborn infant.

35. J. F. Oudet, *ibid.,* 236

36. Velpeau, 'Ophthalmologie', *ibid.,* vol. 22 (1840), 195–6.

37. In all the cases discussed, the list of editors appears at the beginning of the first volume.

38. *Nouveau Dictionnaire de Médecine et de Chirurgie Pratique,* vol. 1, (Paris: Baillière, 1864), v–vi.

39. Neither Londe nor Magendie is listed in Jan Goldstein's index, suggesting their marginality to the developing field.

40. According to Goldstein, Georget had in fact died in 1828.

41. This was Rayer; listed only as doctor of medicine in 1826 he was identified as a physician at Saint-Antoine by 1829.

42. For instance, Georget had been attached to the Salpêtrière as a student and had later worked at Esquirol's private hospital at Ivry. (Goldstein, *Console and Classify,* 389.)

43. George D. Sussman, 'The Glut of Doctors in Mid-Nineteenth Century France', *Comparative Studies in Society and History,* 19 (1977), 296–7.

44. It is worth noting that of the three directories which appeared in the early 1850s, this publication had by a considerable margin the largest number of self-identified specialists.

45. In the earlier directory we found 20 obstetricians among just the first 436 listings.

46. Whether alienism and mental medicine actually comprised a single recognized category at mid-century is not entirely clear but seems likely in view of other evidence.

47. I am basing this discussion on the computerized list of medical periodicals at the National Library of Medicine. A list of French

periodicals which began publication before 1905 was compiled; it was then checked against various other French bibliographical listings.

48. A successor, the *Annales de dermatologie et de syphilographie*, started in 1868, published well into the twentieth century.

49. These were the *Journal de magnétisme* (1845–61) and *Magnétiseur* (1859–72).

50. Poirier, 'La Faculté', 213. It should be noted that opposition to medical specialization was international. Mid and late century American writings on the subject are collected in *The Origins of Specialization in American Medicine*, Charles Rosenberg, (ed.), (New York: Garland, 1989).

51. Jan Goldstein, *Console and Classify*, 346–8 and Poirier, 'La Faculté', 214.

52. George Weisz, *The Emergence of Modern Universities in France, 1863–1914* (Princeton: Princeton University Press, 1983).

53. The clearest expression of these concerns is Léon LeFort, *Rapport sur la création de chaires cliniques spéciales à la Faculté de Médecine*, 4–5, read to the Faculty 18 April, 1878. The report is in Archives Nationales (A.N.) AJ16 6310. The conclusions were voted unanimously. Also see the comments by Hardy to the Faculty Assembly 6 January, 1876, A.N. AJ16 6257.

54. See for instance the faculty discussions of 30 December, 1875, 6 January, 1876 in A.N. AJ16 6357. Poirier, 'La Faculté', 214–18, gives a good account of these discussions.

55. Léon LeFort, *Rapport*, 4–5.

56. *Ibid.*, 7.

57. This has been argued by Poirier, 'La Faculté', 217–18.

58. Our major source for this affair is Pierre Pichot, *Un siècle de psychiatrie* (Paris: Roche, 1983), 25–7.

59. The model of specialization based on new instruments was also consciously followed by otorhinolaryngologists. See the introductory editorial remarks in *Annales des maladies de l'oreille et du larynx*, 1(1875), 1.

60. These were the *Annales de maladies de la peau et de la syphilis* (1843–52), *Annuaire de la syphilis et des maladies de la peau* (1858) and *Annales de dermatologie et de syphiligraphie* (1868–1976).

61. A look in some of the medical dictionaries of the mid-19th century would suggest that the fields were linked by the fact that characteristic venereal lesions appeared on the skin. One could thus not discuss skin diseases without including the venereal variety which were so common; nor could one discuss venereal disease without being able to distinguish their lesions from those of other conditions. The contagiousness of so many conditions constituted yet another link.

62. LeFort, *Rapport*, 13.

63. See Paul Legendre, *Du Quartier Latin à l'Académie (Réminiscences),* (Paris: Maloine, 1930). We know that the minister did not consult the faculty about the appointment due to several letters in Fournier's file in A.N. AJ16 1081.
64. There is some uncertainty about which subjects can be considered real specialties. My own criteria were broadly inclusive. My list of specialty periodicals was initially compiled from the catalogue of the National Library of Medicine and then checked against and supplemented by the catalogue of the Library of the Academy of Medicine in Paris.
65. A. Chéreau, 'Spécialités médicales' *Dictionnaire Encyclopédique des Sciences Médicales,* vol. 10, (Paris: Asselin et Masson, 1881), 797–8.
66. The best discussion of these matters are to be found in the two books by Rosemary Stevens already cited.
67. The newly created Ordre des Médecins made possible the organization of certification.
68. In the 1930s the Paris Faculty of Medicine was awarding seven post-graduate diplomas in: colonial medicine, legal medicine and psychiatry, malariology, hygiene, puériculture, serology, medical radiology and electrology. Unlike the doctorate which was a state degree, these were university degrees with no legal validity for medical practice.
69. G. Roussy, 'L'enseignement de la médecine en France', *Bulletin trimestriel de l'Organisation d'Hygiène de la Société des Nations,* 1(1932), 13.
70. The nomination of Leroy d'Étiolle in 1840 provoked a formal protest from Parisian hospital surgeons. P. Pfister, 'Le phénomène de spécialisation médicale au 19ᵉ siècle', Thèse de doctorat en médecine, Université de Paris-Créteil, 1976, 17. For other cases, *ibid.,* 29.
71. Paul Legendre in discussing his medical student experiences during this period, describes many of those he worked under in hospitals as specialists. Paul Legendre, *Du Quartier Latin.*
72. Despite the creation of specialized chairs, recruitment for junior faculty personnel in the Faculty, the *agrégés,* also did not encourage early specialization since the competitions were very general. In 1904, the competition was divided into the same 4 categories as had existed in the 1860s.
73. See Delaunay, *Du Quartier latin,* 206, and especially, Nadine Lefaucher, 'La résistible création des accoucheurs des hôpitaux', *Sociologie de Travail,* 30 (1988), 323–52.
74. The alienists listed were those in the major Parisian hospitals, the Salpêtrière and the Bicêtre. Those in smaller departmental asylums were part of a different administration which was also evolving. Regulations drawn up at about the same time introduced special competitions for asylum interns. Somewhat later, junior asylum physicians *(médecins adjoints)* also came to be chosen by *concours.*

75. *Bulletin de l'Académie de Médecine*, 17 (1887), 592–645; *Bulletin de l'Académie de Médecine*, 19 (1888), 155–469.

76. What follows is based on Paul Brouardel, 'Création des services pour le traitement des maladies spéciales dans les hôpitaux', in *Conseil des Surveillance de l'Assistance Publique*, session 1897–1898, 931–48. This is located in the archives of the Assistance Publique.

77. *XIIIième Congrès International de Médecine, Paris, 1900, Paris médical, Assistance et enseignement* (Paris: Masson, 1900), 222.

78. Pfister, *Le phénomène*, 38

79. *Bulletin de l'Académie de Médecine*, 42 (1899), 533.

80. Fernet, in *Bulletin de l'Académie de Medecine*, 42 (1899), 575. Also Hallopeau, *ibid.*, 578–9.

81. Panas, *Bulletin de l'Académie de Medecine*, 42 (1899), 577.

82. Faculty projects during the 1870s specifically (but unsuccessfully) excluded venereology from the subject matter of the chair of dermatology that was being created.

83. Robert Debré recounts that as a paediatrician just appointed as a *médecin des hôpitaux* in the early 1920s, his worst fear was that he would be appointed to a geriatric ward. But his luck, as always, held. Some vacancies as well as the willingness of a top hospital administrator to ignore established procedure led to a paediatric service. He did, however, eventually spend several years heading a service for tubercular adults. Robert Debré, *L'Honneur de vivre: témoignages*, (Paris: Herman et Stock, 1972), 139–40.

84. *Annuaire médicale et pharmaceutique du docteur Roubaud* published from 1848 to 1913.

85. *Annuaire des Spécialités médicales et pharmaceutiques*, 1(1880), 61.

86. In his preface to the first edition of the *Guide Rosenwald* (Paris: 1887), viii–ix, the editor, Lucien Rosenwald, insisted that he did not accept just any paid advertising but only for those products which had the confidence of the medical profession or which had 'real intrinsic value'. A brief historical sketch at the front of the centenary edition of the *Guide Rosenwald*, vol. 1 (Paris: 1987) suggests that in starting his publication Rosenwald was motivated in part by the fact that he himself owned several 'pharmaceutical specialties' which could be publicized.

87. *Annuaire des Spécialités médicales et pharmaceutiques*, 1(1880), 40.

88. I shall develop this point more extensively in another paper.

89. Both the centrality of instruments and the somewhat ambiguous status of the nose within the emerging specialty are illustrated by the title of the first journal in the field which appeared in 1875: *Annales des maladies de l'oreille et du larynx: (otoscopie, laryngoscopie, rhinoscopie.*

90. The first journals with *'Gynécologie'* rather than *'Obstétrique'* or *'Maladies des Femmes'* in the title date from the 1870s.

91. Patrice Pinell has suggested to me that part of the reclassification of

surgery expressed by its appearance on this specialist list may have been due to the fact that the law regulating medical practice that was then in the process of being passed (it would do so a year later) eliminated the separate doctorate of surgery, leaving only the doctorate of medicine. That would have weakened the identification of surgery as a constituent element of medicine and facilitated its being treated as another specialty.

92. Another less dramatic indication is in the *Guide Rosenwald* of the early twentieth century which does include the category of mental and nervous diseases but excludes from this category many individuals describing themselves as asylum physicians in the alphabetical listing.

Appendix 1

Specialty	Fac. Med. Chair	Date of 1st Journal[1]	Journals in 1905[1]	Date of 1st Society
Surgery	1795	1848[2]	11	1847
Public Health	1795	1829	10	1877
Legal Medicine	1795	1829	2	1868
Obstetrics	1795	1874	14[3]	1891
Gynaecology	1905	1879	12[3]	1885
Psychiatry	1877	1843	6	1847 *(1889)*
Ophthalmology	1878	1871	11	1883
Paediatrics (paed. surgery)	1878 1905	1883	15	1899
Dermatology/ Venereology	1879	1868 *(1843)*	5	1889
Neurology	1882	1880	4	1899
Urology	1890	1882	4	1896
Otolaryngology		1875	8	1883
Orthopaedics		1887	3	
Physio/Physicotherapy		1898	4	
Nutrition		1893	1	
Odontology		1874[4]	9[4]	1898
Stomatology		1894	2	1888
Electricity		1893	7	1893
Radiology		1890	3	1907
Hydrology		1854	7	1854
Tuberculosis		1888	5	

1. Categories are based on titles.
2. First journal with *only* surgery in the title
3. Most journals in these fields include both obstetrics and gynaecology in the title.
4. Includes dental journals.

5

Doctors and Families in France, 1880–1930: The Cultural Reconstruction of Medicine[1]

Martha L. Hildreth

From the late 1880s to the end of the 1920s French medical practice oriented itself around the family as the subject of primary concern and the focus of medical ministrations. The motif of the family permeates every aspect of professional discourse: in words written for consumption within the profession and in the public pronouncements of physicians. The physiological and biological constitution of the family became central to the construction of disease and was a pervasive theme in the language of diagnosis.[2] At the same time, the family became the basis for the socio-economic organization of medicine, the unit upon which the physician ordered his clientele, and staked a claim to that client-territory. In other words, the family became the object of the medical gaze.[3] Just as the practitioners of the previous generations, influenced by the Paris School, had carefully noted the symptoms of the body's exterior in order to identify the lesions inside, so had the *fin-de-siècle* practitioners studied the family 'body' as defined by its heredity, in order to identify the hidden sources of disease.

During the Third Republic concerns over the family, and in particular over its health, its reproductive capacity and its ability to promote hierarchy and stability, became social and political obsessions, as a number of historians have pointed out.[4] Naturally the relationship of the family and physicians is central to this problem and indeed has received considerable historical notice, by Jacques Donzelot and Robert Nye among others.[5] Nye and Donzelot have traced the medical–social impact of the French version of social Darwinism coupled with population-growth anxieties as they explore the impact of hereditarian ideology on social welfare practices (more important for Donzelot) and medical– welfare discourse (more important for Nye). In both these Foucault-inspired works, physicians are viewed as instruments of a hegemonic discourse, closely identified with state power, seeking to control dissident and non-conformist behaviour by using medical–hygienist notions to create standards of the normal and acceptable versus the deviant and degenerate.

The story of the forceful application of new ideologies of control and normalization captures an important aspect of the social and political realities of new medical ideologies, especially as they were carried out among the poorer and marginal classes. But the deeper cultural origins of these ideas, their acceptance or non-acceptance in the culture in general, and the transformative effects on medicine itself as a system of ideas and actions, needs further consideration.

Medicine is a system of thought/practice consisting of a set of conceptual beliefs (disease etiology), discursive and technical practices (diagnoses, pronouncements and therapies) and social relationships (that of physician and patient). But it is not a closed system; rather medicine is a cultural institution which is the product of broad social forces. It cannot be understood narrowly as the result of scientific systems of thought, or as the product of professional politics, or as the offspring of the socio-political agenda to the state.[6] It certainly reflects the interplay of all these forces, but essentially medicine is a cultural institution whose objects and practices are mediations from and with the general culture.[7] Thus the family-orientation of French medicine at the *fin-de-siècle* must be understood in light of what the general culture felt, feared, expected and rejected from medical ideologies and practices.[8]

A close look at the general culture reveals an extensive social preoccupation with medical issues. The fact that medicine might be profoundly changed by hereditarian as well as bacteriological theories, that new technologies and practices were being brought to bear upon human bodies, and that all of this had profound social, moral and personal consequences, did not escape general notice. A wide variety of cultural expressions ranging from the exaggerations of science fiction to the more subtle dramas of the social–realist theatre reflect these concerns. Taken together, such material reveals not only how society reacted to, but also how it shaped the way medicine incorporated and carried out these new concepts and practices. Central to this discussion is the family practitioner or *omnipraticien* who turns up as an ambivalent icon, hero and anti-hero in one, embodying the hope for relief and cure and the dangers inherent in new theories and practices. Thus we see two reciprocal motifs: the family in medicine, and the family physician in the general culture. The ways in which their respective discourses intertwine reveal how medicine was reconstructed in this crucial period.

The social–realist theatre of the *fin-de-siècle* is an excellent touchstone of social preoccupations. Scores of plays dealt with medical themes, and often physicians figure as major characters. These popular plays were an arena for the expression of immediate cultural concerns and reflect the fears and anxieties, images and ideas, which at that moment caught up the popular imagination.[9] Here playwrights, and presumably their audiences, seem fixated on disease and its ramifications in an era of new scientific knowledge and practices. There is a keen awareness of the impact of a scientific model in medicine which integrated research in bacteriology and chemistry with theory and practice. This new sciences embodied hope, but threats as well.[10] Laboratories and experiments loom large as fearful images, with horrifying implications. Unwary patients could be victimized by physicians experimenting with new therapeutic tools such as antibacterial chemotherapies and X-rays.[11] Equally disturbing were the notions involved in hereditarian ideology. As generally viewed, heredity was simply one more aspect of the new medical sciences including bacteriology, experimental physiology and pharmacology.[12] Along with these conceptual products of the laboratory, the French version of social Darwinisn was equally influential on medical discourse and practices.[13] Hereditarian ideology had a profound effect on how certain important diseases were understood, and it had far reaching and potentially devastating effects on the family. A doctor's diagnosis of one of the dreaded hereditary diseases coloured how the family thought about its past, planned for its future, and how it was perceived by the community.

Hereditarian ideology, like bacteriology, was considered scientific.[14] Physicians realized that scientific knowledge brought both benefits and dangers. Private practitioners sought to distance themselves from the fearful images of science, to portray themselves as 'family friend' and not 'man of science', as family doctor, not scientist–practitioner or, worse yet, as experimenter.[15] The ideal of the family practitioner was the medical profession's answer to the frightening images raised by the laboratory. And it was an answer with great appeal to many within the profession. Private practitioners used the image of the family doctor as a rhetorical tool in their long-standing battle against state and public medicine, against hospitals, clinics, dispensaries, the Pasteur Institutes, the Red Cross, nurses and a whole battery of threats to private practice.[16] But the iconographic image of the family practitioner emerges also from the discourse of the general culture and cannot simply be seen as an ideology forced on patients by the medical profession.

In this popular discourse, the physician is sometimes portrayed as a family friend, protecting the family and shoring up the paternalistic-authoritarian social structure. But more often the physician is a multifaceted character whose position towards the family is highly problematic given his allegiances to the conflicting demands of the individual, the family, society and science. He personifies both the promise and the threat of experimental medicine. He possesses the applied knowledge of what were viewed as the inexorable laws of heredity.

The physician was not only the intermediary between science and the public, but also the very personification of science itself, the only 'scientist' most people would ever come into contact with. In an insightful medical thesis written in 1910, a young physician, Louis-Henri Dejust, commented on how doctors were portrayed in popular culture:

> Le médecin devient l'intermédiaire entre le public et le laboratoire: les théories évolutionnistes, les recherches de bactériologie, la sérothérapie, sont en quelque sorte matérialisés par lui et appliqués par lui sous les yeux des ignorants.[17]

In this quotation, evolutionist doctrine shares equal place with bacteriology and serotherapy as a subject of major social concerns about science. Science was fearful because it seemed impersonal, dogmatic and fatalistic. As Dejust pointed out, 'Science has replaced God as the highest authority.... Science is all powerful ... but Science is not God, it cannot perform miracles.' In other words, the verdict of science was absolute, there was nowhere to appeal for mercy, for forgiveness, no escape from the new rigid diagnoses. The so-called laws of heredity were perceived as an especially heavy social burden, for the doctor's discovery of defects in the family's hereditary make-up was an inescapable verdict. It entailed shame for past transgressions, not only of the current generation of parents, but for their parents and grandparents, and sometimes foretold a doomed existence for their children. Patients looked to the family physician to mitigate their worst fears about scientific medicine, and to make medicine more comfortable. But at the same time that hereditarian concepts made his involvement with the family logical and comfortable, they also created great social tensions.

The desire of physicians to distance themselves from science can be understood if we consider the widespread public fear of victimization by experimenters. The scientific experiment conjured up a variety of troubling scenarios. Patients' fear of becoming the victims of medical experimentation is a prevalent theme in the popular literature of the era. Toby Gelfand resurrected and analysed a notable example of this in Léon Daudet's horror novel, *Les Morticoles*.[18] Gelfand attributes the generally favourable acceptance and popularity of this work as a testament to public anxieties about science. In the novel, the citizens of an imaginary nation ruled by physicians are all 'ill' unless they themselves are physicians. All personal rights over one's body are lost, and the citizen–patients are wholly subject to the medical whims of their physician–rulers. In this context, Daudet describes gruesome and torturous experiments.

A non-fictional work which is a match for Daudet's *Les Morticoles* in its scathing and bitter attack on medicine is *Défends ta peau contre ton médecin*, written by Charles Soller and Louis Gastine and published in 1907. Its themes are similar to Daudet's novel, and indeed *Les Morticoles* is mentioned in the text. Like Daudet, the authors emphasize that patients are defenceless against their doctors and that the encounter of doctor and patient puts the latter in a position of social inferiority.[19] The authors decry the 'martyrs of the hospitals', that is, the victims of experimentation; the mutilated cadavers of the anatomy clinics and autopsy rooms are described as vivid examples of the continuation of victimization after death. Soller and Gastine used the printed records of leading medical congresses and the major medical journals to prove their assertions about medical experimentation. The evidence they found here was very damning, and gives a dimension of reality not only to their work but to *Les Morticoles* as well.

As Soller and Gastine note, there were numerous scandals involving the effects of X-rays on the body, as this new invention was utilized as much for therapy as for diagnosis. At the 1905 Congrès international de l'Ionisation held in Liège, a Dr Lessar candidly reported devastating effects of radiation therapy on several of his patients. From the journal, *Bulletin médical*, Gastine and Soller cited reports of experiments by the dermatologists Gastou and Decrossas. The doctors had treated epithelioma with X-rays, causing extensive facial lesions in their patients. Soller and Gastine pointed to several other articles appearing in the public press, which reported that X-rays were being widely utilized in therapy for a variety of skin diseases. This therapy had often resulted in skin cancer and many deaths among patients who originally suffered from small, benign, skin tumors or simply from psoriasis.[20]

Another questionable practice uncovered by Soller and Gastine involved the frequent experimental treatment of diseases with the injection of other diseases, the rationale being that the one disease somehow prevented the other. In 1905 at the Paris Congrès international de la Tuberculose, as Soller and Gastine reported, 'one of our most renowned savants announced with perfect serenity that he had experimented with inoculating erysipelas to combat lupus.' The evidence backing up such experimental therapy was flimsy and impressionistic. In the *Revue médicale* of 1906 a Dr Bloch reported that he took blood from arthritis sufferers and injected it into tuberculosis patients because 'many doctors had reported that it seemed as if arthritis patients were immune to tuberculosis'.[21]

Now, like Léon Daudet, Soller and Gastine wrote not merely out of a desire to uncover the evil practices of modern medicine. They had a bigger axe to grind. As Gelfand points out about Daudet, Soller and Gastine were likewise opponents of the whole new order of atheistic, positivist, liberal-thinking France. They were part of the conservative reaction that created the Camelots du Roi and Action française. As such it might be tempting to dismiss them as fanatics and as marginal to the overwhelming republican positivist world of medicine. However, Gelfand reminds us that *Les Morticoles* was well reviewed by some of the very sorts of liberal thinkers that Daudet criticized, and that it was well received publicly. Soller and Gastine, although they surely did not find the readership of a Daudet, likewise cannot be ignored. Their evidence is too accurate and the fear of science and the experiment is too readily apparent in other cultural sources.

Daudet and Soller and Gastine are the extreme examples; they have absolutely no sympathy for science or scientists. But there exist more interesting and subtle analyses of the problem of human experimentation elsewhere in the contemporary literature. Here the physician–scientist is given more nuanced treatment. These works examine the cultural stereotype of the devoted man of science, the dedicated experimenter searching for a great medical breakthrough or cure. In the late nineteenth century the Scientist–Discoverer was a hero of French culture, with Pasteur as the archetype.[22] And this archetype shows up in the literature of the *fin-de-siècle* as the physician–scientist, devoted to his patients by day, and ensconced in his laboratory at night. But increasingly, in plays written just after the turn of the century, this character, while retaining his attribute as devoted doctor–scientist is shown to have a dark side. In the popular literature, the doctor–scientist, in order to promote his experimental work, is tempted to rush remedies into production before they are proven, to promote them even though he knows they have serious side effects, or worst of all, to knowingly experiment on his own clients. This is the dilemma faced by Dr Jean Kervil in Paul Adam's *Les Mouettes* (1906), and Dr Hardouin in G. Thurner's *Le Bluff* (1907).[23] The most notable example is François Curel's *La Nouvelle Idole* staged in 1906. Here the main character is Dr Donat, a man portrayed as absolutely devoted to science. He is searching for a cure for cancer and believes he is close to success. To test out his remedy, he inoculates one of his patients with cancer, a young woman whom he believes to be close to death from tuberculosis, (cancer was widely believed to be infectious). Donat's patient gets cancer and dies; his remedy does not work. Donat is absolutely unrepentant, arguing, 'If it is permitted to lose a whole regiment of soldiers to save a country why can't "a grand savant" sacrifice a few lives for a sublime discovery.' Curel, the author, indicates that such logic is widespread among medical scientists.[24]

In the popular literature the doctor–experimenter is sometimes described as a 'savant' or a 'Prince of Science'. He is thus a Paris-based physician–scientist with a faculty and/or hospital position.[25] Or, conversely, he is a man like Donat, a dedicated scientist whom un-favourable fortune has barred from the Paris scientific establishment and cast astray in the countryside. Such men are portrayed as out of their true element, inappropriate practitioners for the isolation of the countryside, and a real threat to their patients: their soothing manner of kindly healer masks a ruthless experimenter. Against these images, the literature contrasts the good family practitioner, the man who is indeed truly dedicated to the welfare of his patients, who is attuned to social and personal needs as well as scientific principles, and who is above all willing to tolerate the ambiguities of real life medical practice. The ideal doctor pays more attention to his patients than to the laboratory.[26] This paragon, as he emerged in the early twentieth century, is educated in all the latest scientific medical discoveries, and especially in bacteriology, hygiene, paediatrics, obstetrics, and the so-called laws of heredity. For as Gastine and Soller pointed out, it was too often true that physicians who portrayed themselves as a 'humble practitioner' and 'not a man of science', used this as an excuse to practise very out of date therapeutics and techniques. This sloppy, dishevelled, unwashed, ageing country practitioner, spreading infection among his clientele, also shows up in the popular media.[27] Conversely, the ideal practitioner embraced the benefits of science, but he de-emphasized the fatalistic, dogmatic and impersonal in favour of the ambiguous and humane.

It is as if French culture, having created the positivist image of the logical scientist ruled by absolute laws of nature as revealed in his laboratory, began to find this image too dogmatic and threatening. In many plays staged from 1900 to 1910, a central character is the doctor–scientist who is shown to have a human side. In these plays, the exacting man of science finds his values and ideals drawn from his scientific world view challenged by his own human fallacies. Usually the challenge has its source in avarice, jealously or sexual desire.

The antithesis of the scientific man and the sexual man is a strong and fascinating undercurrent of social theatre. The play, *L'Instinct*, by Kiestemaekers (1905) has as its central characters two physician–brothers. Dr Jean Bernou has a long string of titles, he is the archetype 'grand savant' and a great surgeon. Dr André Bernou is the humble private practitioner. Jean, the surgeon, discovers that his wife has been having an affair with one of his medical students. He is enraged with jealousy and goes to intercept a rendezvous of the lovers and kill the young man. The student tries to flee, falls, and injures himself gravely. Only the great surgeon can save him, but Jean refuses to operate. The day is saved by the brother, the humble Dr André, who arrives in time to give Jean a lecture on his professional duties. The duly chastised surgeon proceeds with the surgery, saves the young student's life, and emerges with a greater and more humble recognition of his own fallacies and duties. The play is full of other medical–social themes: a sub-plot, for example, deals with the neurasthenia of Jean's wife.[28]

A similar theme is found in *La Femme passa* by Romain Coolus, staged in 1910. Here a young physician–scientist is tormented by his attraction for a coquette. The pull of his desires contradicts his image of himself as a dispassionate scientist and threatens to interfere with his career plans and his scientific values. But he survives the threat, escapes her clutches, and emerges, like Bernou, with a greater appreciation of his humanness and his need to recognize his sensual self. Implicit in these works is the notion that the doctor must recognize his own humanity, as revealed through his sexuality, so that he will be able accept and attend to the humanity of his patients.[29]

The medical community itself was well aware of the cultural attitudes, fears and hopes illustrated by these various images of medical practice. Physicians working to promote private practice within the various professional movements of the era sought concertedly to harness the positive and distance themselves from the negative. This meant putting cultural space between themselves, the private practitioners and the medical savants. The records of the three Congrès des praticiens held in 1907, 1910 and 1914, show this rather clearly.[30] This was the great age of medical congresses, and scarcely a year went by that several national or international congresses were not held within the borders of France. But the Congrès des praticiens were notable for dealing with purely professional issues. The Union of Medical Syndicates still held its own annual membership meetings, but the Congrès des praticiens included practitioners who were not members of the Union movement, as well as dissidents of that movement. Many practitioners felt that the Union of Syndicates, once the leading force in professional issues, had become too establishment-oriented. So these congresses of private practitioners are excellent evidence for the motives and goals of that group.

The primary goal of these congresses was to promote private practice and push the state to enshrine private practice as the mechanism for applying a variety of public and semi-public medical welfare and public health programmes. Consonant with this goal, the Congresses dealt also with the issue of experimentation, condemning this practice and encouraging the view that only a few of the 'savants' and not the ordinary practitioners were involved. The castigation of scientist–practitioners and their disposition to experiment on their patients was a well-established theme in the Union's political discourse. Since 1900, Dr Diverneresse of the Union had been giving lectures on this topic at the *Université populaire,* where he warned workers that if they entered the hospital they would be subject to the experiments of the savants as well as providing practice material for interns.[31] Even earlier than this, in *Le Médecin,* published in 1897, J. M Guardia had warned his fellow physicians that they should distance themselves from the hospitals and other programmes under the Public Assistance Administration because of the association of that bureaucracy with various abuses of the poor, including medical experimentation.[32]

The 1907 Congrès des Praticiens also condemned the educational establishment, the heartland of the savants, for its laxity in reforming medical education to correspond to the modern needs of the *omnipraticien.* Papers presented at the congress cited in particular the need for better training in paediatrics and obstetrics.[33] Critics argued that although these fields were included in clinical training, they were absent in lectures and, most importantly, in examinations. Therefore many students could and did skip them altogether. Only the externs and interns could gain experience in these areas of medical practice. Private practitioners openly admitted at the congresses and elsewhere that typically the first childbirth they witnessed was the first one they were called in to attend.[34]

Treating the whole family demanded, of course, that obstetrics, gynaecology, and paediatrics remain within the purview of the private practitioner rather than becoming the domain of the specialist. For family practice to flourish, the physician had to prove to an often wary clientele that he did indeed know something about the care of women and children. Practitioners' concerns about obstetrics and gynaecology reflected the growing rhetoric in the profession that private practice could be saved by orienting it around the family's medical needs. In 1926, in a preface to a guide for private practitioners, Dr Jean Noir, a leader of the Union movement and editor of *Le Concours médical,* called for better preparation both in paediatrics and *puériculture:*

> Today the doctor must have a serious notion of paediatrics.... If the doctor possesses the art to really know how to examine the child with assurance and with precise indications for the treatment and nutrition of the child, his reputation is made, he has conquered the confidence of the mother and has become the oracle of the family.[35]

A further reflection of professional desires to incorporate paediatrics into general practice is evident from the many guides for the *omnipraticien* published in the early twentieth century.[36] These guides functioned as a ready reference for the private practitioner and contained well-organized advice and diagnostic and therapeutic information for the physician to use with a general family-oriented clientele. These guides are also useful in tracing the incursion of hereditarian ideology into medical thinking and practice.

The guides for general practitioners show that by 1900 hereditarian ideas were deeply embedded in the discourse about a number of diseases which were politically and socially important. In particular, hereditarian thinking was pervasive in paediatrics, and this influence lasted well into the mid-twentieth century.[37]

The Lamarckian influence on French Social Darwinism, that is the notion that the acquired flaws of one generation, such as alcoholism and syphilis, could doom subsequent generations, is well known. This notion had a profound impact on the medical understanding of certain diseases and symptoms. As Linda Clark has demonstrated, physicians were prominently interested and involved in the earliest studies of Darwin in France and with the development of the ideology of *transformisme.*[38] For example, the eminent physiologist and educator, Charles Richet, pioneered efforts to put evolutionist ideology in French school texts. A colleague of his at the Paris Faculty, Dr Jean-Louis de Lanessan, was an early producer of texts on Lamarckian evolutionism. The Société d'anthropologie was founded by physician Paul Broca in concert with a group of physicians from the Paris Faculty and hospitals. Subsequently, physicians figured prominently in the publications of the anthropological movement: *Revue d'anthropologie* and later, *l'Anthropologie* and *Revue anthropologique*. When the Society of Eugenics was formed in 1912, two of the most important physicians of the era were prominent among its leaders. Adolphe Pinard, professor at the Paris Faculty and pioneer in paediatrics and *puériculture*, was a vice-president, as was Louis Landouzy, the Dean of the Paris Faculty. Clark reports that of the original 104 members of the Société, 61 were doctors; the society's meetings were held at the Faculty of Medicine.[39]

Some diseases, and syphilis is the best example, were thought of as the *cause* of a general chain of degenerative inheritance with the possibility of a variety of different clinical manifestations, implying a connection between heredity and infection.[40] Physicians still believed that even cured syphilitics had acquired defects in their heredity which they could then pass along, rendering their children prone to conditions such as rickets and neurasthenia. According to contemporary notions of syphilis, these observations cannot be explained simply as simply misunderstandings of congenital syphilis. Physicians saw the complex in children whose mothers had no apparent infection; they blamed a syphilitic heredity for a wide variety of conditions developing as the child matured; and they believed the origins of the complex could be traced back several generations. Some paediatric experts believed syphilis caused a cluster of hereditary defects. In a prominent 1926 paediatric guide, Blechmann described a 'syphilitic heredity' which, he felt, could produce children with low intelligence, scrofula and cravings for sugar. Blechmann told physicians that if an infant was convulsive, or a young child underweight, they could suspect syphilis in one of the grandfathers.[41] In another guide of the era, U. Dubois' *Le bon médecin de la famille*, the author argued that rickets was the result principally of 'lymphatic' inheritance including scrofula and syphilis in the ancestors.[42]

The belief in the so-called syphilitic heredity prevailed, even though Treponema pallidum was identified as the causal agent of syphilis in 1905 by Schaudin and Hoffman and even though, long before that, for centuries in fact, syphilis had been regarded as a contagious disease. According to the notion of syphilitic heredity, the acquired infection resulted in permanent damage to the family lineage. The explicit connection between microbes and acquired hereditary weaknesses was the subject of several commentaries and ongoing laboratory investigations.[43] The connection between microbes and heredity was also a subject for study within the Société d'anthropologie.

Other diseases were viewed as part of a nexus of diseases afflicting a family with particular heredity defects.[44] This was true of the catch-all diagnosis, neurasthenia, also viewed as a kind of 'red flag' for a number of mental and physical disorders which might plague generations of a family. Cancer was implicated in a wide range of heredity weaknesses. However, whereas syphilis was seen as *causing* hereditary defects, cancer was more commonly viewed as indicative of the existence of pre-existing defects. Blechmann advised, for example, that in a young girl with symptoms including obesity, lethargy and constipation, the physician should suspect 'cancerous antecedents'.[45] Cancer is possibly the most interesting disease through which to study the meeting of microbes and hereditarian ideology, for medical thought held that while cancer was principally hereditary, it could also be microbial in origin.

A variety of so-called nervous disorders, from the ubiquitous and vague neurasthenia to more specific asthma were also seen as results, causes and indicators of hereditary flaws. Dubois pointed out, for example, that asthma was part of a particular hereditary predisposition to certain diseases in which the ancestors' rheumatism or diabetes became asthma in the next generations.[46]

In medical practice, hereditarian dogma reinforced the ideal that medicine was best practised on the basis of a long-term relationship between a single physician and a family. This notion was heavily promoted by physicians, both to the public and among themselves. In the professional guides, successful private practitioners advised young doctors how to gather a steady clientele of loyal families. Dr Frumusan, the author of *Réflexion d'un médecin,* in 1923, claimed that the doctor was most valuable to the family when he possessed at least 'three generations ... of previous facts about the family pathology'.[47] In an earlier advice book, written before the war, Dr Jean remarked that family pathology was the major business of the doctor, whose ... 'deep knowledge will enable him to foresee, advise and perhaps prevent'.[48]

Hereditarian ideology not only pushed the family to the forefront, but also produced deep sources of discord between the physician and his patients. Physicians were quite aware that family heredity was a sensitive topic and realized that great delicacy was required in addressing it. Frumusan told his young colleagues, 'Don't brutally scream out, "well, you have syphilis", this is the best way to lose clients ... an atmosphere of honour and discretion will create a loyal clientele who will not change their doctor like they change their shirts.'[49]

It has been widely noted in the literature that the family physician of the *fin-de-siècle* played a protective and paternalistic role.[50] As one physician wrote, 'The doctor must be considered to be in a special position ... he oversees the confidences and special interests of the family ... his mission entails special duties and delicate tasks, it imposes heavy responsibilities ... the doctor should take the family's anxieties as his own....'[51] Certainly such a posture *vis-à-vis* the family, and women in particular, had oppressive effects. However it is important also to note that this tutelary role, however much it reflected Victorian notions of gender and class hierarchy, was also intrinsically bound up with the medical concepts and social concerns of the era. The doctor's mission was not just to diagnose and cure disease, but to foresee the possible future medical problems of the family members based upon his knowledge of their heredity, and then to do whatever possible to help them or protect them from the awful truth.[52]

The doctor's involvement with family hereditary flaws and the ensuing crises, was a prevalent dramatic theme in contemporary literature. Zola's treatment of the general theme was only the beginning of literary interest in the drama of family, heredity, and degeneracy. Theatre in particular, as part of a vogue of social realism, seized upon this issue. For example, Alphonse Daudet, the liberal pro-medical father of the reactionary Léon, produced several plays and a novel with hereditarian themes. These plays were not very successful, however, since his work was seen as too brutal and realistic, in other words, too fatalistic and pessimistic.[53]

The most famous author of this genre was Eugène Brieux who gave the realist theatre a new beginning. Basically his works had stronger plots than Alphonse Daudet's, and were tied up with neat moral lessons. In *l'Evasion* (1903), the main character is a stereotype of the eminent Parisian savant. Dr Betry is a professor at the Faculty and *chef de clinique*. Betry has a stepson and a niece, both of whom he sees as doomed by heredity. The stepson's father was neurasthenic, the niece's mother was a notorious woman of Parisian high society, and he assumes she had syphilis because of her numerous affairs. Betry prohibits both from marriage and thus ruins their lives. Brieux deals harshly with such action. He does not deny the reality of hereditary diseases, but he argues that physicians need to temper such dogma with some kindness and practical wisdom.

In most of Brieux's other plays, the physician is a central character. The most famous of all his social-medical fiction, which was translated and performed in North America and most of Western Europe, is *Les Avariés* or *Damaged Goods*.[54] The drama was staged in Paris in 1901, immediately closed by the censors, then performed before audiences in Liège and Brussels in 1902, and finally permitted in Paris in 1905. It dealt with a dramatic situation which fascinated contemporary audiences. The dilemma begins when a young man who has been treated for syphilis and seems to be cured, becomes engaged. His family physician, who has overseen his treatment, is faced with an ethical dilemma. He is entrusted with the family secrets and with the responsibility of protecting and promoting the family's interests. What then of his responsibility to protect or forewarn the innocent and unaware fiancée? In Brieux's play, the doctor tries desperately to stop the marriage but does not forewarn the fiancée's family, and the consequences are disastrous. The couple produces three malformed stillborn children, and the young wife goes mad. Brieux's main point was not to disapprove the doctor's behaviour; in fact, in a careful rendering of the play, the physician emerges as the hero. Brieux was arguing not for more aggressive medical action, but for a more honest and open social attitude toward the disease so that medicine might more easily eradicate it. It is clear from a long prologue that Brieux's theme was that cultural shame and secrecy blocked medical efforts to eliminate venereal diseases. This prologue, written in consultation with some of France's leading physician–experts on syphilis, however, was rarely presented in productions of *Damaged Goods*.[55]

The public did not understand Brieux's intended message. Rather the play helped to contribute to a growing national obsession with syphilis and to the belief that syphilis and other venereal diseases were creating a whole generation of children with scarred heredities. It also helped fuel an already intense debate over the duty of the physician to protect family secrets.

In 1909, Jacques Terni's play, *Les Baillonnées*, presented another fascinating drama of hereditary disease involving a woman doctor as the central character. Dr Certel and her former lover, a Russian artist, Serge, have had a child who is severely deformed by hydrocephalus. Accepting the common medical view of her age on the biology of women, Dr Certel attributes her child's deformity to the fact that she was overtaxing her nature by working in a non-feminine domain.

Serge becomes engaged to her niece, and subsequently Serge's father visits Paris from St Petersburg and seeks out Dr Certel's medical advice. The father, a Russian count, proves to be an old reprobate, an alcoholic and former opium user, and the veteran of many sexual orgies. He reveals to Dr Certel that his son, Serge, is a closet melancholic who suffered from suicidal impulses in his youth. Thus Dr Certel learns the true cause of her child's deformity, the hereditary flaws in Serge created by the father's debauchery. She rushes to warn her niece away from a disastrous liaison which will surely result in more flawed children. Dr Certel's conflicting duties as a physician and as an aunt are emphasized, for according to the strictest interpretation of medical ethics, she should not be using her medical knowledge to interfere in the engagement.[56]

As this popular literature shows, the connection of heredity and family created personal and professional dilemmas for doctors. Even the most astute and kindliest physician was likely to become entangled in the moral troubles created by it. But the family was a powerful draw for medicine. As hereditarian notions permeated general and medical culture, the family became the practitioner's central object. As heredity became seen as a powerful influence on the body and a determining factor in many diseases, so too it became imperative that the physician, examining and diagnosing his individual patient, could do so effectively only in the context of the family's medical past. Heredity was the record of the family's past history and the predictor of its future, as indispensable in medical diagnosis as the bacteriological laboratory. Moreover, the emphasis on family involved both the privatization and personalization of medicine and was a successful antidote to the growing fear of medicine becoming overly scientific, or impersonal and mechanical. Looking at the rhetoric of physicians who led the orientation toward the family, we can see that they echoed the fears of laymen that medicine was becoming too laboratory- and experimentally-oriented. The physician commentators thus absorbed and reflected the culturally expressed fears over uncontrolled experimentation with drugs, inoculations and X-rays. Physicians' discourse associated the scientific with the institutional and bureaucratic and thus warned patients to avoid institutional, scientific and bureaucrat care, guiding them instead into the the hands of private, family-oriented practitioners. Nonetheless, the relationship of patients and family practitioners remained highly problematic as the ambivalent motifs of the physician in the literature attests.

Notes

1. Presented at the Conference on 'Researchers and Practitioners: Aspects of French Medical Culture in the Eighteenth and Nineteenth Centuries', Virginia Technological Institute and State University, Blacksburg Virginia, 21 April, 1990.

2. Among the many sources of this discourse within the profession, a discussion of which is outside the boundaries of this paper, are the publications of the Union movement, including journals, newsletters and monographs, biographies and autobiographies of physicians, and the Congrès des praticiens. See: Martha L. Hildreth, *Doctors, Bureaucrats and Public Health in France, 1888–1902*, (New York: Garland, 1987), 36–106.

3. Michel Foucault, *The Birth of the Clinic: an archaeology of medical perception*, trans. A. M. Sheridan Smith, (New York: Pantheon, 1973).

4. Karen Offen, 'Depopulation, Nationalism and Feminism in Fin-de-Siècle France', *American Historical Review* (1984). Francis Ronsin, *La Grève des ventres: propagande néo-malthusienne et basse de la natalité en France* (Paris 1978); Robert Wheaton and T. K. Hareven, (eds), *Family and Sexuality in French History* (Philadelphia, 1980); Jean Meyer, 'La limitation des naissances en France à l'époque moderne, *Histoire sociale* 10 (1977); Angus McLaren, *Sexuality and Social Order: The Debate over the Fertility of Women and Workers in France, 1770–1920* (New York: Holmes & Meier, Inc., 1983); Colin Heywood, *Childhood in Nineteenth-Century France* (New York: Cambridge, 1988); Lee Shai Weissbach, *Child Labor Reform in Nineteenth-Century France: Assuring the Future Harvest*, (London: Louisiana State University Press, 1989).

5. Jacques Donzelot, *The Policing of Families*, trans. Robert Hurley, (New York: Pantheon books, 1979); Robert A. Nye, *Crime, Madness and Politics in Modern France, The Medical Concept of National Decline* (Princeton, N.J.: Princeton University Press, 1984); Yvonne Knibiehler & Catherine Fouquet *La Femme et les médecins: analyse historique* (Paris: Hachette, 1983); Ann La Berge, 'Medicalization and Moralization: The Crèches of Nineteenth-Century Paris', *Journal of Social History* 25 (1991), 65–87; Jane Ellen Crisler, 'Saving the Seed, the Scientific Preservation of Children in France During the Third Republic', Ph.D. Dissertation, University of Wisconsin 1984.

6. My understanding of medicine as socially constructed is drawn in part from Peter Wright and Andrew Treacher, (eds) in their introduction to: *The Problem of Medical Knowledge: Examining the Social Construction of Medicine:* (Edinburgh: Edinburgh University Press, 1982), 1–19; it also derives from my own reading of Foucault, especially *Archaeology of Knowledge*, trans. A. M. Sheridan Smith

(New York: Pantheon Books, 1972) and *The Birth of the Clinic* and of Mary Douglas, especially: *How Institutions Think* (Syracuse NY: Syracuse University Press, 1986).

7. On the concept of cultural institutions see: Mary Douglas, *How Institutions Think.*

8. Jacques Léonard has conceived of French medicine in the late nineteenth century as caught, or torn, between 'les savoirs et les pouvoirs', with the former considered as medical ideology and scientific discovery and the latter as the demands of government and state: Léonard, *La Médecine entre les savoirs et les pouvoirs: Histoire intellectuelle et politique de la médecine française au XIXe siècle,* (Paris: Aubier-Montaigne, 1981).

9. Some of the plays figuring in this analysis are: Henri Bataille, *Les Flambeaux, Petite Illustration* n. 3 [Porte Saint-Martin, 1912; François de Curel, *La Nouvelle Idole* (New York: The Century Company, 1924) [Théâtre Antoine, 1899]; Jules Lemaitre, *Mariage Blanc,* (Paris: Calmann-Lévy, n.d.) [Comédie-Française 1891] also his *Révoltée,* (Paris: Calmann-Lévy, n.d.) [Odéon 1889]; Maurice Donnay, *Le Douloureuse* in *Editions pour toutes les pièces de Donnay* (Paris: Charpentier-Fasquelle, n.d.) [Vaudeville, 1897) and his *L'Eclaireuses* in *Editions pour toutes les pièces de Donnay* (Paris: Charpentier-Fasquelle, n.d.) [Comédie Marigny, 1913]; Lavedan, *Le Marquis de Priola,* (Paris: Flammarion, n.d.) [Comédie-Française 1902] and his *Le Duel,* (Paris: Ollendorff, n.d.) [Comédie-Française, 1905];Pierre Wolff, *Les Marionettes,* (Paris: Librairie théâtrale, 1919) [Comédie-Française, 1910]; Georges Feydeau, *La Dame de Chez Maxim, La Petite Illustration* 1919, 42–74; Sacha Guitry, *Pasteur, La Petite Illustration* 1919, 1–20; Paul Adam *Les Mouettes, La Petite Illustration* 1906/7 1–32; Kistemaeckers, *L'Instinct,* (Paris: Charpentier, 1929) [Théâtre Molière, 1905]; Brieux, *L'Evasion,* (Paris: Stock, 1902) [Comédie-Française, 1896] and his *Les Avariés* (Paris: Stock, 1902) [first staged 1902, then banned]; Romain Coolus, *Une Femme Passa, Illustration Théâtrale* 7 [Théâtre de la Renaissance, 1910). For the history of the social–realist theatre and the role of the Théâtre Libre of André Antoine see: Clifford Bissell, *Les conventions du théâtre bourgeois contemporain en France, 1887–1914* (Paris: Presses universitaires de France, 1930); Barrett H. Clark, *Contemporary French Dramatists* (Cincinnati: Stewart & Kidd, 1915); Pierre de Barcourt and J. W. Cunliffe, *French Literature During the Last Half-Century* (New York: MacMillan, 1923).

10. The important transformation of western medicine towards a laboratory as opposed to bedside orientation of practice is discussed in Russell Maulitz, 'Physician versus Bacteriologist', in Morris Vogel and Charles E. Rosenberg, (eds), *The Therapeutic Revolution: Essays in the Social History of American Medicine* (Philadelphia: University of Pennsylvania Press, 1979), A. McGehee Harvey, *Science*

at the Bedside: Clinical Research in American Medicine, 1905–1945* (Baltimore: Johns Hopkins University Press, 1981) and Mark Altschule, *Essays on the Rise and Decline of Bedside Medicine*, (Bangor, PA: Lea & Febiger, 1989).

11. For a general discussion of therapies see: Hildreth, 'The Influenza Epidemic of 1918–1919 in France: Contemporary Concepts of Aetiology, Therapy, and Prevention, *Social History of Medicine* 4 (1991), 277–94.

12. William Coleman makes this point implicitly in his *Biology in the Nineteenth Century, problems of form, function and transformation* (New York: Cambridge University Press, 1977).

13. Two excellent general discussions of social Darwinism and eugenics in France are: Linda Clark, *Social Darwinism in France* (Birmingham, Alabama: University of Alabama Press, 1984) and William H. Schneider, *Quality and quantity: the quest for biological regeneration in twentieth-century France* (New York: Cambridge University Press, 1990). For genetics in French science and medicine see: Richard M. Burian, Jean Gayon & Doris Zallen, 'The Singular Fate of Genetics in the History of French Biology, 1900–1940' *Journal of the History of Biology* 21 (Fall 1988), 357–402. A general history of hereditarian concepts is found in: Peter J. Bowler, *The Mendelian Revolution: The Emergence of Hereditarian Concepts in Modern Science and Society* (Baltimore, MD: Johns Hopkins University Press, 1989).

14. On the meaning of the natural world in scientific discourse see Wright and Treacher, *The Problem of Medical Knowledge*.

15. J. M. Guardia, *Le Médecin* (Paris: Pedone, 1897), 9; Anon., 'Principes de déontologie', *Le Sud Médical* 51 (1920), 3; and Anon. 'Pour les médecins des campagnes', *Bulletin officiel de l'Union des syndicats médicaux de France* (5 October, 1902), 361.

16. For the medical politics of the era, see Hildreth, *Doctors, Bureaucrats and Public Health in France* and 'Medical Rivalries and Medical Politics in France: The Physicians' Union Movement and the Medical Assistance Law of 1893', *Journal of the History of Medicine and Allied Sciences* 42 (1987), 5–29.

17. Louis-Henri Dejust, *Le médecin dans le théâtre contemporain*, thèse pour le Doctorat en médecine, Faculté de médecine de Paris, (Paris: Ollier-Henry, 1910), 8.

18. Toby Gelfand, 'Medical Nemesis, Paris, 1894: Léon Daudet's *Les Morticoles*', *Bulletin of the History of Medicine* 60 (1983), 155–76.

19. Charles Soller and Louis Gastine, *Défends ta peau contre ton médecin* (Paris: J. Rocques, 1907).

20. *Ibid.*

21. Soller & Gastine, *Défends ta peau*, 42–56.

22. Sacha Guitry's popular play *Pasteur* is an example of the continued idealization of this hero–scientist. Pasteur was seen as the kind benefactor who saved the nation from rabies as well as the dedicated

scientist; people seem to have forgotten that he was not a physician.

23. De Just, *Le Médecin*, 26–34.

24. Jacques Descoust, *La Médecine au théâtre dans les temps modernes*, thèse Doctorat en médecine, Faculté de Médecine de Paris, 1905, 99.

25. An example of the juxtaposition of these two medical archetypes is found in Brieux's *l'Evasion*.

26. For the archetype humanistic, dedicated doctor see: Brieux's *l'Evasion*, Kistemaeckers, *L'Instinct*, and Etienne Rey, *La Belle Aventure*, [first staged Théâtre du Vaudeville 1912] as described in J. Barfield Adams, 'Some Doctors in Recent French Plays', *Edinburgh Review* (1913), 46–50.

27. Soller & Gastine, *Défends ta peau*, 59.

28. De Just, *Le Médecin*, 36–8.

29. Another doctor done in by his sexuality is found in Bataille's *Les Flambeaux*.

30. *Congrès des praticiens* [first] 1907 3 vols (Paris: Maloine, 1907) and *Congrès des praticiens* [third] 1910 (Paris: Maloine, 1910).

31. Charles Diverneresse, *Les Lacunes de la loi sur les accidents du travail* (Paris: Maloine, 1903), 40–3.

32. J. M Guardia, *Le Médecin* (Paris, N. Pedone: 1897), 10.

33. Professor Forgue, 'Le Stage médical', *Le Concours médical* 26 (1904), 680–61; Dr Dumas (de Lédignan), *Le Concours médical* 26 (1904), 648–50.

34. Jules Cyr, *Scènes de la vie médicale* (Paris: Baillière, 1888), 1–13.

35. Dr Jean Noir, preface to Germain Blechmann, *Les Feuillets du Pédiatrie* (Paris: Octave Doin, 1926).

36. In addition to Blechmann, *Les Feuillets*, see: Emile Sergent, L. Ribadeau-Dumas, L. Babonneix, (eds), *Traité de pathologie médicale thérapeutique appliquée* 25 vols, Vol.II: *Pédiatrie* (Paris: Maloine, 1923), 77–95, 379–84, 412–20, 484–93; Jules Comby, *Deux cents consultations médicales pour les maladies des enfants* (Paris: Masson, 1919), 42–5, 72–7, 84–7, 184–7, 200–3, 215–21, 247–9; and Henri Lambert *La pratique médical rurale. Guide de l'omnipraticien*, introduction by Charles Fiessinger (Paris:L A. Maloine, 1924).

37. See for examples: Apert, 'Maladies familiales et héréditaires', Antoine Marfan, (ed.),*Pédiatrie: traité de pathologie médicale et de thérapeutique appliquées*, 3 vols, Vol. II (Paris: Flammarion, 1923). See also in Marfan, *Pédiatrie* Vol. II, 259–61, 379–83, 423–4, 432–3, 725–6; Néhama Braoudé, 'Etude de l'obésité chez les enfants', *Archives de Médecine des enfants* 4 (1901), 696–704; M. R. Morichau-Beauchant, 'Diagnostic des anémies de la première enfance', *Revue mensuelle de gynécologie et de pédiatrie* 1–2 (1906–07), 305–14.

38. Linda Clark, *Social Darwinism in France*. Clark points out that the term 'Darwinism' is a little misleading when applied to hereditarian thought in France, where it was imbued with a heavy dose of

Lamarckianism and where the term most often used was 'transformisme' or less often, 'évolutionnisme'. 'Transformisme' stressed the interaction of the hereditary matter and the environment.

39. Clark, *Social Darwinism in France*, 52–71. Likewise Schneider reports that 51.9% of the early twentieth-century eugenicists in France were physicians: *Quality and Quantity*, 93.

40. For the connections between syphilis and various diseases and symptoms in children see: M. P. F. Armand-Delille, 'Hérédo-Syphilis mongolisme et malformations cardiaques congénitales chez un nourrisson', *Bulletins de la société de pédiatrie de Paris* 10 (1908), 144–6; Albert Mouchet and Jean Rouget 'Arthropathie héréditaire des tibias: arthrites héredosyphilitique' and *ibid.*, 12 (1910), 225; Ribadeau-Dumas et Paul Camus, 'Ostéo-arthrites purulentes et héredosyphilis du nourrisson', *ibid.*, 10 (1908), 223–6; D. E. Gaujoux, 'Hérédo-syphilis à manifestations viscéreles multiples, en particulier avec lésions des surrénales et hypertrophie chez un nourrisson né d'une mère saine en apparence et allaité', *ibid.*, 11 (1909), 282–91; M. Barbier, 'A propos du traitement de l'hérédo-syphilis', *ibid.*, 10 (1921), 137–9; Babonneix, Blum and Sémelaigne, 'Mongolisme infantile-hérédo-syphilis probable', *ibid.*, 20 (1922), 85–101; M. Lance, 'Un cas d'ostéo-arthrite hérédo-syphilitique grave...' *ibid.*, 20 (1922), 143–7 'Péhu, 'La Syphilis infantile', *Revue française de pédiatrie* 1 (1926), 497–517; Péhu, 'La syphilis congénitale des os longs dans la première enfance', *ibid.*, 1 (1925), 261–89. Secondary works on syphilis in France include: Roger L. Williams, *The Horror of Life* (Chicago: University of Chicago Press, 1980); Claude Quétel, *History of Syphilis*, trans. Judith Barddock and Brian Pike (Baltimore: The Johns Hopkins University Press, 1990) and Jill Harsin, 'Syphilis, Wives & Physicians: Medical Ethics and the Family in Late Nineteenth-Century France', *French Historical Studies* 16 (1989). Harsin treats some of the same themes discussed in this article.

41. Germain Blechmann, *Les Feuillets*.

42. U. Dubois, *Le Bon médecin de la Famille, Traité de médecine usuelle* (Lamarche-sur-Saône: J. Martin, 1893).

43. Charrin, Delmarre & Mossu, 'Sur la transmission expérimentale des tares morbides acquises' as discussed in Charles Valentino, *Le Secret professionnel en Médecine, sa valeur sociale*, (Paris: C. Naud, 1903).

44. For examples see: P. Nobécourt, *Les syndromes endocriniens* (Paris: Flammarion, 1923) 47–9, 90–140, 164–96, 269–300 and Georges Schreiber, 'Deux cas d'hérédo-sydtrophie tuberculeuse d'origine paternelle', *Bulletins de la Société de Pédiatrie de Paris* 20 (1922), 359–76.

45. Blechmann, *Les Feuillets*.

46. Dubois, *Le Bon Médecin*, 285.

47. Frumusan, *Réflexions d'un médecin*, 6.

48. Jean, *Confidences d'un médecin de campagne* (Paris: Octave Doin, 1913), 45.

49. Frumusan, *Réflexions d'un médecin*, 66.

50. Knibiehler & Fouquet, *La Femme et les médecins*.

51. J. Vincent (d'Armentières), *Le Médecin, son rôle dans la Famille et la Société* (Paris: Beauchesne, 1911), 37, 40–1.

52. Frumusan, *Réflexions d'un Médecin*, 63–4.

53. Descoust, *La Médecine au Théâtre*, 120–3; Clark, *Social Darwinism in France*, 108–9. Daudet's works deal mostly with syphilis, with which he himself was afflicted. It is interesting that it is Daudet who is credited with originating the notion that physicians were 'les derniers prêtres'.

54. Schneider, *Quality and Quantity*, 52.

55. Decoust, *La Médecine au Théâtre*, 121.

56. Dejust, *Le Médecin*, 59–60.

6

The Uses of Male Hysteria:
Medical and Literary Discourse in
Nineteenth-Century France

Jan Goldstein

In the winter of 1867, Gustave Flaubert wrote to his good friend George Sand that he continued 'to fiddle with' (*tripoter*) his current novel while living in complete solitude in the country. He passed entire weeks, he said, without exchanging a word with another human being and could perhaps best be compared to an anchorite whose 'nights are black as ink' and who was 'surrounded by a silence like that of the desert'. In such an environment, he went on,

> the sensibility becomes inordinately exalted. I experience flutterings of the heart for no reason at all – an understandable thing, moreover, in an old hysteric like me. For I maintain that men can be hysterics just like women, and that I am one.... I have recognized all my symptoms: the ball (rising in the throat), the (sensation of the) nail in the back of the skull.[1]

Some years later, in another letter to Sand, he mentioned with a hint of satisfaction that this self-diagnosis had been confirmed, if partially in jest, by a noted Paris medical authority. In making plans to vacation in the mountains of Switzerland, Flaubert was, he said, 'obeying the advice of Dr Hardy,[2] who calls me "an hysterical woman" – a phrase that I find profound'. So taken was Flaubert with this remark that he repeated it in another letter written the same day: 'Dr Hardy ... calls me an hysterical old woman. "Doctor", I tell him, "you are perfectly right." '[3]

Flaubert's references to himself as hysterical, of which several more instances could be cited, raise the issue of the gender of hysteria in the nineteenth century. Clearly these references depend for their arresting force upon the audience's automatic association of hysteria with women, an association indelibly imprinted on the term by its ancient Greek etymology ('uterus') and its long, subsequent social development. But at the same time Flaubert's self-depictions violate and sever the association they assume. They suggest that if nineteenth-century hysteria was a conceptual space for the conventional, stereotypical definition of femininity, it was also, by that same token, potentially a conceptual space for the subversion of gender stereotypes. Through partaking of the pathological condition 'hysteria', the man Flaubert might also lay claim to the attributes of femininity it had come to epitomize – here, nervous hypersensitivity, vulnerability, self-absorption – and hence implicitly achieve something of the status of androgyny. Applied by men to women, and most typically by male doctors to their female patients, the category 'hysteria' was inevitably bound up in relations of power and generally served a stigmatizing, repressive function. But applied by a man to himself, that same category might disclose radical possibilities.

The purpose of this essay is to explore what might be called a contrapuntal tendency in the nineteenth-century French discourse about hysteria: the manner in which hysteria was used to destabilize the very gender definitions it had helped, and was still helping, to put into place. This contrapuntal tendency made itself heard only occasionally. It derived from the particular relationship between literary and medical discourse in nineteenth-century France, which ensured that hysteria would have a career in each discourse and, moreover, that these two careers would diverge. Hence, before proceeding further, we need to consider that literary–medical relationship and sketch it in broad outline.

We can approach it, or at least one side of it, by observing that Flaubert's flexible and creative manipulation of the category 'hysteria' seems to have depended on his familiarity with technical discussions of the disease. When he announced to Sand that he was a male hysteric in 1867, he bolstered that assertion by citing the medical authorities: 'When I was writing *Salammbô*, I read "the best authors" on that subject, and I recognized all my symptoms.'[4] In fact, Flaubert's researches into the medical literature on psychopathology long antedated the period at the end of the 1850s when he began *Salammbô*. His first 'psycho-medical studies', as he called them, and which he described as having 'so much beguiled' him, accompanied his work on *The Temptation of Saint Anthony* in the latter half of the 1840s; reminiscing on these studies, he could exclaim appreciatively, 'There are treasures to be discovered in that material.'[5]

We know very little about what, exactly, Flaubert read on hysteria at any point in his life, but that he had some direct exposure to the concept of male hysteria, and was aware of its controversial status in the medical community, seems probable. As part of his preparation for *Salammbô*, he consulted Dr Landouzy's *Traité complet de l'hystérie* (1846), a hefty tome that devotes a few pages to a sceptical and ultimately inconclusive review of the evidence for male hysteria offered by other physicians. Flaubert's careful, highly selective notes on Landouzy omit, however, any reference to this section of the text.[6] Flaubert was also in the habit of consulting the vast, multi-volume medical dictionaries that the French produced during the nineteenth century to codify medical knowledge. Replying to Sainte-Beuve's review of *Salammbô*, for example, he protested that the ointment containing 'bitches' milk' that the character Hanno rubs on his diseased skin was 'not a "joke", but is *still* used as a remedy for leprosy; see the *Dictionnaire des sciences médicales*, article 'Leprosy." [7] Hence it is likely that Flaubert read the 1824 article on hysteria in the *Dictionnaire de médecine*, which argues strongly for the existence (though rarity) of hysteria in men.[8]

But whether or not he actually encountered the hypothesis of male hysteria in print, the catalogue of hysterical symptoms that he learned from other technical sources enabled him to interpret as hysterical the disturbing bodily phenomena he experienced firsthand. He practically acknowledged this as his *modus operandi* in a letter of 1859. 'Every time you reflect on yourself, you find yourself sick; it is an axiom, be convinced of it! People beginning to study medicine discover every infirmity in themselves.... I have been through it and can say something about it.'[9]

Flaubert's close relationship with medical knowledge was typical of that of many of his confrères. For reasons that have not yet been fully investigated, the men who became the canonical masters of the nineteenth-century French novel were all unusually well attuned to developments in medical science, especially those in the emergent specialty of psychiatry. Thus Stendhal could be found in the library of the Paris Faculty of Medicine in 1805 reading the recently published treatise on insanity by Dr Philippe Pinel, the founding father of French psychiatry; he subsequently attempted to obtain the book for his personal collection.[10] Honoré de Balzac, who depicted himself as the taxonomist of the social world, read the medical literature voraciously, and his familiarity with the work of the Paris psychiatrist Etienne-Jean Georget, the chief popularizer of the new disease entity of monomania, led to a rather substantial population of monomaniacs among the characters of *La Comédie humaine*.[11] Flaubert's well-documented taste for medical literature seems to have stemmed from two biographical facts: he was the son of a provincial doctor, even growing up in a family apartment within the Rouen city hospital; and from early adulthood on, he was the intermittent victim of convulsive nervous seizures to which no clear diagnostic label could be affixed.[12] Emile Zola learned many of the principles of heredity he subsequently put to use in constructing the Rougon-Macquart series from a treatise by the psychiatrist Prosper Lucas.[13] Finally, Marcel Proust shared Flaubert's background as the son of a physician. In fact, the admissions registers of the Salpêtrière contain diagnoses of hystero-epilepsy signed by Dr Adrien Proust, sometimes on the same page as similar diagnoses under the signature of Dr Jean-Martin Charcot.[14]

Literary discourse and medical discourse intersected repeatedly in France during the nineteenth century, but it is striking that, at the points of intersection, the traffic went one way only. If nineteenth-century French novelists sought in medical texts superior insight into the human psyche, or scientific legitimation of their native intuitions, or a borrowed voice of authority with which to address the reading public, nineteenth-century French psychiatrists remained professionally uninterested in literary resources. One of the few psychiatric comments that I have found on the application of literary to psychiatric method condemns it outright, depicting the literary sensibility as a pitfall rather than a benefit to the psychiatric practitioner. In a discussion of styles of clinical observation in psychiatry, Dr Jean-Pierre Falret noted at mid-century that a highly distortive style resulted when the physician unwittingly imitated the novelist. Seeking to replace the chaos of nature with the order of art, such a physician ended up perceiving and representing each patient he encountered as a 'character' in La Bruyère's sense, a person governed by a single passion or idea. He remained unaware of all the disconfirming clinical evidence screened out for the sake of his artistry. This observational style based on literary models, Falret concluded disparagingly, belonged to the 'infancy' of the psychiatric specialty.[15]

In a formal treatise on hashish and insanity published in 1845, the psychiatrist Jacques-Joseph Moreau de Tours did, to be sure, quote a long account of the effects of smoking that drug written by Théophile Gautier (for whom Moreau had served as supplier). Moreau even initially expressed confidence about admitting the littérateur into the medical sanctum, noting that 'hashish could find no more worthy an interpreter than the poetic imagination of Monsieur Gautier'. But in his very next sentence, he seems to have been assailed by doubts – or by anticipated objections from his medical colleagues – about the propriety of using a literary source as scientific evidence. 'Is there any need to add', he asked defensively, 'that the brilliance of the style, and also perhaps a slight exaggeration in the language, should arouse no distrust about the truthfulness of this writer, who is, after all, only describing sensations already familiar to those who have some experience of hashish?'[16] In a very different context, the psychiatrist François Lélut revealed a quite similar belief in the incompatibility of literature and mental medicine. Bringing a collection of his own poetry before the public in 1840, he noted that its contents had been completed some 12 years before, when he was a young man in his mid-20s just embarking upon a psychiatric career. 'What prevented me from publishing it then was the necessity I felt of making a profession of the science of man, a profession whose seriousness admits of no frivolous diversion.'[17]

Towards the end of the century, as the psychiatric case study began to evolve into a long and complicated narrative form, a French psychiatrist might comment in passing that his account of a particular patient 'savoured of a novel'.[18] But no self-congratulation should be inferred from such a remark, or from the comparable remark of Pierre Janet that a full description of his patients would more nearly approximate 'a novel of manners and morals than it would a clinical observation'.[19] Even Freud, who would later break from the strictly scientific mode of nineteenth-century medicine and tout the ability of psychoanalysis to synthesize science and poetic insight, experienced obvious discomfort with the *Studies on Hysteria* that he produced in the early 1890s. 'Like other neuropathologists', he confessed in the middle of that work, 'I was trained to employ local diagnoses and electro-prognosis, and it still strikes me as strange that the case studies I write should read like short stories and that, as one might say, they lack the serious stamp of science.'[20]

For nineteenth-century psychiatrists, the 'serious stamp of science' entailed avoidance not only of literary modalities but also of subjective evidence. While empathy was a guiding principle of the pioneering psychiatric therapy called the moral treatment early in the century,[21] in matters of the classification and diagnosis of disease, objectivity and distance seem always to have been the unspoken rules. Even after the strict antinomies of mad and sane broke down in the latter part of the century, giving way to the intermediary zone of *demi-folie,* the psychiatrist was not supposed to recognize the 'diseased' aspects of the patient in himself.[22] A psychiatric diagnosis was, in the nineteenth-century, something that a doctor gave to the patient as an 'other'. Not until the advent of psychoanalysis would subjectivity be valorized as an appropriate instrument of medical-scientific investigation.

214

Thus nineteenth-century novelists such as Flaubert might be said to have had a larger repertory, a fuller range, than nineteenth-century psychiatrists. They absorbed and exploited medical knowledge, but even if they professed to emulate scientific objectivity – Flaubert's famous *impassibilité* – the free play of the imagination and the resources of subjective experience were still open to them. This difference between a capacious and a restricted discursive range is reflected in the difference between the literary and the medical handling of the hysteria concept, and especially the handling of the exceedingly 'delicate point' of male hysteria.[23] Whereas the medical classification of disease was an effort to fix, delimit and control disease cognitively, to establish the boundaries and norms that lent both precision and weight to the act of labelling some 'other', the literary interest in disease included as one of its components a fascination with this 'otherness', a tendency to recognize in it aspects of the self and to enlist it in the service of self-discovery. The first modality – objective and boundary-constructing – produced the dominant themes in the nineteenth-century discourse on hysteria; the second modality – premised on the first, but subjective and boundary-blurring – produced the occasional, subversive counterpoint to these same themes. In this essay, I take up each of these discourses in turn. I first explore the uses to which hysteria, and especially its male variety, was put by Flaubert and other nineteenth-century French writers, focusing on the way that diagnostic label could function as a metaphor for androgyny and hence as a challenge to prevailing gender norms. I then look at the far more circumscribed and culturally conservative role that male hysteria played within the psychiatric discourse of the same period.

The Hysteria of Literary Men

Let us turn first to Flaubert. His novels of the late 1850s and early 1860s, *Madame Bovary* and *Salammbô*, are in a sense suffused with hysteria, if one looks at the suggestive descriptions they contain and at the responses they elicited from contemporaries; yet the word *hysteria* never appears in them, or in any of Flaubert's formal literary corpus until his last novel, *Bouvard and Pécuchet*, published in 1880.[24] Even without the cue of a precise label, nineteenth-century readers readily identified the *mal* of Emma Bovary. One critic summed her up as 'that hysterical provincial, surfeited with pleasures (*jouissances*) and nonetheless always famished'.[25] The 1857 review of the novel by Charles Baudelaire saw in Emma the image of the 'hysterical poet' and asked rhetorically, 'Why could hysteria, this physiological mystery, not serve as the central subject, the true foundation, of a literary work?'[26] Some two decades later an article in the *Revue des deux mondes* called Emma 'the most animated, the most authentic of all the hysterics whose stories have been told by novelists' and praised Flaubert for describing her condition in a manner 'so precise and seductive that one does not know whether to admire more the talents of the artist or the science of the observer.'[27]

The case is similar though not as clear-cut with *Salammbô*, Flaubert's exotic novel of ancient Carthage that dismayed so many of its critics. The only explicit disease in *Salammbô* is the gruesome dermatosis that eats away at the body of the magistrate Hanno and seems intended to symbolize the rot and moral decay of Carthaginian society as a whole. But many contemporary reviewers regarded the novel as dominated by pathology – it inaugurated, one said sardonically, 'a new genre that I propose to call the *epileptic genre*'[28] – and they were quick to attribute mental pathology to both of the novel's main characters: Salammbô, a high-born virgin priestess of the cult of Tanit, the Carthaginian deity of love; and Mâtho, the Libyan mercenary 'of colossal stature' who falls in love with her.

The consensus was that Mâtho was frankly insane, 'seized by a kind of furious delirium at the sight and at the name of Salammbô',[29] according to one critic, and gone 'mad (*fou*) with wrath and pain' when Salammbô first disappears from view, according to another.[30] Salammbô, on the other hand, seemed to be suffering from a less flagrant pathology. The critics were struck by her dissociated states of consciousness and, extrapolating from the descriptions in Flaubert's text, they anticipated in uncanny fashion the central link between hysteria and hypnotic trance that Charcot would endeavour to establish two decades later. (Earlier in the nineteenth century, somnambulism enjoyed relatively minor status as a hysterical symptom.)[31] 'One does not know if she is awake or if she sleeps, if she is conscious of her acts or if she is a prey to the hallucinations of the somnambulists', observed Saint-René Taillandier of Flaubert's heroine. Yet surely, he continued, she was a somnambulist, for how else could one make sense of the 'bestial scene' in which she calmly wraps a python around her naked body? Salammbô could be simultaneously 'ecstatic' and 'sensual' precisely because, in her peculiarly dissociated economy, 'mind lacks consciousness of the incitements of the flesh'.[32] While failing to provide such a subtle analysis of Salammbô's trance-like states, another critic explicitly linked them with hysteria. 'Isolated in the midst of the crowd by her ecstasy', he wrote, Salammbô appeared in the opening scene of the novel like a 'somnambulist pursuing I don't know what hysterical dream'.[33]

Contemporaries may have read the figure of Salammbô, 'Madame Bovary's oriental sister',[34] somewhat less clearly as an hysteric than they had read her Rouennaise prototype. But Flaubert's letters together with the notes and rough drafts for his Carthaginian novel leave no doubt as to his intentions. 'A propos of my *Salammbô*, I am busy with hysteria and insanity (*aliénation mentale*)',[35] he wrote to a friend, his pair of preoccupations corresponding well to the diagnoses that critics would later suggest for the characters of Salammbô and Mâtho respectively. To another friend he expressed, a few lines after discussing his progress on *Salammbô*, a wish to go to medical school 'if I were ten years younger', or at least to have sufficient time to attend the 'very curious little course' that the local asylum doctor was then giving for his close friends 'on hysteria, nymphomania, and so on'.[36] (Apparently Flaubert hoped to compensate for his non-attendance of this course by including Landouzy's *Traité complet de l'hystérie* in his broad, preparatory reading programme for *Salammbô*.)[37] Two decades after the publication of the novel, he would even accept a depiction of it as being in some measure 'about hysteria'.[38] Against this background, it is hardly surprising to learn that, in one of his earliest sketches for his Carthaginian novel, Flaubert epitomized the virginal Salammbô as 'intoxicated with the *mystico-hysterical* spirit' of the goddess of love and fertility.[39] Thus his characterization of Salammbô, like his characterization of Emma Bovary, joined hysteria together with two factors long believed to be predisposing causes of that disease: strong sexual impulses and exaggerated religious devotion.

Flaubert underscored the religious factor when he told Sainte-Beuve shortly after the publication of the novel that Salammbô was 'a kind of Saint Theresa', a reference that plays on the long-standing medical identification of that Spanish Carmelite mystic as an hysteric.[40] And if we know from one letter of 1859 that Flaubert was thinking of hysteria as affiliated with nymphomania, we know from another of that same year that he was thinking about the psychopathogenic effects of religious devotion in women and the connection between intense female religiosity and erotic longings.

> It's a sad story that you tell me of that young girl, your relative, gone mad as a result of religious ideas, but it's a familiar one. You've got to have a robust temperament to ascend the summits of mysticism without losing your head. And then, there is in all this (in women especially) questions of temperament that compli-cate the suffering. Don't you see that all of them are in love with

Adonis? He is the eternal husband that they require. Ascetic or libidinous, they dream of love, the great love; and to cure them (at least temporarily), they need not an idea but a fact – a man, a child, a lover.[41]

The link between mysticism, repressed eroticism, and hysteria was apparently axiomatic in Flaubert's mind; it surfaced again when he wrote to Zola in 1874, praising the latter's new novel *La Conquête de Plassans*. In that novel, Zola's heroine Marthe discovers a deep religious sensibility in herself some months after her husband rents a room in their home to the town's new abbé. At about the same time that she begins to experience pious ecstasies, she develops a nervous malady. The two phenomena intensify in tandem, culminating in what Flaubert calls her 'final avowal' of her carnal love for the priest living in her midst. Although Zola's novel leaves Marthe's sickness unnamed, Flaubert matter-of-factly identifies it in his letter as 'her hysterical condition'.[42]

This cursory consideration of the place of hysteria in Flaubert's prose indicates two aspects of his relationship to that disease category that are relevant to us here. First, hysteria was an implicit category in Flaubert's literary works but an explicit one for him when he wrote in the first person. While he seems to have deliberately avoided using the term in his novels, it appears at least a dozen times in his correspondence between 1852 and 1880[43] – a noteworthy tally given the fact that it was not until the early 1880s that, through the rise of Charcot and his school, hysteria gained widespread cultural currency and became 'la question palpitante du jour' in France.[44] As we know from a letter to Sand, Flaubert took the nomenclature of the 'psychological sciences' very seriously.[45] That he was more inclined to call hysteria by name in the relatively private sphere of letter writing than in the public one of novel writing was almost certainly an aesthetic strategy, part of Flaubert's project to create an impersonal, purely mimetic narrator reporting on the thingness of things without colouring them with his own affect, judgements or particular funds of knowledge. But at the same time the selectivity of his usage may have reflected his perception of the category 'hysteria' as existing in immediate relationship to himself.

Second, whatever medical sources he read, some of the views on hysteria that Flaubert absorbed in the 1850s and 1860s were not 'contrapuntal' at all but were instead profoundly conventional. His facile comment that women who fell ill from mystical preoccupations were 'all in love with Adonis' is a version of the old medical and popular representation of hysteria as 'Venus attached to her prey'.[46] It almost seems that in his *Dictionary of Received Ideas*, where he defined 'hysteria' as 'confuse with nymphomania', Flaubert was satirizing not only the vulgar nineteenth-century understanding of the term but also his own earlier banality and *bêtise*. Nor was Flaubert above invoking hysteria explicitly and gratuitously in a way demeaning to women. Writing anxiously to a friend about the forthcoming trial of *Madame Bovary,* he suggested a strategy that might save him from 'ruination': 'What I need especially is men eminent by dint of their high office to vouch that I am not in the business of producing books for hysterical kitchen-maids.'[47]

Yet if hysteria was for Flaubert on one level a tired cliché and a word that in its adjectival form always carried pejorative connotations and always modified women, on another level he found it an intensely interesting concept, one capable of expressive mutation. He seems to have linked it early on with his art and, in particular, with the often agonizing rhythm of his literary creativity. He first applied it to himself – something of a radical act, given the term's strong gender connotations – in 1852, in the context of a writing block of such massive proportions that he felt 'mentally and physically annihilated, as after a great orgy' and had spent five hours lying on his divan in complete torpor, lacking both 'the heart to make a gesture and the mind to have a thought'. Whereas five days before, when his novel was 'not moving', he had described himself as 'having nerves set on edge like brass wires', he was now experiencing, he wrote, 'hysterias of boredom' – a usage that finds support in the contemporary medical literature on hysterical symptoms.[48] And in his 1867 letter to Sand, at a time when he was not blocked in his creativity but was rather 'sculpting my darling novel laboriously like a convict' in solitary confinement, he again linked hysteria to the stresses peculiar to literary labour: 'All this results from our fine occupation.'[49]

Perhaps, given the analogy and the pervasive unconscious association between literary creativity and female biological procreativity, the former was the logical area of discussion in which male appropriation of the hysteria concept could take place during the nineteenth century. From hysteria as a malfunction of the organs of female procreativity (the traditional Hippocratic formulation about the wandering womb still survived), there was only a short step to hysteria as a malfunction of the faculties of male artistic creativity. It is suggestive in this regard that, much like Flaubert, Stéphane Mallarmé applied hysteria to himself in his capacity as a writer, observing in a letter of 1869: 'I have made a vow not to touch a pen from now (mid-February) until Easter.... The simple act of writing installs hysteria in my head.'[50] And it is significant that, when Flaubert ranged through Landouzy's encyclopaedic treatise on hysteria, his note taking on the symptoms of that disease focused on the so-called ball. He jotted down information about the ball's ascendant trajectory from the lower abdomen to the thorax and its failure to return to its place of origin; about the sensations of 'constriction' and 'strangulation' in the throat that accompanied it; about the nonsensical 'repetition(s) of a single word' and the indecipherable animal-like sounds – from 'barks, howls, roars, yelps, down to the grunts of a pig' – that resulted from its obstructive presence.[51] Hysteria, it would seem, presented itself to Flaubert preeminently as an impairment in the capacity for linguistic expression. He was, furthermore, intrigued by those clinical descriptions in which the hysterical blockage appeared as literally displaced from the uterine region to the organs of speech or, figuratively, from the realm of biological procreativity to that of verbal production.

While Flaubert's connecting of hysteria to the labours of male writing can certainly be construed as an implicit assertion of androgyny – I take *androgyny* to mean here that condition under which the affective and behavioural characteristics of the sexes are not rigidly assigned[52] – it hardly makes a strong claim for his use of the hysteria concept as a mediator between dichotomous notions of gender. To bolster that strong claim, we must look at three bodies of evidence: Baudelaire's review of *Madame Bovary*; certain thematic patterns of that novel and of *Salammbô*; and, finally, the Flaubert-Sand correspondence in which Flaubert's announcement of his male hysteria was embedded.

Flaubert regarded Baudelaire's review of *Madame Bovary* as the only fully satisfactory one the novel received, and it elicited his grateful encomium, 'You have entered into the secrets of the book as though my brain were yours.'[53] The review in fact turns on the issues of androgyny and hysteria, which are addressed in its final, climactic sections. Baudelaire characterizes *Madame Bovary* as a last-ditch effort to reinvigorate the moribund genre of the nineteenth-century novel, to shake up a complacent reading public by substituting icy detachment for engagement in the authorial voice and banality for deep significance in the subject matter. In carrying out this strategy, or artistic,'wager', much depended upon the realization of the title character. Flaubert had to pour himself into Emma Bovary, or in Baudelaire's words,

> to divest himself of his actual sex and make himself into a woman. The result is miraculous, for despite his zeal at wearing masks he

could not help but infuse some male blood into the veins of his creation.... Like weapon-bearing Pallas issuing forth from the forehead of Zeus, *this bizarre androgyne* houses the seductiveness of a virile soul within a beautiful feminine body.

To prove his point, Baudelaire enumerates the 'virile qualities' with which the author has 'perhaps unconsciously' endowed Emma, and it is at the end of this enumeration that he introduces, or rather slips in, hysteria, relating that nervous disease to the subject of androgyny not so much by logical argument as by allusive juxtaposition. Emma's gender ambiguity emerges, he says, even during her adolescent convent days, when she exhibits both the 'astonishing aptitude for life' that marks the 'man of action' and the typically girlish tendency 'to get intoxicated from' the lush trappings of Catholicism, 'to gorge herself' on stained-glass windows and vespers music. But Emma offers an embellishment on this latter, passive, and characteristically feminine posture. She converts the true Christian God into 'the God of her fantasy', one equipped 'with spurs and moustaches'; and this eroticized transformation, entirely attributable to the condition of her 'nerves', renders her the 'hysterical poet'.[54]

The meaning Baudelaire gives to *hysteria* here is itself ambiguous. The term seems to have two referents. First, there is the familiar equation of female mystical tendencies with hysteria and the contention that both serve as a screen for erotic longings – ideas to which Flaubert also gave credence, as we have already seen. But Baudelaire's *hysteria* seems to refer not merely to the supposedly feminine component of Emma's behaviour in the convent but, more broadly, to her very coupling of male and female traits; it seems to be the expression of her 'bizarre' androgyny. After all, what qualifies Emma as an hysteric in Baudelaire's view is the unorthodox metamorphosis of God that she enacts in fantasy; and Baudelaire had, earlier in the review, identified the faculty of 'imagination' as 'supreme', 'tyrannical' and preeminently masculine.[55]

That Baudelaire intended to link hysteria with androgyny is borne out as well in the paragraph of the review devoted entirely to that nervous pathology. Here, consigning hysteria to the status of a 'mystery' as yet unsolved by the Academy of Medicine,[56] he casually makes the controversial move of assuming its existence in both men and women. This move probably had autobiographical resonance: elsewhere in his writings, he, like Flaubert, depicted himself as an hysteric.[57] Developing the gender theme, Baudelaire ends his brief discussion of hysteria on a cryptic but highly evocative note. The principle symptom of the disease in women, the well-known 'rising and strangulating ball' is, he tells us, 'translated' in men into a symptomatology which combines various forms of 'impotence' with a 'proclivity to excess'.

Read metaphorically, this clinical description could be taken to mean that hysteria represents in each sex an aspiration to androgyny – that is to say, a protest against conventional gender definitions and an (ultimately failed) attempt to transcend them. In women, according to Baudelaire's rendition, hysteria problematizes the organs of speech; the effort to escape the self-absorbed interiority of that pure bodily life to which society relegates women, to address the outside world in the 'masculine' mode of language, is both highlighted and foiled. In men, hysteria problematizes the 'masculine' mode of action through a vacillation between the desire to resign that mode utterly and embrace the 'feminine' mode of impotent passivity and the compensatory desire to exaggerate action beyond measure.[58] The structure of Baudelaire's review at this juncture further indicates that he intended an integrative discussion of hysteria and androgyny, for immediately after the paragraph devoted to hysteria he returns quite explicitly to the androgyny motif. '*Intellectual* women', he asserts, 'owe (Flaubert) a debt of gratitude for having (in the character of Emma Bovary) elevated the female to a position of such efficacy, so far from the pure animal and so close to the ideal man, for having made her participate in that double nature of rational calculation and of dreaming that constitutes the perfect human being.'[59]

Many twentieth-century commentators have elaborated upon the theme of androgyny in *Madame Bovary* first announced by Baudelaire, most notably Jean-Paul Sartre, who turned this aspect of Flaubert's novel into a fascinating, and vastly ambitious, research programme:

> One problem then – without leaving the work itself; that is, the literary significations – is to ask ourselves why the author (that is, the pure synthetic activity which creates *Madame Bovary*) was able to metamorphose himself into a woman ... what the artistic transformation of male into female means in the nineteenth century ... and finally, just who Gustave Flaubert *must have been* in order to have within the field of his possibles the possibility of portraying himself as a woman. The reply is independent of all biography, since this problem could be posed in Kantian terms: 'Under what conditions is the feminization of experience possible?'[60]

But these discussions by Sartre and others do not pick up Baudelaire's suggestion that Flaubert uses hysteria as the vehicle of androgyny, as the liminal ground where ordinary gender boundaries can be transgressed.

While *Salammbô* has elicited far less commentary – both in general, and as a novel about hysteria – it, too, is amenable to interpretation in terms of the conjoint theme of hysteria and androgyny. Certainly the novel plays on the binary opposition of male and female and on attempted mediations between the two.[61] This pattern is set forth in the opening scene when the rowdy, brawling, barbarian mercenaries – almost caricatures of masculinity – are suddenly interrupted by the ecstatic, virginal, lyre-playing Salammbô; she is accompanied by the 'mediators', a corps of pallid, beardless and hairless eunuch priests. Later in the novel, Flaubert explicitly underscores this mediation, noting of Schahabarim, the eunuch priest who oversees Salammbô's religious training, 'His condition established between them something like the equality of a common sex.'[62]

That hysteria is another candidate for the mediating function in the novel can be inferred from a recent essay by Benjamin Bart that presents persuasive textual evidence for the proposition that Flaubert endowed Mâtho, the strapping Libyan mercenary, with the traits of an hysteric.[63] Building upon this suggestion, one can argue that both Mâtho and Salammbô are afflicted with hysteria: looking at the python, she experiences the hysterical ball ('another serpent slowly coming up in her throat to choke her'),[64] and confronted with her father's wrath, that same symptom condemns her to speechlessness ('She did not dare open her lips, yet she was choking with the need to voice her sorrow').[65] The common ground of hysteria thus mediates the polar opposition between these stereotypically male and female protagonists. Indeed, it helps to explain why the crucial scene in the tent, the supposed consummation of their passion, has been left so oddly ambiguous and unrealized. After all, Flaubert saw hysterical desire as essentially self-contradictory in its nature and hence not amenable to fulfillment. 'In search of love and not of a lover', he laconically characterized Salammbô's 'vague hysteria' in his notes for the novel.[66]

The early years of Flaubert's correspondence with George Sand provide another, more direct way to demonstrate the strength of the connection between androgyny and hysteria in Flaubert's mind. The friendship of these two writers, which effectively began in 1866 when he was 45 and she 62 has long puzzled critics, for the aesthetic philosophies of the two were (and would always remain) antithetical, and in his younger days Flaubert had even made contemptuous remarks about the flabby romanticism of Sand's novels and about the mindless 'seamstresses' who read them.[67] A few months into the relationship, Flaubert was as puzzled by it as the critics later were. 'Under what constellation were you born', he exclaimed to Sand, 'that enabled you to unite in your person such diverse, numerous, and rare qualities! I don't know what kind of sentiment I bear for you, but I know that I feel a *specific* tenderness and one that I have never, up to this time, felt for anyone.... All the doors between the two of us are not yet open.'[68]

What brought the two writers together for the first time was Flaubert's gratitude for the review of *Salammbô* that Sand published at the beginning of 1863 – one of the few favourable assessments which that novel received. With her masculine pseudonym and intermittent assumption of a masculine demeanor, the bountifully maternal Sand was a kind of nineteenth-century French incarnation of androgyny. 'That hermaphroditic writer', one critic had called her in the 1830s, reflecting the fact that she deliberately, and provocatively, insisted upon a male authorial identity despite the public's awareness of her actual gender. Another, pronouncing her 'an enigmatic man and a phenomenal woman', speculated that Sand's power as a writer derived precisely from these 'two opposing natures within a single being' – a being that would, he added, 'honour whichever sex it deigned to choose'.[69] Thus a shared fascination with gender definition, including a questioning of traditional gender boundaries, seems to have been an important, though tacit, factor underlying the soul union that Sand and Flaubert eventually forged. At least the letters leading up to and immediately following Flaubert's declaration of his hysterical pathology persistently reflect this theme.

At first, a spelling problem implicitly announces the theme. Flaubert addresses Sand as 'cher maître', using the masculine form of the adjective – a mistake with respect to Sand's gender, though an accurate usage with respect to the masculine noun he has chosen for her ('master' instead of 'mistress') in recognition of her senior status as a writer. The next time, he produces the spelling *chère maître* (the feminine form of the adjective), and twice after that, grown self-conscious about the gender confusion that reflects itself in the orthography of this particular phrase as applied to Sand, he underlines the final *e* in *chère.*[70]

There is much play on the simulacrum of a cloistered life that Flaubert has arranged for himself, a motif that is important for us here for several reasons: because monks and nuns represent a particular variant on ordinary gender identity; because the enforced

224

sexual abstinence and the religious exaltation of the formal cloistered life were routinely linked with female hysteria (*Salammbô*, as priestess of Tanit, falls into this category Carthaginian style); and because Flaubert would, in the critical 1867 letter, depict himself as an 'anchorite'. Thus, after her first visit to Flaubert at his home in Normandy, Sand writes, calling stark attention to her own female corporeality, 'I was truly touched by the warm welcome I received in your monastic environment (*milieu de chanoine*), where a wandering animal of my species is an anomaly that could be found troublesome.' A few weeks later, she calls Flaubert 'my Benedictine, all alone in your ravishing monastery (*chartreuse*), working and never going out'.[71] By return mail, Flaubert picks up the theme from another angle, informing her that he is reading through the ten volumes of her autobiography, and that 'what struck me the most is the (section on) convent life. I have a lot of observations about all that to submit to you'.[72] In *Histoire de ma vie*, Sand had described her early adolescent years in a Paris convent as a typical female experience ('More than one person of my sex will recognize (in this account) the sometimes good and sometimes bad effects of religious education'). She had passed through a series of stages: total rebellion against the institution; then an 'ardent and agitated' mysticism; and finally, a 'calm, firm, and lively devotion'.[73] It seems likely that Flaubert was interested in her ability to move beyond the mystical stage, the one that he had portrayed as a kind of developmental impasse conducing to hysteria in both Emma Bovary and Salammbô. Indeed, as Flaubert could not have helped noticing, Sand mentions hysteria near the conclusion of her account of her convent days, explicitly distinguishing it from the 'calm devotion' that she eventually achieved:

> Whoever has passed that way knows well that no terrestrial affection can give comparable intellectual satisfactions. This Jesus, as the mystics have interpreted and remade him for their purposes, is a friend, a brother, a father, whose constant presence, untiring solicitude, tenderness, and infinite patience can be compared to nothing in the realm of the real and the possible. I don't like the fact that nuns have made him their husband. *There is in that something that is bound to feed a hysterical mysticism, the most repugnant of the forms that mysticism can take.* This ideal love for Christ is without danger only during that period of life when the human passions are silent.[74]

To the motif of monastery and convent is joined the metaphor of literary creativity as biological procreativity which Sand contributes

225

to the correspondence. She refers to a work in progress as 'my foetus.'[75] Regaled with details about the anguish that accompanies Flaubert's literary endeavours, she tells him that he has 'the pains of childbirth' and that she empathizes with him as thoroughly as when 'my daughter-in-law brings dear infants into the world', a process that causes Sand to become 'more sick, and seriously so' than the woman actually in labour.[76] Another time, 'astonished' by Flaubert's accounts of his difficulties as a writer, she does not use metaphors of female reproduction, but she counsels him to adopt a more passive, perhaps implicitly a more female, stance. 'Ah well, when we are absolutely only instruments, it is still a pleasant condition and a sensation matched by no other to feel ourselves vibrate. Let the wind run up and down your strings a little, then. I think you make greater efforts than necessary, and that you ought more often to give free rein to the *other*.'[77]

Even more striking are the two writers' explicit statements about a wish for, or about the actuality of, gender transformation. In the course of making plans to meet in Paris for the opening of a friend's play – a meeting that was, in effect, to be their first date – Sand writes, apparently alluding to her advanced age and the cessation of her menstrual cycle, 'Since at present I am no longer a woman, if God were just I would become a man. I would have physical strength and would say to you, "Let's go and take a trip to Carthage or some other place." But, behold, one progresses toward a child-hood which has neither sex nor energy....'[78] Musing about his own ageing process some four months later, Flaubert presents Sand's mirror image with respect to gender fantasies. 'I believe that the heart does not grow old. There are even some people in whom it expands with age: I was more dried up and crabbed 20 years ago than I am today. I have been feminized [*je me suis féminisé*] and softened with wear and tear, as others become callous.' The feminization Flaubert imputes to himself has thus been initially depicted in wholly positive terms: the feminine vulnerability he has acquired is equated with true vitality, with a capacity for openness and continued emotional growth. But Flaubert immediately renders his assessment of it ambiguous by injecting a negative note. 'And that makes me indignant. I feel I'm becoming too soft. I am moved by nothing at all. Everything troubles and agitates me.'[79]

Thus Flaubert begins by positing androgyny, that fluidity of gender definition which enables the integration of selected feminine traits into himself, as a desirable end. But he then partially retreats, fearfully enthralled, it would seem, by the low value placed on those traits by the culture at large, the general tendency to view female emotion as a sign of weakness, as intrinsically excessive and slightly ludicrous. At the time that he announced his identity as a male hysteric, Flaubert did so with an ambivalent commitment to the ideal of androgyny. Not surprisingly, he was much more able to appreciate the marks of Sand's androgynous condition than to affirm and cultivate that condition in himself. As he wrote in the very same letter in which he waffles on the value of his own feminization, 'I, too, ask myself why I love you. Is it because you are a great Man, or because you are a charming being?'[80]

This affirmation of the androgynous ideal achieved by distancing that ideal from himself and displacing it onto a woman was not an entirely new emotional motif for Flaubert. Rather, it recalls a disappointed longing that had already coloured his protracted sexual relationship with the writer Louise Colet. 'I believed from the beginning that I would find in you less feminine personality, a more universal conception of life', he wrote to Colet with exasperation in 1846, going on to describe a personal ideal of 'hermaphroditism' to which he imagined she could conform:

> I should like to make of you something entirely apart, neither (male) friend (*ami*) nor mistress. Both of those are too restrictive, too exclusive. One does not love one's friend enough, and one is too silly with one's mistress. It is the intermediate term I seek, the essence of those two sentiments combined. What I want, in short, is that, *like a new kind of hermaphrodite*, you give me all the joys of the flesh with your body, and *all those of the soul with your mind*.[81]

Flaubert feared that this concept was unclear, poorly articulated, even self-contradictory ('It's strange how bad my writing is in these letters to you.... Everything comes into collision, as if I wanted to say three words at once'),[82] but it persisted in his mind as an *idée fixe*. In the spring of 1854, a year before ending their liaison, he voiced it again to Colet in a more despairing tone. 'I have always tried (but it seems to me that I failed) to make a sublime hermaphrodite of you.'[83]

Sand's commitment to androgyny was, in her letters to Flaubert, much more inclusive and whole-hearted than her correspondent's. It tended to take the form of so thoroughly undermining conventional distinctions between properly masculine and properly feminine traits that the category of gender nearly disappeared altogether.[84] Sand expressed this view quite succinctly in her reply to Flaubert's letter on his male hysteria. In the first place, she doubted that hysteria could be a gendered malady:

What does it mean to be hysterical? Perhaps I've also been so, perhaps I am now, but I know nothing about it, having never examined the matter thoroughly and having only heard about it second-hand without studying it. Isn't it a malaise, a great distress, caused by the desire for an impossible *something?* In that case, all of us who have imagination are afflicted with it, with that strange sickness. And why would such a malady have a sex?[85]

Thus, like Baudelaire in his review of *Madame Bovary,* Sand identified hysteria with the overreaching tendency of imagination; but since, unlike Baudelaire, she declined to identify imagination as a masculine faculty, hysteria became for her not a condition that mingled gender attributes but rather one simply without gender. In the next sentence of the same letter, she went on to question the validity of the very category of gender:

And then, for people knowledgeable in anatomy, *there is only one sex.* A man and a woman are so much the same thing that it is difficult to comprehend the heap of distinctions and subtle arguments about the subject that societies have fostered. I observed the infancy and the development of my son and daughter. My son was me, and consequently much more a woman than was my daughter, who was an unrealized man [*un homme pas réussi*].[86]

Medical Men Deploy Hysteria

This consideration of Flaubert and, to a lesser extent, Sand and Baudelaire, shows the use to which the hysteria concept could be put by French creative writers in the 1850s and 1860s. Construed metaphorically, it became the springboard for free-ranging and unorthodox ruminations about gender definition. Such ruminations were, in the case of Flaubert and almost certainly in the case of Baudelaire,[87] nourished by contact with the technical medical literature. But other factors must have nourished them as well. For example, if one accepts the claims of Freudian psychoanalysis, these writers may have been especially sensitive to the pervasive, unconscious fantasy of androgyny as expressed in the young child's belief in a phallic mother. Or, on the historical plane, they may have been influenced by the articulation of an androgynous ideal by such early nineteenth-century intellectual movements as Saint-Simonianism and Comtean positivism, which sought to achieve post-Revolutionary social stability by synthesizing the rational (and 'male') element with the sentimental (and 'female') one and which invented personifications of the desired synthesis.[88] At mid century Flaubert's close friend Maxime Du Camp even found this desirable androgynous synthesis embodied in the creative writer, a position consonant with that literary application of *hysteria* to the trials of male writing that we have noted. 'The artist, and especially the poet', Du Camp asserted in a novel, 'should be a sort of androgyne who combines in himself serenity and sensitivity, strength and tenderness'; he ought to be 'a man in terms of intelligence, a woman in terms of heart.' Interestingly enough, Du Camp attributed this opinion to his main character – a troubled young man, on the verge both of serious writing and of suicide, whom he described as a 'hystero-melancholic'.[89]

But what about nineteenth-century medical discourse itself? Although the medical community had furnished the discursive pre-conditions for the 'discovery' of male hysteria and in fact engaged in intermittent debate about its existence throughout the nineteenth century, the medical supporters of that new category were not in a position to perceive or exploit its implications for the definition of gender. The field of vision of physicians and psychiatrists was effectively limited both by the discursive norms of medical science and by the nexus of power relations that enmeshed medical doctors as professional men who actively sought to increase the authority they commanded in society and whose expertise was, in turn, often sought after and applied by political agencies. These two factors combined to contain the cultural iconoclasm that might seem to have existed in the male hysteria concept.

Throughout the nineteenth century, male hysteria entered medical discourse as the by-product of one or another more general scientific hypothesis. It was, consequently, regarded as far less inter-esting as a datum in itself than as evidence in support of that larger hypothesis. Thus the boldly inventive young Paris psychiatrist Georget propounded the existence of male hysteria in the 1820s in connection with his conviction, inspired by pioneering work in brain dissection, that all mental disease resulted from cerebral lesions. From this new theoretical perspective, hysteria became for Georget 'an idiopathic affection of the brain ... observable in both sexes'. The long-standing belief that its locus was the female reproductive organs could, he said, be disproved both by documenting cases of hysteria in men and by showing that the uterus and ovaries simply lacked the neural 'sympathies' necessary to spread a pathological condition throughout the organism as a whole.[90]

During the 1830s and 1840s, articles occasionally appeared in medical journals in Paris and the provinces painstakingly detailing the symptoms of a putative case of male hysteria and citing Georget as an authority on the theoretical possibility for such a clinical finding. But, as had been true for Georget himself, the subject really under discussion in such accounts was the bodily seat of hysteria.[91] The doctors failed to recognize – or, perhaps, automatically suppressed as irrelevant and inconvenient their unarticulated recognition – that their clinical findings might have implications for the definition of gender in the larger culture.

Some awareness of these general cultural issues was demonstrated by Dr Pierre Briquet, whose monumental treatise on hysteria appeared in 1859. In affirming the existence (though extreme rarity) of hysteria in men and jettisoning the uterine theory of that disease, Briquet made clear that he hoped to contribute to the eradication of certain negative cultural stereotypes of women. Despite the connotations its name carried in the non-medical world, hysteria was not, he said, a 'shameful malady'. It was not caused by unsatisfied sexual desires – a widespread belief that, according to Briquet, 'tends to degrade women' – but rather by 'the existence in women of the noblest and most most admirable sentiments, ones which they alone are capable of feeling'.[92] Denying hysteria all anatomical determinants, Briquet championed a psychophysiological theory of the disease that rooted it in the emotions mediated by the nervous system and which rendered it, if not exclusively female in its incidence, still an expression of characteristics that he regarded as feminine by nature.[93] 'Woman has a noble mission of the greatest social importance – that of raising children, looking after the welfare of adults, and taking care of the elderly. To this end, she has been endowed with a special kind of sensibility, very different from that of men; and it is in this kind of sensibility that lies the source of hysteria.'[94] The kind of sensibility to which Briquet was referring was in fact 'an excess of sensibility', a disposition to feel intense and 'incessant' emotion. Existing in women with 'nothing to counterbalance it', it moved them to socially indispensable outpourings of tenderness and pity and also shaded by degrees into pathology.[95] Thus, with his particular slant on the social meaning of hysteria, Briquet valorized male hysteria as part of his project of desexualizing that disease while at the same time leaving it resoundingly gendered.

With the rise of Charcot and his Salpêtrière school in the 1870s and 1880s, everything about hysteria in France increased in scale[96] – the number of people diagnosed as afflicted with it, the popularization of knowledge about it, and, of particular interest here, the number of diagnosed male hysterics. A recent study has examined this last point in depth, ascertaining that some 20 to 25 per cent of Charcot's published case studies of hysterics were in fact

230

about men.[97] What are we to make of such avid interest in male hysteria on the part of Charcot and his disciples? Does it show that Charcot was free of the anti-female bias that had marked earlier medical research on hysteria, that his clinical gaze was, in this respect at least, a truly objective one? Might Charcot's erosion of the classically female nature of hysteria even mean that, like Flaubert, he entertained unconventional notions about gender definition?

Such a Charcot is not a very credible creature. For while Charcot's project entailed the affirmation of male hysteria, the doctor's real interest lay elsewhere. Much like Georget, he wanted to make a general theoretical point, one which happened to carry male hysteria along in its wake. In Charcot's case, that point concerned the universality of the clinical picture that hysteria presented and hence, ultimately, the legitimacy of hysteria as a diagnostic entity. Where his predecessors had found only a chaotic and chameleon-like bevy of symptoms, Charcot's much-hailed scientific achievement was to have found an orderly array; he had delineated four phases, or periods, of hysteria that, he asserted, 'follow one another with the regularity of a mechanism'. In other words, he had gained cognitive control over that disease (he still did not know how to cure it) by subsuming it under positive laws, and he made the supremely confident claim of the positivist – that the laws he had discovered and which governed hysteria were 'valid for all countries, all times, all races' and 'consequently universal'.[98] Demonstrating the universality of hysteria thus became one of Charcot's continuing scientific preoccupations; and just as it led him to make retrospective diagnoses of that disease on the basis of the visual evidence contained in the paintings and woodcuts of past centuries, so·it led him to emphasize the existence of hysteria in men.[99] The discussions of male hysteria in Charcot's lectures bear out this interpretation, for they are larded with explicit assertions about hysteria's 'unity' – the single clinical picture that it presented in varied contexts.[100]

Other aspects of Charcot's work and public persona support this conclusion that his championing of male hysteria was not indicative of a revisionist attitude toward gender definition. For one thing, he appears to have barely tolerated the entrance of women into the medical profession. A late nineteenth-century French feminist journal reproduced his remarks at the 1888 public dissertation defence of a young Polish woman aspiring to a degree from the Paris Faculty of Medicine. The first of the jurors to speak, Charcot unabashedly acknowledged that he had not read the thesis, a statistical study entitled 'The Woman Doctor in the Nineteenth

Century'. But he nonetheless proceeded to develop a case against women doctors. 'The special physiology of their sex', he said, including their monthly 'indispositions', rendered them unsuitable to care for patients; but since French law had granted them the right to practise medicine, they should be confined to the humble position of country doctor rather than competing with men for lucrative and prestigious urban posts. Their career accomplishments must never be superior to those of their husband, for such a situation rendered a man 'piteous alongside his wife'. Charcot even invoked as relevant to the question at hand the natural 'beauty of woman and the ugliness of the male sex'. Women with careers, he noted, tended to 'neglect their toilette', a dereliction of duty apparently countenanced by the Anglo-Saxons but unacceptable to the French as an 'aesthetic people'.[101]

Second, while Charcot's rendition of male hysteria was in many ways explicitly patterned on its female prototype, in certain details the disease also differed in its male and female victims – and the chief difference noted by Charcot paralleled and thus reaffirmed the most stereotypical notions of the difference between the sexes. Among the majority of female hysterics, 'instability, mobility of symptoms' preponderated, and 'the capricious course of the ailment is frequently interrupted by the most surprising strokes of theatricality'. In the male, however, hysteria displayed none of this flightiness but presented an appropriately sober clinical picture 'remarkable in the permanence and tenacity of the symptoms'.[102]

Finally, looking at the social and ethnic backgrounds of the men whom Charcot judged to be hysterics, we find that male hysteria was a highly selective diagnosis. While female hysterics could be found in all social strata, male hysterics – at least those identified by Charcot – were, if French and Christian, almost invariably members of the working class or of the unemployed underworld. They might also be Jews or Arabs, in which case they could be either middle class or working class.[103] In other words, from the vantage point of the male, bourgeois, Christian doctor who made the diagnosis, the male hysteric remained the 'other', as radically foreign and as extruded from the self as the female hysteric. Rather than introducing a fundamentally novel, non-stigmatizing element into the hysteria diagnosis, or seriously problematizing gender definition, or rendering the psychiatric doctor vulnerable to his own labels, Charcot's male hysteria was a variant on a familiar nineteenth-century rhetorical theme: it conflated forms of otherness, linking the characteristics of women with those of the lower classes or, alternatively, with those of the Orient.[104]

That Charcot's advocacy of male hysteria should respect rather than violate the *status quo* with respect to gender was in the first place dictated by the norms of medical scientific discourse, which sought to restrict the meanings of terms rather than to exploit their connotative or metaphorical possibilities. Charcot even paid obeisance to those norms when, in the course of affirming the positivity of hysteria as a diagnostic entity, he took the opportunity to denigrate the productions of literary men. Hysteria, he asserted, was 'not one of those unknowns where one sees whatever one wishes'. It was, in other words, '*not a novel:* hysteria has its laws'.[105] But the fundamental conservatism of Charcot's male hysteria was also dictated by the complex of power relations in which his medical scientific discourse was involved.

As my earlier research has shown, Charcot's emphasis on hysteria was in part instrumental, serving to enhance the professional power of the psychiatric specialty and to facilitate psychiatry's collaboration with the anti-clerical politics of the early Third Republic.[106] Most relevant here, a politics of gender went hand in hand with this professional expansion and republican entrenchment. It had long been axiomatic in French anti-clerical thought that priests exercised their most tenacious control over the minds of women; hence the warning issued by the prominent republican politician Jules Ferry in 1870 that 'women must belong to science, or else they will belong to the Church'.[107] Now among the several ways to make women 'belong to science' and, by extension, to the Republic, was to medicalize their bouts of indeterminate emotional distress, defining them as illnesses that required the consultation of a physician, rather than as moral failings or spiritual crises that required the guidance of a priest. From this perspective, disease categories such as hysteria or its cousin neurasthenia were permeated with political significance.

But the republican politics of gender extended further, furnishing a response not only to the traditional bonding of woman and priest but also to the new historical phenomenon of feminism. Although French feminism was a numerically unimpressive movement in the closing decades of the nineteenth century, Frenchmen typically perceived it as a serious threat to traditional gender relations and hence to that network of alliances between liberals and conservatives upon which the still fragile republican synthesis had been founded.[108] In the face of such a threat, the utility of the hysteria diagnosis was unmistakable. For hysteria confirmed, in the supposedly neutral language of science, the weakness and vulnerability of women and thus their congenital lack of fitness for the traditionally male social roles that feminism sought to obtain for them. After all, French psychiatric doctors routinely described the victims of hysteria as deceitful, contrary, and capricious and sometimes even characterized the *normal* female character as 'mildly hysterical'.[109]

Given Charcot's thoroughgoing commitment to *fin-de-siècle* republican politics – a commitment that had redounded to his professional benefit, resulting in the creation of the first chair in nervous disease at the Paris Faculty of Medicine and the naming of Charcot as its first occupant – he could hardly have deployed his psychiatry to redefine gender. Or, more strongly put, discursive and political constraints combined to place gender redefinition outside Charcot's possibilities as a thinker, even when he was advancing as seemingly transgressive a category as male hysteria. If the dominant themes of the discourse on hysteria figured prominently in his repertory, their counterpoint eluded him.

A comparative remark is in order here. Wolf Lepenies recently suggested that the new discipline of sociology was in the nineteenth century caught between two rival epistemologies: the positivistic orientation that led it to imitate the natural sciences and the hermeneutical attitude that shifted it in the direction of literature.[110] The same cannot, however, be said of the new discipline of psychiatry, at least in France. There is nothing in the disciplinary experience of nineteenth-century French *médecine mentale* comparable to those 'literary' moments that Lepenies has located for its sociological counterpart: Auguste Comte's love affair with Clotilde de Vaux, which led him to integrate emotion and poetry into his sociology, for example, or the utopian novel written by the *fin-de-siècle* sociologist Gabriel Tarde. Firmly wedded to the scientific ethos of the Enlightenment, psychiatry remained insulated and aloof from the literary sensibility and counter-Enlightenment 'culture of feeling' that periodically captivated sociology. As a result, the discourse of hysteria underwent quite separate developments in the literary and medical domains. Flaubert's male hysteric and Charcot's male hysteric were roughly contemporaneous constructions which bore the same name, but there was a radical disjunction between them.

The Parameters of Gender Redefinition through Androgyny

Just how radical was the disjunction between literary and medical male hysteria, and how are we to construe its meaning? At the beginning of this essay, I called the nineteenth-century literary use of male hysteria a 'subversive counterpoint' to its medical use in the same period. Now that I have presented my evidence in support of that proposition, it is appropriate to step back and consider what the evidence really amounts to. Have I perhaps exaggerated my initial claim, been hornswoggled by a surface appearance of gender redefinition that masks a fundamental perpetuation of traditional stereotypes?

A case for the *lack* of subversiveness of male-hysteria-as-androgyny is in fact relatively easy to make. It rests upon the contention that, at least at the hands of Flaubert, the metaphorical identification of male hysteric and androgyne neither revalues the feminine nor alters the old hierarchy that subordinates the feminine to the masculine. After all, what Flaubert has done by declaring himself a male hysteric is to take upon himself a pathology, and a concept of the feminine as the pathological – fragile, hypersensitive, debarred from effective expression or action. In one of his letters to Sand, he did, to be sure, give a highly positive assessment of the female emotionality associated with hysteria, depicting it as inherently more vital than the phlegmatic rationalism that causes men to 'dry up' as they advance in age. But, as we have seen, he turned against that idea almost as soon as he had given voice to it.

Hence (such an argument might continue), if Charcot used the hysteria concept, including its male variant, in the service of a kind of professional imperialism, expanding the patient population of the psychiatric doctor to include the partly as well as the fully mad, Flaubert's use of that concept, though very different in substance, was equally imperialistic – and in its way as benighted as Charcot's with respect to gender issues. Flaubert enacted his imperialism in the personal as well as the professional realm. By defining himself as suffering from hysteria, he expanded the scope and aesthetic possibilities of his own personality, adding female modalities to his repertory without sacrificing male prerogatives. He thus exemplifies what Elaine Showalter has pejoratively called 'critical cross-dressing', a form of self-representation as female by a literary man that shares the psychodynamics of literal male transvestism. In both its literary and its literal manifestations, according to Showalter, the assumption of a female persona functions psychologically not as a genuine tribute to the feminine but as a covert promotion of male power. The female impersonator takes great pride in the fact that he ultimately retains his masculinity and hence is able to shift back and forth between gender identities or to occupy both simultaneously, in the latter case incarnating a phallic woman. He regards himself as having the wherewithal to be, if he so chooses, a better woman than any biological female.[111]

Showalter's incisive critique of the strategy of critical cross-dressing doubles as a more general critique of the emancipatory potential of the androgyny concept. In this latter respect, her argument is part of a current in feminist thinking inaugurated in the mid 1970s in reaction against Carolyn Heilbrun's *Toward a Recognition of Androgyny*. Instead of seeing the ideal of androgyny as transcending dichotomous gender stereotypes and thus offering liberation to both women and men, feminist critics of androgyny have analyzed it as a deceptive and fundamentally male-centred ideal, either subsuming the feminine into the already dominant masculine (Showalter's point) or, in the form of the couple-as-androgyne, precluding the independent functioning of women in society.[112]

How then do these late-twentieth-century strictures against androgyny as an emancipatory ideal affect the thesis of this essay? They certainly call into question any implication that androgyny à la Flaubert can be held up today as an unassailable *normative* ideal for feminism. But they do not, I think, much affect the *historical* point that I have attempted to make: that in the nineteenth century and as a result of divergent epistemological norms, a single discursive object, male hysteria, underwent different developments in medical and literary discourse; that the medical usage conformed to the gender stereotypes enshrined in the nineteenth century's prevailing ideology of domesticity, while the literary usage challenged the dichotomous notion of gender. In the minds, conscious and unconscious, of the literary men who articulated it, male-hysteria-as-androgyny may not have been a completely laudable or revolutionary doctrine by some absolute, transhistorical standard. But in relative, historical terms – which is to say, within the bounds of its nineteenth-century context – it nonetheless retains its credentials as subversive. It opened up possibilities and alternatives otherwise hidden by the prevailing domestic doctrine that held that 'nature' had made the sexes to fit a pattern of strict opposition, with rational, active men commanding the public life and passive but feelingful women consigned to a sheltered private sphere.

Notes

Copyright © 1991 by the Regents of the University of California. Reprinted by permission of the University of California Press from *Representations* 34 (Spring 1991): 134–65.

Earlier versions of this paper were presented at an interdisciplinary symposium on *Representing Hysteria* held at Trinity College, Hartford, Connecticut in May 1988, at a meeting of the Workshop on the History of the Human Sciences at the University of Chicago in January 1990 and at a conference on Aspects of French Medical Culture in the Eighteenth and Nineteenth Centuries held at the Virginia Polytechnic Institute in April 1990. I am grateful to friends and colleagues for the helpful comments, criticisms and suggestions they made on these and other occasions. In particular, I wish to thank Keith Baker, Janet Beizer, Priscilla Ferguson, Stephen Gabel, Robert Morrissey, Peter Novick, Lawrence Rothfield, Barbara Sicherman, George Stocking and the editors of *Representations*.

1. Gustave Flaubert to George Sand, 12–13 January, 1867 in Flaubert and Sand, *Correspondance,* Alphonse Jacobs (ed.) (Paris: Flammarion, 1981), 117–18. The portion of the letter cited was omitted from the standard twentieth-century edition of Flaubert's *Correspondance,* that published by Editions Louis Conard, 13 vols (Paris, 1926–54). Unless otherwise indicated, translations are my own.
2. The reference is to Dr Alfred Hardy, a highly respected Paris internist with a hospital appointment and a professorship at the Paris Faculty of Medicine. Like many experts in *pathologie interne* at this date, Hardy included mental and nervous pathology within his purview.
3. Flaubert to George Sand, 1 May, 1874, *Correspondance,* 7:134; to Mme Roger des Genettes of the same date, *ibid.,* 137. By 1879, the doctor had changed but the diagnosis remained the same. As Flaubert wrote to his niece Caroline: 'You know that I gorge myself on shrimp everyday, being no longer able to eat meat. Fortin (Flaubert's local physician in Croisset) calls me more than ever "a big hysterical girl"'; 25 April, 1879, *ibid.,* 8:261.
4. Flaubert to Sand, 12–13 January, 1867, Flaubert and Sand, *Correspondance,* 118.
5. Flaubert to Mlle Leroyer de Chantepie, 18 February, 1859, *Correspondance,* 4: 314. In the same letter Flaubert declares, 'The anatomy of the human heart has not yet been discerned. How, then, can you expect anyone to heal the heart? The unique glory of the nineteenth century will be to have begun these studies.'
6. The Bibliothèque nationale in Paris recently acquired a photocopy of Flaubert's undated 'Notes de lecture pour *Salammbô',* a manuscript of 63 pages that includes two pages on Landouzy; see BN Manuscrits Don 37287, 34–5. Hector Landouzy's discussion of 'hystérie chez l'homme' occupies 218–24 of his *Traité complet de l'hystérie* (Paris, 1846).
7. Flaubert to Charles-Augustin Sainte-Beuve, reprinted as an appendix in Sainte-Beuve, *Nouveaux Lundis,* 13 vols (Paris, 1885), 4:437. The *Dictionnaire des sciences médicales* also appears in *Madame Bovary* and serves in that novel as the emblem of nineteenth-century medical knowledge; see the excellent analysis of this point by Lawrence Rothfield, 'From Semiotic to Discursive Intertextuality: The Case of

237

Madame Bovary', *Novel* 19 (1985), especially 59–60.

8. See Etienne-Jean Georget, 'Hystérie' (1824), *Dictionnaire de médecine*, 21 vols (Paris, 1821–28), ll: 532, 541. The comparable article in the *Dictionnaire des sciences médicales*, written by Jean-Baptiste Louyer-Villermay and published in 1818, acknowledged the occurrence of hysteria-like symptoms in men but insisted that they were distinguishable from true hysteria; 60 vols (Paris, 1812–22), 23:229–30. Implicit in the author's discussion, however, is the fact that the existence of male hysteria was already a reputable hypothesis, if a controversial one, within the medical community.

9. Flaubert to Mlle Leroyer de Chantepie, 15 June, 1859, *Correspondance*, 4:320.

10. See Stendhal's journal of 1805, cited in Jules C. Alciatore, 'Stendhal et Pinel', *Modern Philology* 45 (1947): 118; and a letter Stendhal received in 1806, cited in V. Del Litto, *La vie intellectuelle de Stendhal* (Paris: Presses universitaires de France, 1959), 289 n. 76. For the full range of Stendhal's medical interests, see Jean Théodoridès, *Stendhal du côté de la science* (Aran [Switzerland]: Grand Chêne, 1972), ch. 5.

11. On Balzac's reading in technical medical sources, see, e.g., Madeleine Fargeaud, *Balzac et 'La Recherche de l'absolu'* (Paris: Hachette, 1968), 138–45. Monomania and monomaniacs make appearances in *Le Peau de chagrin*, *La Recherche de l'absolu*, *Eugénie Grandet*, *La Vieille Fille*, *Illusions perdues*, and *Pierrette*; on this point, see J.-L. Tritter, *Le langage philosophique dans les oeuvres de Balzac* (Paris: Nizet, 1976), 365.

12. A biographical sketch of Flaubert stressing his connections with the world of medicine can be found in Roger L. Williams, *The Horror of Life* (Chicago: University of Chicago Press, 1980), ch. 3.

13. See F. W. J. Hemmings, *Emile Zola*, 2nd edn (Oxford: Oxford University Press, 1966), 56–9.

14. See, for example, Archives de l'Assistance publique de Paris, Salpêtrière 6Q2–66 (5 March, 1880 to 18 February, 1881), nos 37691, 37717. Proust did not have a position at the Salpêtrière but in these and other instances functioned as the referring physician, arranging for the transfer of mentally ill patients from the Lariboisière Hospital.

15. Jean-Pierre Falret, 'Leçons faites à la Salpêtrière, 1850–51', reprinted in his *Des maladies mentales et des asiles d'aliénés* (Paris, 1864), 109–10, 139–40.

16. Jacques-Joseph Moreau (de Tours), *Du Hachisch et de l'aliénation mentale: Etudes psychologiques* (Paris, 1845), 20–1. Théophile Gautier's account, the feuilleton 'Le Hachisch', was originally published in *La Presse*, 10 July, 1843, and was subsequently reprinted in his *L'Orient*, 2 vols (Paris, 1877), 2:47–56.

17. Louis-François Lélut, *Poésies* (Paris, 1840), ix.

18. The phrase comes from Philippe Tissié, *Les Aliénés voyageurs: Essai médico-psychologique* (Paris, 1887), 58, in the context of a particularly baroque tale of the exploits of one of the 'travelling' lunatics referred to in the title.

19. Pierre Janet, *Etat mental des hystériques*, 2 vols (Paris, 1894): vol. 1: *Les stigmates mentaux*, 224–5.

20. Sigmund Freud and Josef Breuer, *Studies on Hysteria*, trans. James Strachey (New York: Avon, 1966), 201. The quotation comes from the 'Discussion' of the case of Elisabeth von R., one of the cases written by Freud.

21. See my discussion of the moral treatment in Jan Goldstein, *Console and Classify: The French Psychiatric Profession in the Nineteenth Century* (Cambridge and New York: Cambridge University Press, 1987), ch. 3.

22. One exception is the early nineteenth-century psychiatrist Charles-Chrétien-Henri Marc, who acknowledged that he experienced, though only on a single occasion during his life, feelings that helped him to develop the concepts of instinctive impulsion and transitory madness. 'I remember that, passing over the Pont-au-Change one day, and seeing sitting on the parapet a young stonemason who swung to and fro while eating his lunch, I was seized by the appalling desire to make him lose his balance and to hurl him into the river. This idea was only a flash; yet it inspired such horror in me that I rapidly crossed the street ... thus promptly distancing myself from the object that had given rise to that hideous passing fancy'; quoted in René Semelaigne, *Les Pionniers de la psychiatrie française avant et après Pinel*, 2 vols (Paris: J.-B. Baillière, 1930–32), 1:122.

23. The phrase is a doctor's: Landouzy, *Traité complet de l'hystérie*, 223, calls male hysteria 'un des points les plus délicats de la science'.

24. This information was supplied by a computer scan of the ARTFL (American and French Research on the Treasury of the French Language) textual database at the University of Chicago. The database includes the Louis Conard edition (Paris, 1926–54) of Flaubert's *Oeuvres complètes*.

25. Alcide Dusolier, 'M. Gustave Flaubert', in *Nos gens de lettres: Leur caractère et leurs oeuvres* (Paris, 1864), 59. The essay, primarily a review of *Salammbô*, first appeared in the *Revue française* on 1 January, 1863.

26. Reprinted in Charles Baudelaire, *Oeuvres complètes*, 15 vols (Paris: Conard, 1923–48), 4:404.

27. Charles Richet, 'Les Démoniaques d'aujourd'hui', *Revue des deux mondes* 37 (1880): 340–72, especially 348.

28. Ed. Dargez, 'La quinzaine d'un liseur', *Le Figaro*, 4 December, 1862, italics in the original. Dargez was not playing cruelly on Flaubert's own vulnerability to epileptoid seizures; this detail of Flaubert's biography was not made known to the public until Maxime Du Camp's

revelations in the *Revue des deux mondes* in 1881; see Williams, *Horror of Life*, 124. Nor was Dargez's usage entirely idiosyncratic; by the 1880s epileptic had become a term associated with the artistic style of the performers at the café concert. See Rae Beth Gordon, 'Le Caf'conc et l'hystérie', *Romantisme*, 64 (1989): 53–66.

29. Elme-Marie Caro, 'Gustave Flaubert', in his *Poètes et romanciers* (Paris, 1888), 266. The article was originally published in *La France*, 9 December, 1862.

30. René-Gaspard-Ernest Saint-René Taillandier, 'Le Réalisme épique dans le roman', *Revue des deux mondes*, 15 February, 1863, 852.

31. See Louyer-Villermé, 'Hystérie', 242, which mentions it last in a paragraph devoted to 'accidental symptoms'; and Pierre Briquet, *Traité clinique et thérapeutique de l'hystérie* (Paris, 1859), 412–4. On the other hand, neither Landouzy, *Traité complet de l'hystérie*, nor Jean-Louis Brachet, *Traité de l'hystérie* (Paris, 1847) include it in their chapters devoted to symptomatology.

32. Saint-René Taillandier, 'Réalisme épique', 854–5.

33. B. Jouvin, 'M. Gustave Flaubert: Salammbô', *Le Figaro*, 28 December, 1862.

34. Caro, 'Flaubert', 261.

35. Flaubert to Mlle Leroyer de Chantepie, 18 February, 1859, *Correspondance*, 4:314.

36. Flaubert to Ernest Feydeau, 29–30 November, 1859, *Correspondance*, 4:149.

37. Flaubert, 'Notes de lecture pour *Salammbô*; the reading programme also included ancient and modern works on slavery, astronomy, political economy and even serpents.

38. See Flaubert to his niece Caroline, 18 April, 1880, *Correspondance*, 9:23. Learning second-hand about Richet's 'Les Démoniaques d'aujourd'hui' (see note 27 above), which a friend had accurately described to him both as being 'about hysteria' and having 'praised me as a physician', Flaubert here accepts the friend's misinformation that Richet had 'cited *Salammbô* as proof'. In fact, the article discusses hysteria in *Madame Bovary* and makes no mention of *Salammbô*.

39. Quoted in Anne Green, *Flaubert and the Historical Novel: Salammbô Reassessed* (Cambridge, Cambridge University Press, 1982), 36, my italics.

40. Flaubert to Sainte-Beuve, December 1862, reprinted in Sainte-Beuve, *Nouveaux Lundis*, 4:437. The hysteria of Saint Theresa is mentioned in two medical sources with which Flaubert was almost certainly conversant: the article 'Hystérie' in the *Dictionnaire des sciences médicales* (23:235) and Briquet, *Traité clinique*, 409.

41. Flaubert to Mlle Leroyer de Chantepie, 18 February, 1859, *Correspondance*, 4:313. The same letter, cited earlier, goes on to mention Flaubert's researches into hysteria in connection with

Salammbô. Flaubert was very much a certain type of nineteenth-century Frenchman in the anticlericalism that marked his belief in the connection between piety and psychopathology. See his letter to Mlle Leroyer de Chantepie, 15 June, 1859: 'In rereading your last two letters..., I was sorry to see you so sad. Why do you persist in wanting to go to confession when the mere idea of it troubles you and the confessional itself occasions your relapses? Be, then, your own priest.... If I were your physician I would order an immediate visit to Paris, and if I were your spiritual director, I would forbid you access to the confessional.' (4:320).

42. Flaubert to Emile Zola, 3 June, 1874, *Correspondance,* 7:143.

43. My information is based on a computer search of the ARTFL database. I have added the critical letter to Sand of 1867 (not included in the Conard edition) to the tally.

44. The phrase comes from Pierre Giffard, *Les grands bazars* (Paris, 1882), 157.

45. See Flaubert to Sand, 29 September, 1866, in Flaubert and Sand, *Correspondance,* 81: 'The psychological sciences will stay where they lie – that is to say, in darkness and folly – insofar as they lack a precise nomenclature and the same expression can be employed to signify the most diverse ideas. When the categories are jumbled up, farewell moral philosophy!' (italics in the original).

46. The quoted phrase comes from the physician Pierre Briquet, who explicitly represents it as a hoary stereotype in need of renovation. See his *Traité clinique,* vii.

47. Flaubert to Emile Augier, 31 December, 1856, *Correspondance,* suppl. vol. l, 213–14.

48. Flaubert to Louise Colet, 8 April, 1852, *Correspondance,* 2:386–7. For the nerve-brass wire analogy, see Flaubert to Colet, 3 April, 1852, *ibid.,* 2:283. The 'lethargic' form of hysteria, as a variation on the standard form of the disease, is discussed in Brachet, *Traité de l'hystérie,* 285.

49. Flaubert to Sand, 12–13 January, 1867, Flaubert and Sand, *Correspondance,* 117–18.

50. Stéphane Mallarmé to Henri Cazalis, 18 February, 1869, in Mallarmé, *Correspondance, 1862–1871* (Paris: Gallimard, 1959), 301.

51. Flaubert, 'Notes de lecture pour *Salammbô',* 34.

52. I am here following the definition of androgyny set forth by Carolyn G. Heilbrun, *Toward a Recognition of Androgyny* (1973; New York: Norton, 1982), especially ix–x.

53. See Francis Steegmuller, *Flaubert and Madame Bovary: A Double Portrait,* rev. edn (Chicago: University of Chicago Press, 1977), 339, 341.

54. Charles Baudelaire, review of *Madame Bovary, Oeuvres complètes,* 4:400–4. I have combined elements of Paul de Man's translation of

this essay in the Norton Critical Edition of *Madame Bovary* (New York, 1965; see especially 339–41) with my own translation from the French.

55. *Ibid.*, 402. Imagination, says Baudelaire, is the masculine 'substitute' for 'what are called feelings' (*coeur*); the latter, entirely lacking a rational component, are 'generally predominant in women, as they are in animals'.

56. His use of the Academy to stand for professional medicine suggests that he may have been reading the two treatises on hysteria that had received prizes from that august institution and, hence, that he shared the taste for medical knowledge demonstrated by so many of his literary confrères. The relevant treatises, the most up-to-date books on the subject of hysteria before the appearance of Briquet's treatise in 1859, are Landouzy, *Traité complet de l'hystérie,* and Brachet, *Traité de l'hystérie* ; both bear on their title pages the notation 'Ouvrage couronné par l'Académie royale de médecine'. (Recipient of an award from the Royal Academy of Medicine.)

57. See, e.g., *Fusées* 23: 'J'ai cultivé mon hystérie avec jouissance et terreur' (I have cultivated my hysteria with pleasure and terror), an autobiographical note of 1862 in which hysteria is identified as a physical and psychological sensation of dizziness in face of an abyss (*gouffre*) and the latter is associated with such experiences as action, dreaming, memory and desire; Charles Baudelaire, *Ecrits intimes,* Jean-Paul Sartre (ed.) (Paris: Editions du point du jour, 1946), 32.

58. That Baudelaire would later point to the hysterical potentiality of action in *Fusées* (see note above) squares with this characterization of male hysteria in his review of *Madame Bovary.*

59. Baudelaire, review of *Madame Bovary,* 404–5, italics in the original.

60. Jean-Paul Sartre, *Search for a Method,* trans. Hazel E. Barnes (New York: Vintage, 1968), 140–1, italics in the original. Other commentators who have developed the androgyny theme are Dominick LaCapra, *Madame Bovary on Trial* (Ithaca, N.Y.: Cornell University Press, 1982), 179–82; and Naomi Schor, 'For a Restricted Thematics: Writing, Speech, and Difference in *Madame Bovary',* in her *Breaking the Chain: Women, Theory, and French Realist Fiction* (New York: Columbia University Press, 1985), 3–28.

61. Flaubert's own commentary on his novel stresses the super-masculinity of Mâtho and the super-femininity of Salammbô. In an early sketch for the novel, he succinctly described Mâtho as 'the real man' (*le vrai homme*); see Green, *Flaubert and the Historical Novel,* 37. In a letter to a critic after the publication of the book, he depicted the deity Tanit, of whom Salammbô is a devotee, as 'the goddess ... of love, of the female, humid, fecund element'; see Flaubert to Guillaume Froehner, 21 January, 1863, in *The Letters Of Gustave Flaubert,* Francis Steegmuller (ed. and trans.), 2 vols (Cambridge, Mass.: Harvard University Press, 1980–82), 2:55.

62. Gustave Flaubert, *Salammbô*, trans. A. J. Krailsheimer (Harmondsworth: Penguin Books, 1977), 169. I have altered the translation slightly.

63. B. F. Bart, 'Male Hysteria in *Salammbô*', *Nineteenth-Century French Studies* 12 (1984): 313–21.

64. Flaubert, *Salammbô*, 166.

65. *Ibid.*, 123.

66. BN Manuscrits, Nouvelles acquisitions françaises 23662, 198. On the ambiguity and 'undecidability' of the scene in the tent, see Bart, 'Male Hysteria in *Salammbô*', 317–19; and Naomi Schor, '*Salammbô* Unbound' in *Breaking the Chain*, especially 118–19.

67. The remarks, from Flaubert to Colet, 16 November, 1852, and an 1843 draft of *The Sentimental Education*, respectively, are quoted by Alphonse Jacobs, Flaubert and Sand, *Correspondance*, 49–50. The letter to Colet is particularly vicious in its sexual characterization of Sand's prose: 'In George Sand one perceives vaginal discharge (*fleurs blanches*); it oozes, and the idea runs between the words as between thighs without muscles.'

68. Flaubert to Sand, 12–13 November, 1866, in *ibid.*, 91–3.

69. The quotations come from an unsigned review of *Heures du soir, livre des femmes* – an anthology of women's writing to which Sand contributed under a male signature! – in *Le Figaro*, 20 May, 1833; and Jules Janin, 'Georges Sand', in *Biographies des femmes auteurs contemporaines françaises* (Paris, 1836). Both are cited in Leyla Ezdinli, 'George Sand's Literary Transvestism: Pre-texts and Contexts' (Ph.D. Dissertation, Princeton University, 1988).

70. For the four usages, see Flaubert to Sand, 12 February, 1863, March–May 1866, 15 May, 1866, and 8 September, 1866 in Flaubert and Sand, *Correspondance*, 55, 60, 63, 74.

71. Flaubert to Sand, 31 August, 1866, 21 September, 1866, in *ibid.*, 72, 75.

72. Flaubert to Sand, 22 September, 1866, in *ibid.*, 78.

73. George Sand, *Histoire de ma vie*, in Sand, *Oeuvres autobiographiques*, G. Lubin, (ed.) 2 vols (Paris: Gallimard-Pléiade, 1970) 1:869.

74. *Ibid.*, 964, my italics.

75. Sand to Flaubert, 23 October, 1866, in Flaubert and Sand, *Correspondance*, 86.

76. Sand to Flaubert, 8 December, 1866, in *ibid.*, 108.

77. Sand to Flaubert, 29 November, 1866, in *ibid.*, 102–3, italics in the original. Sand never mailed this letter, but instead sent another version of it, parallel in content, the next day.

78. Sand to Flaubert, 1 October, 1866, in *ibid.*, 84.

79. Flaubert to Sand, 23–24 January, 1867, in *ibid.*, 122.

80. *Ibid.*, 122, capital letter in the original.

81. Flaubert to Colet, 28 September, 1846, in *Correspondance*, 1:343, my italics. I have in most respects followed the excellent Steegmuller

translation, *Letters,* 1:81–2.

82. *Ibid.*

83. Flaubert to Colet, 12–13 April, 1854, in *ibid.,* 4:58.

84. For a typology of different varieties and subvarieties of the androgynous ideal, see Joyce Trebilcot, 'Two Forms of Androgynism', in Mary Vetterling-Braggin, (ed.), *'Femininity', 'Masculinity', and 'Androgyny': A Modern Philosophical Discussion* (Totowa, N.J.: Littlefield, Adams, 1982), 161–9, especially 164.

85. Sand to Flaubert, 15 January, 1867, in Flaubert and Sand, *Correspondance,* 120. A survey of the ten published works of George Sand included in the ARTFL database revealed two references to the term *hysteria,* both in the context of female religious experience: the reference in the *Histoire de ma vie* of 1855 (see note 73 above) and a similar one some 20 years before in the novel *Lélia* (1833): 'The naive poetry of primitive ages, the voluptuous canticles of Solomon ... sometimes seemed to me more religious in their sublime nakedness than the mystical pantings and fanatical hysterias of Saint Theresa.'

86. Sand to Flaubert, 15 January, 1867, in *ibid.,* 120.

87. *Fusées* 14, for example, indicates that Baudelaire had been reading the 1856 monograph of the psychiatrist Alexandre-Jacques-François Brierre de Boismont, *Du suicide et de la folie suicide.* See also my speculative gloss on his reference to the Academy of Medicine in his review of *Madame Bovary,* note 56 above.

88. See, on this point, A. J. L. Busst, 'The Image of the Androgyne in the Nineteenth Century', in Ian Fletcher, (ed.), *Romantic Mythologies* (New York: Barnes & Noble, 1967), 1–95, especially 3–4 and, on early nineteenth-century France, 12–39.

89. Maxime Du Camp, *Mémoires d'un suicidé* (1853; new edn Paris, 1876), 256. Du Camp's diagnosis of Jean-Marc, the *suicidé* of the title, is found in the 1876 'Avertissement de cette nouvelle édition', vii, but it is entirely consistent with the description of Jean-Marc's malady in the original text. For the hysterical component, see, e.g., his dreaminess, mild catalepsy, sense of being inhabited by a demon, and tendency to ecstasy (46–7).

90. See Georget's dictionary article 'Hystérie', 541. On the scientific influences on Georget, see Goldstein, *Console and Classify,* 245–57.

91. See, e.g., Dr Mahot, 'Observation chez l'homme des phénomènes dits hystériques', *Journal de la section de médecine de la Société académique de Nantes et du Département de la Loire-Inférieure* 15 (1839): 114–23, which cites Georget (115) but in the end comes out in favour of the uterine theory of hysteria, regarding the hysteria in a 20-year old mason as the result of a spinal lesion caused by a work accident and pointing out 'the close sympathies by which the spine is linked to the uterus' (120); Dr Mouchet, 'Note sur un cas d'hystérie chez l'homme', *Gazette médicale de Paris,* 3rd ser., 3 (1848): 167–8, which concludes, 'The careful observation of this patient seems to decide in

favour of Georget, who placed the seat of hysteria in the brain'; and H. Desterne, hospital intern, 'De l'hystérie chez l'homme', *Union médicale* 2 (28 September, 1848): 455–7, which depicts its project as using clinical data to defend the thesis of Georget *et al.* against proponents of the 'dogmatic' uterine hypothesis.

92. Briquet, *Traité clinique*, vii, 126

93. *Ibid.*, 598–604.

94. *Ibid.*, 51.

95. *Ibid.*, 47, 48.

96. These points are discussed in Jan Goldstein, 'The Hysteria Diagnosis and the Politics of Anticlericalism in Late Nineteenth-Century France', *Journal of Modern History* 54 (1982): 209–39; an expanded version of that discussion appears in *Console and Classify*, ch. 9.

97. Mark S. Micale, 'Diagnostic Discriminations: Jean-Martin Charcot and the Nineteenth-Century Idea of Masculine Hysterical Neurosis' (Ph.D. Dissertation, Yale University, 1987). Some of Charcot's published work on male hysteria was recently collected and reprinted; see Michèle Ouerd, (ed.), *Jean-Martin Charcot, Leçons sur l'hystérie virile* (Paris: Le Sycomore, 1984).

98. Jean-Martin Charcot, 'Leçon d'ouverture', *Progrès médical* 10 (1882): 336.

99. The link between Charcot's claims of universality and his emphasis on male hysteria is made by Kenneth Levin, 'Freud's Paper "On Male Hysteria" and the Conflict between Anatomical and Physiological Models', *Bulletin of the History of Medicine* 48 (1974): 377–97, especially 381–2. I built upon Levin's argument, explicitly tying it to Charcot's commitment to positivism and to the political connotations of positivism, in 'Hysteria Diagnosis', 234.

100. See, e.g., Jean-Martin Charcot, *Leçons du mardi à la Salpêtrière*, 2 vols (Paris, 1889), 2:36, 50.

101. C. R. (Mme C. Renooz), 'Charcot dévoilé', *Revue scientifique des femmes* 1 (December, 1888): 241–7, especially 241–5. The dissertation in question was written by Caroline Schulze. Charcot likewise used the occasion of the January 1889 defence of Blanche Edwards' dissertation, 'De l'hémiplégie dans quelques affections nerveuses', to remark that female doctors should confine themselves to the treatment of women and children; see Mélanie Lipinska, *Histoire des femmes médecins depuis l'antiquité jusqu'à nos jours* (Paris: G. Jacques, 1900), 426, n. 2.

102. Jean-Martin Charcot, *Leçons sur les maladies du système nerveux faites à la Salpêtrière*, 3 vols (Paris, 1877), 3:252–3. Charcot notes here that all female hysteria does not follow the 'capricious' model. But he made his point about the basic difference between male and female hysterics repeatedly, observing more than a decade later, 'I have already remarked many times that one should not expect to encounter in men that morbid brio so frequent in reality in women';

Leçons du mardi, 2:50.

103. Michèle Ouerd, introduction to Charcot, *Leçons sur l'hystérie virile,* stresses the class background of Charcot's male hysterics; so does Micale, 'Diagnostic Discriminations', which also discusses Charcot's Jewish and Arab cases. One late-nineteenth-century medical student researching male hysteria at the Necker Hospital found the disease most common among members of the liberal professions; see Auguste Klein, 'De l'hystérie chez l'homme' (Doctoral diss., Paris Faculty of Medicine, 1880), 14. But although Charcot cited Klein's work in support of the male hysteria diagnosis, Klein's specific sociological results did not, tellingly enough, affect the way Charcot represented the population of male hysterics.

104. Michèle Ouerd makes the fascinating point that the wandering uterus motif of traditional hysteria was replicated by the unrooted, vagrant and marginal social status of the male hysterics that predominated in Charcot's late case studies; see her introduction to Charcot, *Leçons sur l'hystérie virile,* 27–8. On the linkage of women and the lower classes in the context of a scientific and stigmatizing rhetoric in nineteenth-century France, see Susanna Barrows, *Distorting Mirrors: Visions of the Crowd in Late Nineteenth-Century France* (New Haven: Yale University Press, 1981), ch. 2; and Ruth Harris, 'Murder under Hypnosis in the Case of Gabrielle Bompard: Psychiatry in the Courtroom in Belle Epoque Paris', in W. F. Bynum, Roy Porter and Michael Shepherd, (eds), *The Anatomy of Madness: Essays in the History of Psychiatry,* 2 vols (London: Tavistock, 1985), 2:219–20. On the linkage of women and the Orient in nineteenth-century French discourse, see Edward W. Said, *Orientalism* (New York: Vintage, 1979), 182, 186–8.

105. Jean-Martin Charcot, 'Contracture hystérique et aimants' (1878), in *Oeuvres complètes,* 9 vols (Paris, 1888–94) 9:277, my italics.

106. Goldstein, 'Hysteria Diagnosis'; and *Console and Classify,* ch. 9.

107. Quoted in Louis Legrand, *L'influence du positivisme dans l'oeuvre scolaire de Jules Ferry* (Paris: Rivière, 1961), 118.

108. This argument is made by Debora L. Silverman, *Art Nouveau in Fin-de-Siècle France: Politics, Psychology, and Style* (Berkeley and Los Angeles: University of California Press, 1989), ch. 4.

109. See, e.g., Jules Falret, 'Discussion de la folie raisonnante', *Annales médico-psychologiques,* 4th ser., 7 (1866): especially 404–7; Charles Lasègue, 'Les Hystériques, leur perversité, leurs mensonges', *ibid,* 6th ser., 6 (1881): 111–18; and, on the mild hysteria of normal women, Richet, 'Les Démoniaques d'aujourd'hui', 346. Richet's point was cited in the work of Charcot's student Henri Huchard, 'Caractère, moeurs, état mental des hystériques', *Archives de neurologie* 3 (1882): 206.

110. Wolf Lepenies, *Between Literature and Science: The Rise of Sociology,* trans. R. J. Hollingdale (Cambridge: Cambridge University Press,

1988), especially introduction. Lepenies makes this case for France, England and Germany.

111. See Elaine Showalter, 'Critical Cross-Dressing: Male Feminists and the Woman of the Year', *Raritan* 3 (Fall 1983): 130–49, especially 138.

112. An overview and bibliography of this debate can be found in William Veeder, *Mary Shelley and Frankenstein: The Fate of Androgyny* (Chicago: University of Chicago Press, 1986), 234–5.

7

From Religious to Bio-Medical Anti-Semitism: The Career of Jules Soury•

Toby Gelfand

> Je voudrais bien vous répondre, mais je n'ose. Vous ne consentirez
> pas à discuter avec moi. Et comme vous êtes médecin – car vous
> êtes tout, vous savez tout, et c'est ce qui m'effraye, – vous voudrez
> me guérir au lieu de me pursuader.[1]

> ...a short man with piercing eyes under white eyelashes, the fresh
> face of a child, a mouth twisted by the crooked smile of a wicked
> puppet: 'Monsieur,' he says to me, 'I am a psychologist of history,
> that's who I am ... my life is given over entirely to experiments....'

Thus, Edmond de Goncourt described his introduction to Jules
Soury in February, 1879.[2] At age 36, Soury was a well-known writer
and literary and scientific journalist for several leading Paris
newspapers and reviews.

Two decades later, at the turn of the twentieth century, Soury
had become the most knowledgeable authority in France on the
anatomy and physiology of the central nervous system, a reputation
consecrated by his publication in 1899 of a monumental work. *Le
système nerveux central, structure et fonction. Histoire critique des
théories et des doctrines* (two volumes totalling nearly 2,000 pages)
brought together the substance of lectures Soury had been giving
since 1881 at the Ecole Pratique des Hautes Etudes. After reviewing
the development of knowledge of the nervous system since antiquity,
Soury devoted detailed discussion to recent decades and especially to
the vast literature on cerebral localization since 1870. The aim of the
book, he announced, was to lay bare the 'anatomical and
physiological history of intelligence ... it is the natural history of the
human mind'.[3] It was also, perhaps not surprisingly given the exhaus-
tive synthesis it represented, his last major scientific publication.

But Soury was not quite finished writing. While the author of *Le système nerveux central* was still collecting plaudits for his magnum opus, including prizes from the academies of sciences and medicine, he launched a second rather different intellectual last testament. *Campagne Nationaliste 1899–1901* (1902) consisted of essays and letters Soury had written at the height of the Dreyfus Affair as well as a revealing autobiography entitled 'Ma vie'. Dedicated to General Mercier, 'for contributing more than any other Frenchman to the two condemnations ... of the Jew traitor Alfred Dreyfus', *Campagne Nationaliste* situated Soury in the company of the most virulent anti-Semites of the day, anti-Dreyfusards such as Edouard Drumont, Maurice Barrès and Charles Maurras to whom he addressed the published letters and essays.[4]

To a greater extent than these non-academic writers and journalists, Soury insisted upon theories of biological and racial inferiority of Jews. His aim to anchor anti-Semitic polemic in biomedical discourse was underscored by a display of academic credentials unusual in a personal work of this sort. Soury included his academic rank and affiliation as *directeur d'études* at the Sorbonne under his name on the title page, along with a long list of scholarly oeuvres on the facing page. He made use of recondite neurological 'facts' about Jews, such as recently identified Tay-Sachs disease (which had escaped mention three years earlier in the immense *Le système nerveux central*) to buttress his argument.

Campagne Nationaliste had a certain shock impact, not so much for its racial opinions (which could be found elsewhere), but for its disconcerting and ostentatious deployment of medical science and its exploitation of the author's position in a *grande école.* Previously regarded as someone who eschewed public issues in favour of abstract ideas, one who preferred à retreat within the university to worldly interests, Soury came out of his anti-Semitic closet with a vengeance. In a book-length rebuttal of *Campagne Nationaliste,* the socialist Eugene Fournière expressed regret that an uncontested master of science had strayed from laboratory and library.[5] Joseph Reinach, a leading Dreyfusard and author of a multi-volume history of the Affair, condemned Soury's abuse of his role as a 'high mandarin of letters' and classed him among the 'doctors of nationalism' who had embraced the false science of race.[6] Reinach noted Soury's long-standing materialism and atheism. He also speculated, basing himself on hearsay, that Soury's anti-Semitism arose from professional spite.

We shall see later that this rumour was probably well-founded.

But, whatever the personal roots of Soury's hatred of Jews, I shall argue that the significance of his case lies in the intimate and logical grounding of Soury's anti-Semitism in his conception of science. Both Reinach and Fournière suggested the linkage, but then fell back on explanations in terms of 'false science', misapplication of biology to social and political questions, or simply the idiosyncratic and perverse ideas of a bizarre individual who happened to be a savant as well.

Late nineteenth-century Frenchmen, especially those of liberal Republican and positivist convictions, had difficulties associating the rebirth of anti-Semitism in their country with the putatively neutral, progressive and universalist realm of science. Whatever particular explanations they offered for the recrudescence of anti-Semitism – economic, political, religious or ethnic – the causes and furthering conditions were assumed to be socio-cultural. Theories of race, to the extent that they were taken into account, tended to be seen as epiphenomenal and, in any case, as importations from Germany rather than indigenous to France.[7]

In 1898, however, Ferdinand Brunetière, the influential conservative editor of the *Revue des Deux Mondes*, blamed 'intellectuals' (a recent and pejorative group designation) as a whole and scientists in particular for the rise of anti-Semitism. Over the course of the century, anthropologists and ethnographers, followed by linguists and then historians and literary critics, had invented and propagated the concept of race and racial hierarchies to the point where 'animal hatreds, physiological hatreds, blood hatreds' had become commonplace. They were responsible for the virulent anti-Semitism that had escalated the case of the arrest, trial and condemnation of an obscure Jewish army captain into the *Affaire Dreyfus*. Its most recent manifestation, the crisis following Zola's *J'accuse* (13 January, 1898) and his trial, divided France and threatened to bring down the Republic.[8]

Brunetière, who had built a reputation for deploring the cultural consequences of science, lacks credibility as an objective critic. He coupled his attack on science with a political denunciation of the intellectuals who, as individuals, he thought, had no right to challenge the collective authority of army, state and church, nor to assert a privileged capacity as scientists to weigh evidence and make rational judgements. He was effectively countered by the sociologist Emile Durkheim and the chemist Emile Duclaux, both active Dreyfusards.[9]

Nevertheless, Brunetière's general point, if not the way he argued it, deserves consideration. We know little about how professional scientists or medical professionals aligned themselves with respect to race and specifically to the rise of anti-Semitic ideology. As Durkheim himself might have approached it, the problem is one where the sociology of the professions and anti-Semitism intersect, and it is in principle susceptible to empirical investigation.

Medical scientists, as a group, cannot be expected to have been as outspoken about race as public leaders or men of letters. But ample sources, such as the various petitions and subscription lists published during the Dreyfus Affair, are available from which medical opinion could be sounded.[10] One might further inquire, as has been done for the literary field, whether and how doctors' opinions on the Jewish question during the Dreyfus Affair related to the content of their science and the career niches they occupied within their profession. Who employed, for example, concepts of hereditary determinism in an anti-Semitic context?[11]

I examine Soury's career to see how he came to forge his synthesis of science and racial anti-Semitism. Using the case study approach, I seek to raise the general problem of the relationship between science and racism and their respective practitioners in *fin- de-siècle* France (as has been done for example with the milieux of literary writers and academic historians at the time of the Affair).[12]

Such questions are easier put than even to begin to answer. Soury's biological racism admittedly represents an extreme example, and he was in many ways a bizarre figure whose personal idiosyncrasies cannot be pursued here. Yet, despite the atypicality of Soury's career, it suggests more than a casual connection between medical epistemology of the period and the constitution of racial beliefs about Jews during the last decades of the 19th century. And he was not without influence on his contemporaries, notably on Maurice Barrès, the foremost proponent of nationalism and anti-Semitism at the time of the Dreyfus Affair.[13]

In what follows, I reconstruct Soury's career using his early writings and unpublished correspondence; I suggest that Soury's doctrines came from three principal sources: first, a consistent commitment to a universally applicable determinism and extreme reductionism evident from his earliest publications; second, adventitious circumstances resulting in an abrupt mid-life career transition; and third, his immersion in a bio-clinical discourse on race in the broader context of the rise of anti-Semitism in France during the 1880s.[14]

Jules-Auguste Soury was born in 1842 into an artisan family living on the Rue Saint-Julien-le-Pauvre in what is now the V⁽ᵉ⁾ arrondissement of Paris.[15] The son and grandson of glass workers, Soury, at first a recalcitrant student, began an apprenticeship in the family métier. But, at age 17, he embarked on an academic career, entering the lycée Louis le Grand and going on to complete his university degree in 1863. In 1867, he earned a diploma of archivist palaeographer from the Ecole des Chartes with a thesis on hebraic studies in medieval Western Christendom. A student of Ernest Renan (1823–1892), Soury followed his master in focusing on the history of the ancient Middle East and comparative religion. In return for service to Renan, the famous scholar helped his disciple obtain a modest librarian's job at the Bibliothèque Nationale.[16]

After the events of 1870–71, Soury, who had been sympathetic to the Commune but absent from Paris, returned to the Bibliothèque Nationale. Renan's continuing patronage and that of Léon Gambetta, the leading politician on the left in the Third Republic, secured him affiliations as a critical reviewer with newspapers such as *Le Temps, La Republique Française,* Gambetta's newly-founded daily and elsewhere.

By the end of the 1870s, Soury could claim authorship of 12 volumes of criticism ranging over an impressive array of scholarly disciplines and languages. Widely respected for his erudition and prose style, his flamboyant atheism and materialism made him a controversial figure as well.[17]

Although Soury's interests included the biological sciences, the bulk of his writings at this stage of his career dealt with the historical criticism of religion. Here one can find his early views on the subject of the Jews and race. 'The miserable race of Israel', Soury exclaimed in a note to Renan, had suffered persecutions through the centuries. He pitied the Jew but he could never bring himself to love the eternal exile whom he viewed as parasitic upon all nations.[18] In his *Etudes historiques sur les religions* (1877), Soury evoked the millennial struggle between Aryan and Semite and the inferiority of the latter, by then a banal thesis that Renan had popularized in the mid-1850s. 'Our race, [is] the Aryan race which has created science and quickly conquered the entire earth from the other human races';[19] the following year in his *Essais de critique réligieuse,* he urged readers not to forget 'our spiritual ancestors, the fathers whose language we speak and whose spirit lives again in us were Aryan peoples, Romans, Greeks, Germans, and Slavs – and not the Semitic horde of Israel. For those who possess Homer, Aristotle and Lucretius, the Bible is a useless thing....'[20]

While patently anti-Semitic, Soury's views and the idiom in which they were expressed, were scarcely innovative. They reflected earlier Biblical criticism and, beyond that, the anti-clericalism of the Enlightenment which enjoyed popularity with Republican intellectuals. Elsewhere in his literary reviews, Soury could write of the Jews of the German ghetto with something approaching nostalgia.[21] As a competent historian, he recognized that the Graeco-Roman pagan religions inherited much from their earlier Semitic counterparts and that the Aryan and Semitic races had enjoyed 'fertile contacts'.[22] The young Soury appears to have stridently disliked contemporary Jews, and he was prepared to claim that the hereditary distinctiveness of Jews outweighed any changes in their character that new social and political conditions might bring.[23] His mature anti-Semitic doctrine, however, would incorporate sources beyond these vulgar prejudices mixed with historical erudition. The discourse of the natural sciences provided the basis for his later biological anti-Semitism.

Ernest Renan once declared that if given the opportunity to begin his career again, he might have chosen the natural over the religious sciences. After 1881, Jules Soury, in a sense, lived out Renan's wish.[24] But Soury did not need to begin a second career; his critical essays from the early 1870s extended to the realm of the biological and medical sciences. 'The Ecole des Chartes leads to everything', he wrote, in praise of the school that had taught him how to analyse documents 'whether it be a question ... of a cartulary, an animal or vegetable cell, a crystal, etc., the method remains the same for all sciences based upon observation'.[25] To those who accused Soury of being a mere compiler and critic of the research of others, he replied rhetorically by asking whether Aristotle had ever done anything other than synthesizing the knowledge of his time. And he compared his relationship to Renan with that of Aristotle, the scientist, to Plato, the philosopher.[26]

Soury's exposure to science in fact went beyond the confines of archives and library. In the mid-1860s, concurrently with his training at the Ecole des Chartes, he attended clinics and laboratories at the Salpêtrière Hospital. There, under the tutelage of two physicians, the alienist, Auguste Voisin and, especially, the neurologist, Jules Luys, Soury had opportunities for direct study of the nervous system and mental diseases such as would be available to advanced medical students.[27]

His long critical review of Hippolyte Taine's *De l'Intelligence* (1870) demonstrated Soury's commitment to extreme reductionism in psychology. The study of the soul, he wrote, belonged to the physiologist, not to the philosopher: the causes of all manifestations of intelligence were to be sought in the 'gray substance of the convolutions of the encephalon'.[28] In subsequent years, Soury would continue to probe these convolutions with the dissecting knife and examine them under the microscope as well as keep abreast of the scholarly literature. Already, in 1873, he was prepared to fault Taine for not devoting enough attention to the organic neuro-anatomical foundations of intelligence; he thought it a 'great shame' that Taine had failed to use Jules Luys' *Recherches sur le système nerveux cérébro-spinal.*[29]

From at least the early 1870s, then, as he remarked to a correspondent in 1874, Soury kept himself 'au courant of everything going on in the domain of comparative anatomy and physiology'.[30] His reviews for *Le Temps* reflected a command of the scientific literature; at *La République Française,* the science editor, Paul Bert, claimed Soury's services from the historical section. When Ernst Haeckel, the German champion of Darwin visited Paris in 1878, it was Jules Soury who delivered the after-dinner speech at the banquet in Haeckel's honour, and who in the next few years translated three of his biological works.[31]

Thus poised between the religious sciences and the sciences of life, the future direction of Soury's scholarly career would have been difficult to predict at the outset of the 1880s. His most controversial work to date, the scandalous *Jésus et les Evangiles* (1878), which portrayed the founding figure of Christianity as a victim of general paralysis of the insane, attempted to synthesize religious history with neurology.[32] Although, by this time, Soury had achieved recognition in diverse fields, he earned his living as a minor functionary and sometime journalist who had to cope with economic hardship and, perhaps more gravely from his perspective, the fragmentation of his intellectual energy.

Such problems found a sudden favourable resolution in 1881 when he was named to the seminar course he would teach for more than 30 years, until virtually the end of his life. At the time Soury expressed satisfaction with his appointment at the Ecole Pratique des Hautes Etudes.[33] And he continued at various times to boast of his priority in introducing the 'practical study of physiological psychology' into French higher education. Destiny, it would appear, and he explicitly asserted, had dictated an original role for him in the domain of the natural sciences rather than a continuation of his work in the history of religion, a field where the accomplishments of illustrious predecessors made a pioneering impact impossible.[34]

Yet Soury's career transition was not nearly as smooth as the public record suggests. He had in fact suffered a humiliating rejection of his bid for a much more prestigious chair which he badly wanted at the Collège de France. And even the modest appointment to the

Ecole Pratique des Hautes Etudes met with concerted initial opposition and enduring isolation from his colleagues.

In 1879, Soury's left-wing patrons, Gambetta and Paul Bert, secured funds for a new chair in the history of religions at the Collège de France, an appointment whose anti-clerical mandate appeared all the more provocative as the nomination was known to be promised to the author of *Jésus et les Evangiles*. During a debate within the Chambre des députés which resulted in approval of a budget for the post, Paul Bert joked that the chair ought really to be called the 'history of comparative mythologies'; his opponents on the right railed against the designation of a 'savant notorious for his anti-religious passions' and identified Soury without naming him by quoting the opening sentence from his *Essais de critique réligieuse* (1878): 'atheism and scientific materialism have inspired these studies: that is the spirit that pervades them and the breath which animates them'.[35] Again, a few months later, in the Senate, Jules Ferry, the minister of Public Instruction, had to defend the establishment of the chair against opposition from the right wing, including a spokesman from the Collège de France, by promising to name a prestigious scholar and not a polemicist.[36] Meanwhile, a private note, probably written by Paul Bert, addressed to a friend in the ministry, sought to allay anxieties over how Soury might conduct the course and vouched for his scholarship: 'he read me his programme, which is excellent and consists in a truly new interpretation of the title of the chair'.[37]

Nevertheless, in January 1880, the Ministry of Public Instruction named someone else to the chair at the Collège de France. Soury's fury at his own rejection is fully conveyed in an extraordinary letter he addressed on 20 March, 1880, evidently to Jules Ferry, himself. 'M. le ministre', he began: 'recall, if you would, recall, if you have already forgotten it, that in taking away my chair at the Collège de France, in breaking my career, you have done me as much harm as one man can do to another, short of dishonouring him.'[38] Soury continued that he considered himself 'one of the countless victims of your article 7', this a reference to a controversial provision in Ferry's global educational reform project that would have forbade members of religious orders to teach in the university. To placate clerical opposition to his educational reforms, Ferry had sacrificed article 7 and, Soury believed, his promised appointment as well.[39] Alternatively beseeching and threatening the minister, Soury demanded 'some compensation in your vast province of public instruction', a post commensurate with his intellectual abilities and prolific record of scholarly achievement. Specifically, he suggested that ministerial reparation should take the form of 'a modest chair of psychology' at the Ecole des Hautes Etudes:

> if not, I tell you very frankly, as a gallant man who salutes his adversary before striking, – if not I shall bring all these facts before the public – the complete dossier on the *Histoire d'une chaire*, and I shall do it with so much simplicity and eloquence, inspired by justice and rectitude, that, minister and legislator though you may be, I shall break you like glass under my pen.[40]

Soury ended his long harangue by urging the minister to create a new course for him without further delay, 'with a stroke of the pen', and to ignore the objections which were sure to come from the directors of the Ecole des Hautes Etudes. For his part, he would be ready to begin teaching 'psychology or the history of philosophy' within two weeks.

Soury in fact had to wait another 20 months before his patron, Paul Bert, who had succeeded to the post of Minister of Public Instruction in the new Gambetta ministry, came through with an appointment. On 30 November, 1881, 14 days after the advent of the Gambetta government, Soury was named *maître de conférences* responsible for a course on 'history of psychological doctrines' at the Ecole Pratique des Hautes Etudes.[41] In the interval between rejection and success, he strengthened his academic status as well as his credentials in the natural sciences by earning a doctorate, sustaining two theses on biological subjects, which attracted favourable attention.[42] In early December he began the bi-weekly seminar course which served as the basis for a growing reputation as an avant-garde professor and from which all his subsequent publications on the nervous system flowed. With a spartan but secure annual salary of 4,000 francs from the Ecole, Soury was able to abandon the despised marginal position at the Bibliothèque Nationale, (although he managed to keep his stipend of 3,000 francs there too).[43] He curtailed his contributions to the popular press and ceased publishing on the history of religion. All seemed to have ended well.

But the events of 1879–81 revealed and doubtless exacerbated a capacity for violent invective replete with metaphors of physical violence and revenge in Soury. He continued to vituperate privately in a letter to Anatole France a decade later and finally publicly in his autobiography of 1902 over the injustice he felt over the deprivation of 'his chair'.[44] Although he had escaped the disaster of the 'broken career' he had feared, Soury believed he still did not enjoy due recognition from his colleagues.

Nor were these feelings of discrimination entirely without foundation. As he had predicted, the Ecole des Hautes Etudes did not welcome him into its ranks. Within days of Soury's appointment, the members of the section to which he had been assigned protested *en bloc* against the nomination of the new historian of psychology. The petition to the minister of public instruction signed by 22 distinguished members of section IV of the Ecole (section of history and philology) opposed the mode of nomination by ministerial fiat, the subject matter of psychology and the likelihood that his proposed 'course' would attract too many students; they suggested that Soury be assigned to another section, that of the natural sciences.[45] Soury himself hoped to find a more congenial home in the Ecole, perhaps a new section of 'philosophical and sociological sciences'.[46] But he remained attached to the IVᵉ section, 'annexed' rather than officially recognized, not promoted until 1897 nor even listed until then in the section's annual reports or its course notices.[47]

The ambitious Soury thus remained in a marginal position professionally. Was this the basis for the 'pedantic rancour' Joseph Reinach later associated with Soury's anti-Semitism?[48] It is, of course, not possible to say for sure. But among the scholars from the Ecole who petitioned against Soury's appointment, there were at least five influential Jewish signatories.[49] Perhaps more telling was the naming of the liberal Protestant minister and scholar, Albert Réville (1826–1906) to the chair at the Collège de France originally intended for Soury. In his letter to Ferry, Soury denounced the successful candidate as 'an ignorant and unknown pastor'. The assumed conspiratorial link between Jews, Protestants, and Freemasons would shortly become a staple of French anti-Semitic discourse, then in germination.[50] Ironically, Réville, who made a great success of the chair of History of Religions at the College and became president of the new Vᵉ section of Religious Sciences at the Ecole des Hautes Etudes a few years later, emerged as a prominent Dreyfusard just before Jules Soury came out publicly on the other side at the end of the century.[51]

Soury, as we have seen, held and published anti-Semitic views before 1880. In Taine's famous tripartite formula – race, milieu, and moment – Soury's deep-rooted and commonplace prejudices against Jews, probably 'inherited', that is to say, learned from his family Catholic background, may be likened to the racial component as a determinant of his anti-Semitism. The milieu – an emerging bio-medical discourse on the Jewish race – presented Soury with a novel terrain and, ultimately, a powerful expressive idiom for his anti-Semitism.

This discourse was available at the outset of the 1880s when the anti-Semitic movement began to gather strength in France launched by economic hard times and reacting against the first substantial influx of Eastern European Jews who appeared strikingly different physically as well as culturally from assimilated French Jews. Soury's definitive career move from religious sciences to an exclusive devotion to the history of the biological and, specifically, the neurological sciences, thus mirrored in microcosm and coincided in time with similar changes within the discourse on Jews.

Perhaps, as I have suggested, a sense of personal grievance, hostility and professional isolation following the traumatic rejection in 1880, contributed to Soury's anti-Semitism. In any event, there was no turning back on the career shift, nor, if we can trust Soury's later testimony, no regrets for a 'destiny' now linked to the study of the natural sciences. Soury's manuscript notes introducing his inaugural lecture in December 1881 at the Ecole des Hautes Etudes made explicit his intention to follow a rigorously biological approach to the subject at hand.[52] He now had a forum to put into practice the advice he had given in the review of Taine's *L'Intelligence* eight years earlier.

The third element, Taine's 'moment', the timely, but in a deeper sense fortuitous, occasion for the public espousal of anti-Semitism came for Soury, as for many others, with the explosion of the Dreyfus Affair at the end of the century. For our purpose, the basic problem for interpretation is the move from milieu to moment. What was the connection between the two and how can one offer a plausible reconstruction of Soury's merger of the 'moment' of the Affair, which triggered the raging anti-Semitism of his *Campagne Nationaliste,* with the 'milieu' of his previous two decades of scholarly devotion to knowledge of the central nervous system? To understand Soury's conflation of scientific knowledge and racial anti-Semitism, one must locate him in the context of bio-medical discourse on the Jews during the 1880s. Only then does his particular case take on meaning, and, more important, it provides entrée into the scientism of the early Third Republic, an aspect of that culture which conferred upon Soury considerable status and even fashionability in intellectual circles.

The association of Jewish difference with essential biological differences had venerable antecedents going back at least to the race's supposed immunity to the Black Death in the fourteenth-century.[53] With the ascendancy of the concept of race in science after about the mid-nineteenth century, a systematic bio-medical discourse on Jews made its appearance. Demographers and statisticians examined the question of superior Jewish vitality while medical geographers discussed characteristic immunities or enhanced resistance to certain infections. On a darker note, anthropologists and clinicians debated the dangers of consanguineous marriage, which was prevalent among Jews, and noted increased tendencies towards a wide range of pathological conditions including skin and eye diseases, diabetes, and a variety of nervous and mental ailments.[54]

The anthropological society of Paris tended to resist biological constructs of a Jewish race, citing the extensive intermingling of Aryans and Semites over the centuries.[55] As well, anatomical measures, such as the famous cephalic index, proved an inconsistent guide to racial difference despite efforts by anthropologists like Georges Vacher de la Pouge to construct racial psychologies from the data of physical anthropology.[56] By the early 1880s other scholars in the historical sciences like Ernest Renan were turning away from stereotypes they had helped to create. Renan, deeply concerned over the spectre of rising mass anti-Semitism, lent his tremendous prestige to defending the contribution of the Jewish religion to history and to denying validity to the notion of contemporary Jews as a race. Even in his famous distinction between Aryan and Semite propounded three decades earlier, and often cited by anti-Semites, Renan had rejected physiological differences between these two races.[57]

Bio-clinical evidence appealed strongly to those who saw race as the primordial category with which evident cultural diversity might be reduced to differences in nature. Diseases, particularly those of a serious chronic nature, could be read as manifestations of a person's or a people's otherwise secret bodily nature and organization. The inner language of pathology, transmitted by heredity over the genera-tions, seemed a more reliable affirmation of race doctrine and sign of racial identity than either philology or visible anatomical conformation. Causal factors intrinsic to the blood or to the organization of the central nervous system were more powerful (and certainly more difficult to challenge) than crude and increasingly dubious evidence from physical anthropology. On this view, disease, an otherwise inexplicable, seemingly arbitrary event, gained meaning as a revealer of constitutional type, familial, and, at times, racial identity.[58]

Among French clinicians who linked Jews as a race with a pattern of pathology, the most influential was Jean-Martin Charcot (1825–1893), one of the world's most respected authorities on diseases of the nervous system. In 1881, Charcot consolidated his medical faculty professorship with the hospital courses in neuropathology he had been teaching for 15 years by obtaining appointment to a new Faculty chair in diseases of the nervous system.

Custom designed to suit his needs at the Salpêtrière, an enormous hospice for women, many of whom suffered from chronic nervous and mental ailments, Charcot's new chair, like Soury's, originated by ministerial fiat rather than from collegial or institutional demand. Indeed the coincidences between the two foundations of teaching chairs dealing with the nervous system within several months of one another and the government personalities involved in each – Gambetta was a personal acquaintance of Charcot's, and Paul Bert, his professional colleague – are striking.[59]

Whatever similarities there may have been between the consecration of an international medical celebrity and the placating of an irascible philosopher should not obscure the fact that Charcot's enterprise at the Salpêtrière was of an altogether grander magnitude, and endowed with correspondingly vast material as well as human resources. Under the leadership of Charcot, the Salpêtrière developed into a 'school', to use the label most contemporaries accorded to its conceptual as well as institutional dominance over the field.

Charcot's reticence on matters of scientific theory and political ideology also contrasted with Soury's hostility towards Jews and his formulation of racial biology. Unlike Soury, Charcot never published anything overtly anti–Semitic, and he died before the Dreyfus Affair might have provoked him into one camp or the other.[60] But, at the same time as Soury shelved his explicit racialism, to devote himself wholly to doctrines of neurophysiology at the Ecole des Hautes Etudes, the new professor of clinical diseases of the nervous system began to mention Jews. Charcot's first clinical observations on Jewish patients appeared soon after he inaugurated his new chair at the Salpêtrière.[61] This vein of research was aided or even made possible by the fact that in 1880 Charcot's rapidly expanding research and teaching empire finally acquired an outpatient clinic where, for the first time male, as well as female patients, young as well as the elderly, and the acutely ill as well as those suffering from chronic and advanced nervous disease, could be received.

Among the arrivals at the Salpêtrière clinic were a sprinkling of Eastern European and Russian Jews. Charcot, a hidebound positivist, unsympathetic to scientific theory or to animal experiment for that matter (unlike Soury, who had a sophisticated understanding of the epistemology and history of science), became persuaded on clinical grounds that Jews as a race exhibited marked predispositions toward hysteria, neurasthenia, diabetes and in fact the entire spectrum of neurological and arthritic disease. Beginning in the early 1880s and continuing until his last lectures shortly before his death in August, 1893, the famous neurologist peppered his clinical lectures with observations on Jewish neuropathology.[62] Such observations were particularly conspicuous in the two volumes of informal bedside lectures, the *Leçons du Mardi* published toward the end of his career; in the *Leçons*, Charcot's intention to use the Jews as both illustration and paradigm for his conception of the neuropathic family, a constellation of pathological entities tied together and propagated by heredity, became explicit.[63] Although such notions concerning Jews, in particular the assumed link with mental illness, were not original with Charcot, his personal prestige and the reputation of his Salpêtrière school contributed enormously to their acceptance as standard medical knowledge and the basis for further inquiry.[64]

The assumption of inherited pathological tendencies among Jews became a commonplace in medical literature of the *fin-de-siècle* and beyond. These ideas had immediate resonance outside learned circles as well. Even before Charcot's *Leçons du Mardi* were published, Edouard Drumont had seized upon the neurologist's testimony. In *La France Juive* (1886), the call to arms of an organized anti-Semitic movement in France, Drumont cited 'Dr Charcot's curious revelations on Russian Jews' at the Salpêtrière.[65] These provided impeccable authority for widespread Jewish 'neurosis' and fuel for Drumont's polemic that physiological and pathological differences of Jews constituted a contagious menace to native Frenchmen.

What Jules Soury thought of these developments can only be surmised, but he doubtless kept abreast of the literature.[66] Comfortably ensconced in the small library in the old buildings of the Sorbonne where he taught his seminar to an élite group of auditors as well as several dozen students of the Ecole des Hautes Etudes, Soury kept silent, at least publicly, about the escalating Jewish question. After being promoted at long last on 30 December, 1898 to *directeur d'études* at the Ecole, Soury attended the second Dreyfus trial at Rennes the following year and took his place in the camp of the anti-Dreyfusards. In *Campagne Nationaliste* he praised Drumont as the 'precursor and prophet' of racial anti-Semitism and he cited Charcot's name several times, noting that his 'clinical genius placed the cornerstone for knowledge of the special neuropathology of the Jew'.[67] Distancing himself from Renan (he thought the death of his old master prior to the Dreyfus Affair a timely demise that had prevented him from joining the Dreyfusards), Soury nevertheless agreed that a philological argument for race, an argument both men had formerly advocated, was no longer tenable. But his conclusion was diametrically opposed to Renan's retreat from race. For the scholar of physiological psychology, 'it [race] is not a question of language: it is a matter of ethnic, anthropological, anatomical and physiological elements, derived from the structure and texture of the tissues of various organic systems and the central nervous system in particular; in short, hereditary elements'.[68] So-called educated people (*des lettrés ignorants*) might speak of an *esprit sémitique* but anthropologists, physiologists and clinicians knew that this implied a corresponding *cerveau sémitique*. Aryans and Semites were in fact irrreducibly different races, 'perhaps two human species'.[69]

Soury's essay 'La Race. Juifs et Aryans' in *Campagne Nationaliste* envisaged a new science of comparative human ethology in which racial differences would become as securely established as inherited differences between lower animal species. His survey of current knowledge focused on clinical evidence that he believed supported the conclusion of hereditary degeneration of the central nervous system in Jews: high frequencies of neurasthenia, dementia praecox, general paralysis of the insane, and amaurotic family idiocy (Tay-Sachs disease).[70] Jews did not suffer from alcoholism, Soury conceded, an advantage they used against Aryans by promoting the distribution of 'the most profound and extensive cause of our national and ethnic degeneration'.[71]

Soury held out the prospect that recent progress in techniques of staining tissues would reveal differences in the fine structure of the nervous system between Semites and Aryans. Although the older studies comparing the weight and volume of the brain had proved inconclusive, these crude measures would be superseded by histological and biochemical investigations. Such studies had scarcely begun on Aryans, and were non existent for Semites because of religious prohibitions of autopsies. But Soury had confidence that laboratory science provided the ultimate means for demonstrating irreducible differences between the two races.[72]

On the eve of the First World War, the right wing polemicist Léon Daudet paid tribute to Soury as the first to have placed the Jewish question in proper perspective, that of biological heredity.[73] Such an assessment coming from a leading anti-Semite of the Action Française, himself a medical student in the late 1880s, who had likeiy attended Soury's course, was not surprising. Léon Daudet also had intimate knowledge of the Salpêtrière and, although filled with ambivalence towards Charcot, he continued to invoke his name to legitimate notions of Jewish pathology well into the 1930s.[74]

But, Daudet's bio-medical anti-Semitism was not widely shared, even by other leading French anti-Semites, of the post-Affair period. Charles Maurras, for example, admired Soury's scientific achievement and his devoted service to the anti-Semitic cause, but he did not see any positive contribution of the former to the latter.[75] By the time of his death in 1915, Soury and his version of biological determinism were remembered by Maurras and others mostly as relics of an earlier generation's naive confidence in the applicability of positivist natural science to human affairs.[76]

Certain aspects of Soury's thinking could, of course, be pursued to a more sinister denouement in twentieth-century racial anti-Semitism, and Zeev Sternhell has, with reason, likened Soury's world view to that of the Nazis.[77] But Soury's historical significance, I think, lies not so much in his legacy as in his remarkable appeal to his contemporaries and his stature among intellectuals of the 1890s. Moving from historical criticism of religion to a preoccupation with neurological science, Soury's career trajectory epitomized changing cultural values and a strand of medical reductionism that had become deep as well as broadly shared at *fin-de-siècle*.[78]

Soury's reputation as a 'master' philosopher of the natural sciences led contemporaries to compare him with the cultural giants Renan and Taine, who had dominated the philological, historical and literary sciences of the preceding generation.[79] In retrospect, the linking of the now-obscure Soury with such figures may appear incongruous, but it testified to the prestige of the subject matter as much as or perhaps more than the scholar. After his career shift, Soury assimilated doctrines and techniques enabling him to establish impressive credentials as critic and historian of science. But he continued to use to advantage the knowledge and skills of his first career, notably the scholarly tools of the historian, philologist, philosopher and, perhaps above all, the talents of a gifted prose stylist and speaker.[80] As his remark at the height of his career, that 'the Ecole des Chartes leads to everything', indicated, Soury had not so much abandoned letters for science but managed to apply the former to the latter. In a cultural context that worshipped science but lacked a professional cadre of science historians or philosopher critics of science (an activity assumed partially and imperfectly by practitioners of science themselves on the one hand and by essentially literary people like Brunetière on the other), the fusion of the two in a single personality, who had a teaching forum, made for a potent combination.

By the early 1890s, Soury had established his niche as the humanist's scientist, not so much a popularizer but a mediator of doctrines and values to an educated but non-scientific élite. The writer Maurice Barrès, who at the age of 20 began to follow Soury's course at the Ecole des Hautes Etudes in 1883, spoke of it a decade later as 'sublime poetry and the highest philosophy' for those who, like himself, could not follow the intricacies of cerebral anatomy and physiology.[81] Barrès confessed that he had initially regretted Soury's career shift, fearing that the 'great mind' would be 'imprisoned in special investigations', but he had come to appreciate Soury's 'supreme poetry of science' and to accept his claim of the aesthetic as well as cultural superiority of great scientific literature over standard literary classics:

> in the midst of the explanations which constituted the subject matter of the course, I used to wait for those flashes of fancy with which he at times burst forth. Rather than going home to write up these notions that he had let us hear, he remained ever so late to sketch on the blackboard, for three or four initiates, the luxuriant dendrites and the networks of axon cylinders of the neurons ... 'doubtless [Soury said] there is more great poetry in the theories of Newton, of Kant, of Laplace, Lamarck and Darwin, than in all those epics of India, Greece, and Rome'.[82]

Instead of losing a poet, Barrès gained in Soury a *maître à penser*, 'the sublime madman' who makes repeated and lengthy entries into the pages of Barrès' first three volumes of *Cahiers* covering the period 1896 to 1904. Here the character of Soury clearly provides the intellectual inspiration for Barrèsian notions of the neurophysiological basis of race and nationalism, and even specific conceits such as 'decerebration' and automatism.[83] One almost feels from the *Cahiers* that if Soury had not existed, Barrès would have had to invent him.

But the extensive unpublished correspondence from Soury to Barrès beginning in 1888 and continuing until nearly his death confirms that Soury in fact had a close relationship with the younger disciple whom he referred to as 'one of the sons of his mind' and whom he defended when Barrès was accused of simply copying his ideas.[84] Barrès reciprocated by bringing his mentor into the political arena and eventually to active involvement with the anti-Dreyfusard cause at Rennes.[85]

Barrès may have been Soury's most ardent champion, but he was not alone among influential men of letters who came under his spell and who witnessed the cultural relevance of the scientism he epitomized. Anatole France, a successful author of Soury's own generation, re-introduced readers of *Le Temps* to the former journalist, now 'one of the most comprehensive and audacious minds of these days, a soul at once artist and savant'.[86] France faithfully reproduced in his literary column of 8 November, 1891 the materialist perspectives and biographical details Soury had provided in three long recent letters. Like Barrès he judged Soury's treatment of the central nervous system to have 'a stronger romantic and dramatic interest than all the fictions of poets'. France wrote of the impact of the Sorbonne instructor, 'scalpel in hand, brain on the table ... [who] taught an élite group of students the complexities of cerebral innervation and developed the theory of cerebral localization ... hands plunged in the prodigious white or gray matter....'[87] For France, the writer of psychological novels, Soury was willing to go beyond the classroom:

> I thought that it would perhaps not displease you to see close up and to touch the living mechanism of intelligence, in short to examine ... with its filaments and its large ganglions, the marvellous tapestry, which the vulgar know only by its location ... I offer, then, M. France, to give you at your place, and for you alone, the performance [comédie] of a necropsy, an autopsy of the brain, such as I interpret and practice it.[88]

Whether France accepted the invitation is not clear, but he apparently did attend Soury's course, and he consistently represented him as one of the leading spokesmen for scientific determinism; Soury was for Anatole France 'our Gassendi', a philosopher–scientist whose melancholy appreciation of the implacable laws of the universe, stood in opposition, on the one hand, to the empty formalism and notions of free will of the older generation of Sorbonne philosphers and, on the other, to a rising current of anti-scientism becoming fashionable in literary circles, particularly among younger writers and artists around 1890.[89]

As the naturalist school of literature yielded to symbolists, decadents, spiritualists and other trends sceptical of science, Soury appeared as a champion of scientism, as well as a philosopher who had a sophisticated, critical, and deeply pessimistic view of the limits of all human effort to gain knowledge of the external world. Here was someone who could view Zola's novels as simplistic, and who could express his congratulations to Edmond de Goncourt for the account of his dying brother in his *Journal:* 'a masterpiece of sorrowful but implacable analysis. It leaves far behind all clinical descriptions of general paralysis', but nevertheless fault the patriarch of naturalist literature for several technical scientific errors and express his wish that 'certain aspects of the death of Jules Goncourt had been more rawly exposed'.[90]

By the early 1890s Soury had published three volumes based on his courses of physiological psychology, including the substantial and well-received history of the 'functions of the brain' in 1891. Despite continuing marginality in a strictly professional sense at the Ecole des Hautes Etudes, his reputation as the philosopher– historian of the brain was secure. The ground-swell of anti-science only served to underline Soury's stature. Paul Bourget's sensational and deeply anti-scientific novel of 1889, *Le Disciple,* presented a harrowing picture of how the academic doctrines of a master of deterministic psychology might lead an admiring disciple to apply them in ways both experimental and criminal. Although *Le Disciple* has received a good deal of scholarly attention from literary historians, it seems curious that no one, to my knowledge, has noted the remarkable resemblance of Adrien Sixte, Bourget's amoral philosopher–scientist anti-hero, to Jules Soury. To a much greater extent than Hippolyte Taine, who is usually taken as the model for Sixte (despite the fact that Taine himself explicitly rejected Bourget's creation as a wicked caricature) the 'modern philosopher' of *Le Disciple* is transparently based on Jules Soury. A master of 'the natural sciences and par-ticularly the physiology of the brain', so detached from mundane affairs that he did not even read the daily newspaper, Adrien Sixte in these and numerous details of his life, works and habits matches the savant whose course Bourget, too, attended.[91]

Nor was Soury's image simply one which had resonance in lay literary circles. When, in 1895, scientists replied to the attacks on their enterprise, which had found a rallying point in Brunetière's slogan of the 'bankruptcy of science', the normally reclusive Soury took a public stance among the leading academic apologists for science.[92] He drew disciples and auditors for his course not only from the likes of Barrès, France, Bourget, and other literary figures, but from medical men as well. Georges Clemenceau, who had a medical training, fell into this category, to some extent, although Clemenceau also knew Soury from their early years together in journalism and radical politics; he remained Soury's friend and follower until the Dreyfus Affair divided them.[93]

Perhaps Soury's most enthusiastic medical follower and booster was Maurice de Fleury (1860–1931). Dr Fleury, a well-trained neuropathologist who met Soury through Barrès and sat in on his course, also had literary aspirations but they were largely confined to medical popularization. Fleury celebrated the schools of Charcot and Pasteur, served as unofficial consultant on medical subjects to his friend, Emile Zola, and official correspondent to the daily *Le*

Figaro where he discussed medicine and, especially, élite doctors under the pseudonym 'Bianchon'. In Fleury's judgement, written under his own name in a *Figaro* piece of January 1895 entitled 'Un Maître', Jules Soury ranked as one of the leading intellectual luminaries of the republic: 'he is the historian, the critic, the one who understands what others do'. Working to compile, interpret and synthesize investigations 'at the frontiers of human knowledge ... of the science of life', Soury had established himself as 'the bard of this epic'; his 'modern poem', the book entitled 'the functions of the brain' presented nothing less than the *raison d'être* of the brain.[94] Fleury persisted in his florid praise of Soury when, a few years later, he called for the creation of a new chair of physiological psychology at the Paris medical faculty for the savant he called 'my master, how greatly do I admire him'.[95]

On the eve of the Dreyfus Affair, Soury's status with the dominant intellectual élite, including members of the medical profession, transcended differences between political ideologies, because he symbolized in a particularly striking and unambiguous manner the master ideology of science. Praise for the author of *Le système nerveux central*, such as that lavished by Louis Liard, director of French higher education, who called the book 'a unique monument of erudition and science' or by the prestigious academies in their prize citations, was in effect praise of science.[96]

When Soury subsequently launched his nationalist and anti-Semitic credo, the consensus around him collapsed. As a public anti-Dreyfusard, Soury immediately lost the allegiance of those on the other side like Anatole France and Clemenceau, and the respect of many colleagues in the university. He became the object of attacks in the popular press which matched in their aggression those he began to write regularly in *Action Française*. Most political commentators like Joseph Reinach, assumed that Soury's anti-Semitism had nothing to do with science, that it was, on the contrary, an aberration or perversion of the ethos of science; they attributed Soury's abrupt shift to the right, and his sudden conversion to anti-Semitism to idiosyncratic if not completely irrational private motives.[97]

The attacks on Soury tended to be partial and superficial. By reading his discourse entirely in political and personal terms, its potential for ideological suasion could be limited. In seeking to discredit and marginalize the man, a tactic that in some measure succeeded,[98] Soury's opponents, perhaps intentionally, misconstrued a message that drew its coherence and power from melding science with race. In this respect, as I have argued, Soury underwent no conversion; his supporters perceived him accurately as one who had derived his political position from a scientific ideology he had espoused for decades.[99]

In September 1899, less than two weeks after the second condemnation of Dreyfus, Soury declared in a letter to Barrès, published at the time by the disciple and later reprinted in *Campagne Nationaliste,* that he had been moved to enter the public controversy over the Affair not so much from political concerns but because of 'questions of race and national conscience', which he went on to discuss in terms of 'the enormous heterogeneity of the elementary structure and functions of the central nervous system'.[100] This was not a conversion. Five years earlier, before he became politically active, Soury had explicitly reaffirmed to Barrès his long-held position that differences in religion and culture probably depended upon biological differences in the nervous system.[101]

Barrès popularized these doctrines on behalf of the anti-Dreyfusard cause during the Affair. Although he was an eminently political creature, who needed no coaxing to enter the fray, Barrès followed Soury in relegating politics to an epiphenomenal position with regard to deeper racial structures embedded in the collective nervous systems of Aryans and Semites. One illustration, among the many invocations of this doctrine by Barrès, was his appeal to a 'nationalist literature'. That literature, which in 1902 Barrès saw coming to fruition with new reviews and publications, including Soury's *Campagne Nationaliste,* 'a magnificent psalm' by a 'universally respected savant', was not fundamentally political. It dealt with 'our land, our dead ... but also with art, morality and even hygiene'.[102]

Soury's peculiar career trajectory and professional niche within but on the margin of the Parisian scientific establishment enabled him to construct a biological anti-Semitism that exceeded religious and earlier versions of racial anti-Semitism in its claims to philosophical determinism and materialism. Not all biological determinists, of course, followed the path to anti-Semitism; nor can Soury's peculiar background, experience and psychology be ignored in the aetiology of his racialism. But, as I have sought to show, Soury's anti-Semitism flowed from his scientific ideology and was a logical and consistent, if speculative, extrapolation from science to culture. Soury argued that the domain he knew supremely well – the nervous system, its anatomy, physiology and pathology – was constitutive of racial difference. Confronted with the implications of such doctrines, those who took a stand against anti-Semitism had to disjoin scientism from the realm of politics and culture, or at least conduct themselves as if such a disjunction obtained.

By using building blocks from medicine and biology to construct race, and specifically Semitism, Soury was more radical than a Drumont and most others in the anti-Semitic movement who dreamed of at most a social science of anti-Semitism. He also appealed to a more intellectual and necessarily much more restricted following. On the other hand, unlike his former journalistic colleague, Drumont, Soury held considerable prestige as a savant during the last decade of the century. His case serves as a cautionary reminder of the compatibility between scientism and Semitism in the period before the Dreyfus Affair, a period when in the words of one historian of modern racism: 'France rather than Germany or Austria ... seemed likely to become the home of a successful racist and National Socialist movement.'[103] Along with much else about French society, the Affair exposed the potential dangers of a slippage from science to race and for Dreyfusards, especially those of a scientific bent, the urgent need to separate one from the other.

Notes

This is a revised and expanded version of a paper presented to the 32nd Annual Meeting of the Society for French Historical Studies, Quebec City, 22 March, 1986. I wish to thank George Weisz, for his critical comments on that occasion which in part inspired this revision. I also draw upon two subsequent unpublished papers: 'The French Medical Profession and the Jews on the Eve of the Dreyfus Affair', Virginia Tech, Blacksburg, VA, 20 April, 1990 and 'Language of Pathology: Medical Discourse and the Jews', University of Wisconsin, Madison, 17 April, 1991.

My current research deals with the confluence between theories of pathology and race in late nineteenth-century France. The present paper derives from that larger project.

1. The spiritualist professor of philosophy at the Sorbonne, Elme-Marie Caro, to Jules Soury on the occasion of Soury's doctoral thesis defence in 1881. Anatole France, *Le Temps*, 17 July, 1887, 2. There is no evidence that Soury ever took a degree in medicine but see below and n. 27.
2. Edmond de Goncourt, *Journal. Mémoires de la vie littéraire*, Robert Ricatte (ed.), 20 vols, (Monaco: Fasquelle and Flammarion, 1956), t. 12, 14–15 (21 February, 1879).
3. Jules Soury, *Le système nerveux central, structures et fonctions. Histoire critique des théories et des doctrines* [hereafter *Système nerveux*](Paris: Carré et Naud, 1899), x. Earlier publications by Soury based upon his lessons were the enormous article 'Cerveau' in *Dictionnaire de Physiologie*, C. Richet (ed.), (Paris, 1897), 547–976; *Histoire des*

doctrines de psychologie physiologique contemporaines. Les fonctions du cerveau, doctrines de l'école de Strasbourg, doctrines de l'école italienne (Paris, 1891); *Histoire des doctrines psychologiques contemporaines. Les fonctions du cerveau. Doctrines de F. Goltz* (Paris, 1886); and *Des doctrines psychologiques contemporaines* (Paris, 1883). On Soury's reputation and the favourable reception of *Le système nerveux central,* see Maurice Barrès, 'Note sur Jules Soury', *Le Journal* (24 November, 1899), 1 and *Revue de l'Hypnotisme et de la psychologie physiologique* 15 (1901), 200–3. Francis Schiller considers Soury 'the first and to this day the greatest and most voluminous writer on the history of neurology' and accords him an entry in the revised edition of *The Founders of Neurology,* 2nd edn W. Haymaker and F. Schiller, (Springfield, Ill., Thomas, 1970), 573–6, where he appears as the only non-medical 'founder'. Schiller, who uses a quotation from *Système nerveux* as an epigram for his collection, notes that Soury's magnum opus weighs 'nearly nine pounds'.

4. *Campagne Nationaliste, 1899–1901* (Paris: Imprimerie de la cour d'appel, 1902). A second edition (Plon) also appeared in 1902.

5. Eugène Fournière, *L'Artifice Nationaliste* (Paris: Charpentier, 1903), especially 2, 67–8, 81, 87, 120–5, 257–9 Fournière's 300-page rebuttal originally appeared as a series of articles in *Revue socialiste* (July–October 1902).

6. Joseph Reinach, *Histoire de l'Affaire Dreyfus,* t. 4 (Paris, 1904), 445–6 and t. 5 (Paris, 1905), 495; see also Jean Serc, 'Un clerical athée. M. Jules Soury', *Mercure de France* 56 (1905), 215–30.

7. Henri Dagan, *Enquête sur l'Antisémitisme* (Paris: Stock, 1899). For a comprehensive study, see Stephen Wilson, *Ideology and experience. Antisemitism in France at the time of the Dreyfus Affair* (London and Toronto: Associated University Presses, 1982).

8. F. Brunetière, 'Après le procès', *Revue des deux mondes* 146 (1898), 428–46, especially 429.

9. Emile Durkheim, 'L'individualisme et les intellectuels', *Revue politique et littéraire* 10 (1898), 7–13; Emile Duclaux, *Avant le procès* (Paris, 1898).

10. Examples on the anti-Dreyfussard side are lists from *La Patrie Française* (BN Lb 57 12316) and the Henry subscription list from P. Quillard, *Le Monument Henry* (Paris, 1899), both of which contain names of physicians from the Académie de Medecine and other medical leaders and students. See also S. Wilson, 'Le Monument Henry: La structure de l'antisémitisme en France 1898–1899' *Annales ESC* 32 (1977), 265–91.

11. See Robert A. Nye, *Crime, Madness, and Politics in Modern France. The Medical Concept of National Decline* (Princeton, N. J.: Princeton University Press, 1984). For literary fields, see Christophe Charle, 'Champ littéraire et champ du pouvoir: les écrivains et l'affaire Dreyfus', *Annales ESC* 32 (1977), 240–64, and more generally the

work of Pierre Bourdieu.

12. *Ibid.* and Madelaine Rebérioux, 'Histoire, historiens et Dreyfusisme', *Revue historique* 205 (1976), 407–32; Robert J. Smith, 'L'Atmosphère politique à l'Ecole Normale Supérieure à la fin du XIXe siècle', *Rev. d'Hist. Mod. et Cont.* (1973), 248–68.

13. On Soury and Barrès, see Zeev Sternhell, *Maurice Barrès et le nationalisme français, Cahiers de la fondation nationale des sciences politiques* (Paris: Armand Colin, 1972), 253–67, and Camille Vettard, 'Maurice Barrès et Jules Soury', *Mercure de France* 170 (1924), 685–95.

14. On the anti-Semitic context in France see Wilson, *Experience and Ideology* and Jeannine Verdès-Leroux, *Scandale financier et Antisémitisme Catholique* (Paris: Centurion, 1969).

15. The fullest account of Soury remains his autobiographical essay 'Ma vie' in *Campagne Nationaliste*, 17–71. See also Mousson-Lanauze, 'Jules Soury' *Paris Médical* (1927), 30–5.

16. Soury was reputed to have been Renan's secretary ('Chez. M. Jules Soury' *La Presse*, 11 May, 1898), but he explicitly denied having served in this capacity, (*l'Aurore*, 14 May, 1898) and 'Ma vie', 31. For his indebtedness to Renan intellectually and for helping him obtain posts in 1872 as correspondent with the *Revue des Deux Mondes* and *Le Temps*, see *ibid.*, 26–32.

17. Soury's monographs and regular contributions to *Le Temps* and *La République française* on religious, literary, and scientific subjects as well as occasional publications in the *Revue des Deux-Mondes, Revue philosophique* and *Revue scientifique* were sufficient to earn notice in Gustave Vapereau, *Dictionnaire universel des contemporains* (Paris: Librairie Hachette, 1880), 1685.

18. Bibliothèque Nationale, NAF, 11495, fo. 224–7, ms note to Renan (n.d.). Jules Soury, *Morbid Psychology. Studies on Jesus and the gospels* (London, 1881), 71 note. (translated by Annie Bessant from *Jésus et les Evangiles* (Paris, 1878)).

19. Soury, *Etudes historiques sur les religions, les arts, la civilisation de l'Asie antérieur et de la Grèce* (Paris, 1877), 200, 248–9.

20. Soury, *Essais de critique religieuse* (Paris, 1878), 138.

21. See Soury's review, *Le Temps*, 25 August, 1874, 4.

22. *Etudes historiques*, 213–14.

23. *Le Temps*, 25 August, 1874.

24. Maurice Barrès, 'M. Jules Soury', *Le Journal*, 11 May, 1894, 1. Renan's declaration appeared in 'Les sciences de la nature et les sciences historiques, lettre à M. Marcellin Berthelot (1863)' in *Oeuvres complètes*, H. Psichari (ed.), (Paris: Calmann-Levy, 1947), 633.

25. Soury, 'Ma vie', 34.

26. Letter to Gaston Paris, 18 December, 1881, BN NAF 24457, ff. 437–8.

27. Soury, 'Ma vie', 34–8. Soury also claimed to have done two years of clinical surgery at the Hôpital Saint-Louis. BN NAF 15438, fo. 573. Letter to Anatole France (25 Oct. 1891).

28. *Le Temps* (3, 8, 12 August, 1873). See especially 12 August, 3.

29. *Ibid.* 8 August, 3 Luy's text (1865), as the title suggests, was a histological study of the nervous system. For Taine's reply to Soury protesting the latter's extreme reductionism and insisting on the autonomy of psychology as a science, see Taine, *Sa vie et sa correspondance* (Paris, Hachette, 1904) t. 3, 252–5, especially 255 (letter to Soury, 13 August, 1873).

30. Letter to Eugène Müntz, 23 January, 1874, NAF 11311, fo. 157. In this letter, Soury referred to his 'article of *physiology* on Taine'. (emphasis mine).

31. *Le Temps,* 30 August, 1870, 3. The translations were *Les Preuves du Transformisme* (1879), *Le Règne des protistes* (1879) and *Essai de psychologie cellulaire* (1880).

32. Soury began his book: 'Après le dieu et l'homme, le malade' and believed that Jesus' early death had been timely from the point of view of his illness: 'le gibet lui épargna la démence', *Jesus et les Evangiles,* preface, 1, 7. Soury conceived his work as following a medical tradition of 'historical psychology' then fashionable in France and Europe, but he soon regretted the popular misunderstanding of the book and its harmful effect on his reputation. Letter to G. Paris, 18 December, 1881 and Soury, 'Ma Vie', 38.

33. Letter to Paul Bert, 4 December, 1881, BN NAF 17379, fo. 211–12.

34. Letter to Anatole France, 26 October, 1891 and Soury, 'Ma vie', 52–3.

35. *Journal Officiel de la république française* (Chambre) (20 July, 1879, 23 July, 1879).

36. Jules Ferry, *Discours et opinions,* P. Robiquet (ed.), (Paris, 1855), t. 3, 232–41, especially 237, 241. The Senate debate took place on 11 December, 1879. In the earlier debate in the Chamber when the opposition claimed that Soury was 'publiquement désigné', Ferry interrupted: 'Désigné par qui?' *Journal officiel* (23 July, 1879).

37. Archives Nationales F17 23521, Soury dossier [hereafter AN Soury]; the signature on the letter dated Paris, 17 December, 1879 has been excised. The author remarked of Soury: 'Je l'aime beaucoup, malgré ou peut-être à cause de ses défauts.' The salutation, 'Monsieur et ami' was probably addressed to Albert Dumont (1842–1884), a scholar and archaeologist, named *directeur de l'enseignement supérieur* in July 1879. Soury, apparently an old friend and colleague, immediately addressed a letter of congratulations to his exact contemporary in which he asked for Dumont's support with Jules Ferry for his nomination to the Chair of history of religions: 'j'ose compte sur votre bienveillance pour l'[Ferry] amener, au besoin, à faire ce que désirent MM Gambetta et P. Bert.' AN Soury, 22 July, 1879.

38. AN Soury, 20 March, 1880. Soury began his five-page letter by demanding why he had been refused an audience with Ferry to whom he had been sent by Paul Bert.

39. Soury later claimed Albert Dumont had told him that his nomination had been sacrificed in exchange for Senate approval of the chair. Letter to Anatole France, 26 October, 1891, fo. 576.

40. AN Soury, 20 March, 1880. Soury added: 'méfiez-vous des critiques, M. le ministre, c'est notre métier de disséquer les gens – souvent tout vifs.' Soury's threatening imagery appeared all the more bizarre in contrast to his diminutive stature, just slightly over five feet tall, and normally retiring manners. 'Soury transformé en homme de combat m'a un peu fait sourire', Paul Bert commented, alluding to the Senate debates over his friend's reputation. AN Soury, 17 December, 1879. Although Soury apparently did not proceed with his threat against Ferry, a university report noted that following his rejection for the chair, Soury had been guilty of 'une conduite étrange' toward the minister which had given rise to 'toute une légende.' AN Soury, 31 May, 1881.

41. AN Soury, 30 November, 1881. Letter to Soury and note. In his letter of 4 December, 1881 to Bert, Soury commented: 'c'est l'épilogue de la chair de la Collège de France que M. Jules Ferry ne peut me donner, quoi qu'elle dut été fait pour moi.'

42. AN Soury. Reports on Soury's theses, 31 May, 1881 in which the ministry expressed concern that Soury might now propose a chair for himself in History of Religions at the Faculty of Letters. See also *Le Temps*, 27 May, 1881, 2.

43. AN Soury. Various records and letter of 22 November, 1881; of his situation at the BN, Soury wrote: 'Je suis en effet le seul homme possédant une instruction générale et des titres universitaires supérieurs qui se trouvent au département des imprimés. La reste est une tourbe de garçons de service.' Soury's job designation at the BN for more than 15 years (1869–1885) remained that of 'employé'; for the following 24 years until he was obliged to retire in 1909, he was a 'sous-bibliothécaire'.

44. Letter to Anatole France, 26 October, 1891; Soury 'Ma vie', 50–1. Soury used the phrases 'cette chaire, qui est et restera ma chaire' and 'la perte de ma chaire' in the letter of 20 March, 1880 to the Minister.

45. AN Soury. Letter to minister from members of IVe section of EPHE, 4 December, 1881.

46. Letter of Soury to Gaston Paris, 9 December, 1881, BN NAF 24457, ff. 433–5.

47. A eulogist recalled: 'Soury supporta pacifiquement la tacquinerie un peu mesquine que consista à l'exclure de l'affiche générale et à l'isoler dans une petite affiche particulière.' Maurice Vernes, *Journal des débats* 18 August, 1915; His promotion to *directeur adjoint* came on

10 December, 1896, and to *directeur d'études* two years later; see also J.-J. Weiss, 'L'esprit philistin' *Revue politique et littéraire (Revue Bleue)* (6 May, 1882), 547; Maurice Barrès, *Le Figaro* (19 May, 1888).

48. Reinach, *Histoire de l'affaire Dreyfus*, t. 4, 446: 'il [Soury] est devenu antisémite par quelque rancune de cuistre, disait-on....'
Mousson-Lanauze, 'Jules Soury', 31, writing of Soury's rejection for the Collège de France chair, says that he 'garda de cet échec une rancune profonde'.

49. These included one of Soury's earliest mentors, Michel Bréal, and the Darmesteter brothers, Arsène and James. Soury described his treatment by the Collège de France as being sacrificed to 'tout un consistoire, tout un sanhédrin', 'Ma Vie', 51. Yet, like most antisemites, he claimed to have great respect for individual Jews among scholars he had known. *Campagne Nationaliste*, 7.

50. See Edouard Drumont, *La France Juive*, (Paris, 1886), vol. 2, 307–81; Maurice Barrès, *Scènes et doctrines du Nationalisme*, (Paris: Plon, 1925), t. 1, 67.

51. On Réville, see *Dictionnaire des Lettres Françaises*, G. Grente, (ed.) (Paris: Fayard, 1972), 321–2 and his Dreyfusard tract, *Les étapes d'un intellectuel* (Paris, 1898).

52. AN Soury: 'J'estime que la psychologie, qui est devenue un chapitre de la physiologie générale, appartient aux naturalistes, aux savants voués à l'étude des sciences biologiques, et non aux philosophes.' See also the excerpt of Soury's lesson of 22 November, 1882 in *l'Encéphale* (1883), 62–85. Soury referred to his course as 'physiological psychology' in the letter to Anatole France in 1891, but the Ecole did not formally employ the term until 1898.

53. For an informative, if polemical, review see Bernard Lazare, *L'Antisémitisme son histoire et ses causes* (Paris, 1894), especially 94–6 and Joshua Tractenberg, *The Devil and the Jews: The Medieval conception of the Jew and its relationship to modern anti-Semitism* (New Haven: Yale University Press, 1943).

54. For examples from the French literature, both of which translated older stereotypes into medical language, the first positive and the second negative, see Alfred Legoyt, *De certaines immunités biostatiques de la race juive* (Paris, 1868) and J. C. M. Boudin, *Traité de géographie et de statistique médicales et des maladies endémiques* (Paris, 1857), 140–2; see also 'De certaines immunités de la race juive', *Revue scientifique* 27 (1881), 530–3, 618–27.

55. See discussions in *Bulletins de la Société d'Anthropologie de Paris* 2 (1861): 410–13; 4 (1863): 386–8, 552–8; 6 (1865): 515–22; 7, 3 ser. (1884): 698–701; 2, 4 ser. (1891): 539–49.

56. See Leon Poliakov, *The Aryan Myth*, trans by E. Howard, (New York: Basic Books, 1971), 269–85.

57. E. Renan, *Histoire des Langues Sémitiques* in *Oeuvres Complètes*, H.

Psichari (ed.), (Paris: Calman-Lévy, 1958), t. 8, 576–7. See also, Wilson, *Ideology and Experience*, 468–72.

58. See Sander L. Gilman, *Difference and Pathology: Stereotypes of sexuality, race and madness* (Ithaca, N.Y.: Cornell University Press, 1985).

59. For opposition among his colleagues to the tailor-made establishment of the new chair for Charcot, see Archives Nationales, AJ 16 6260 (12 May, 1881). I plan to discuss Charcot's concept of and efforts on behalf of this innovation in a forthcoming publication based on manuscript holdings in the Bibliothèque Charcot, Salpêtrière Hospital, Paris. See also J. L. Signoret, 'La création de la Chaire de Charcot', *Revue Neurologique* 138 (1982), 887–92.

60. See Jan Goldstein 'The Wandering Jew and the Problem of Psychiatric Anti-semitism in Fin-de-Siècle France', *J. Contemporary Hist.* 20 (1985), 521–52, and T. Gelfand 'The French Medical Profession and the Jews on the Eve of the Dreyfus Affair'.

61. The earliest published references to Jewish patients at the Salpêtrière which I have found were a 15-year-old girl and a 13-year-old boy, both Russians whose parents brought them to Charcot's outpatient clinic in 1882. See *Le Progrès Médical* (10 June, 1882), 441 and (23 December, 1882), 1003–4.

62. Jane B. Henderson, 'Personal reminiscences of Charcot', *Glasgow Med. J.* 40 (1893), 297. Henderson attended Charcot's Tuesday lessons in the autumn of 1892.

63. Charcot, *Leçons du mardi à la Salpêtrière: Polyclinique 1887–1888*, I, 2e edn (Paris, 1892), 6, 110, 408, 477 and, II 1888–89, (Paris, 1892), 11–12, 347–55.

64. Several of Charcot's students, including Joseph Babinsky, Paul Berbez and M. A. Dutil alluded to Jewish patients at the Salpêtrière, but the major publication on the subject was that by Henry Meige, *Etude sur certains névropathes Voyageurs. Le Juif Errant à la Salpêtrière*, Thèse de Médecine, (Paris, 1893). Meige's thesis, directly inspired by Charcot, was also published with photographs as a monograph (Paris: Bataille, 1893) and serialized in *Nouvelle Iconographie de la Salpêtrière* (1893). Widely reviewed by the medical and lay press, including favourable comment by Drumont in his daily, *La Libre Parole*, Meige's thesis presented anti-Semitic stereotypes in medical language. See Goldstein, 'The Wandering Jew'.

65. *La France Juive*, vol. 1, 106. See also Drumont, *La fin d'un monde* (Paris, 1889), xv for another example of his recourse to Charcot's authority on Jewish pathology.

66. Thus he wrote in *Campagne Nationaliste*, 140: 'Les caractères différentiels du Sémite et de l'Aryen ont été souvent étudiés en ethnologie, en anthropologie, en épidémiologie, en clinique.'

67. *Ibid.*, 124, 147.

68. *Ibid.*, 127.

69. *Ibid.*, 140–1.
70. *Ibid.*, 143–4. In addition to invoking Charcot as authority for Jewish predisposition to neurasthenia, degenerative diseases of the brain and spinal cord, congenital nervous diseases, tuberculosis, and diabetes (*ibid.*, 130–1), Soury cited the work of Pilz of Vienna on 'psychoses in Jews', which in turn provided a host of prestigious German and British references. Soury believed the prognosis was also much worse in Jews than in 'our race, French, Germans, English, Italians, Russians'. *Ibid.*, 143.
71. *Ibid.*, 144–5.
72. *Ibid.*, 141–2.
73. Léon Daudet, *Devant la douleur* (Paris: Nouvelle Librairie Nationale, 1915), 44.
74. Léon Daudet, 'La question Juive', *L'Action Française*, 19 January, 1934, 1; Daudet, *Panorama de la IIIe République* (Paris: Gallimard, 1936) 88 in which Daudet remarks a contrast between Charcot's clinical lessons on Jews and his 'philosemitism'. See Toby Gelfand, 'Medical Nemesis, Paris 1894: Léon Daudet's *Les Morticoles*', *Bull. Hist. Med.* 60 (1986): 157–9, 164.
75. Charles Maurras 'Jules Soury' in *Tombeaux* (Paris: Nouvelle Librairie Nationale, 1921), 80–5, especially 82–3. Originally published in *Action Française* (13 August, 1915). Maurras likened biological and pathological explanations of human history to astrological causes; they were possible but irrelevant. Soury, for his part, violently criticized Maurras' spiritualism. Ms Letter to Maurice Barrès, in BN NAF Fonds Barrès, 25 July, 1904.
76. Mousson-Lamauze, *L'Echo de Paris*, 16 August, 1915, 'Jules Soury', 34; *Revue philosophique* 30 (1915), 384. André Rouveyre, 'Jules Soury heurté' in *Souvenirs de mon commerce* (Paris: Gres., 1921) 254–5.
77. Sternhell, *Maurice Barrès*, 254.
78. See Nye, *Crime, Madness, and Politics*.
79. Maurice de Fleury, 'Un Maître', *Le Figaro* 2 January, 1895, 4–5. Vernes, 'July Soury'; Rouveyre, 'Jules Soury heurté', 253–4.
80. His eulogist at the Ecole pratique commented: 'Il eût pu, avec son titre de doctorat, briguer une chaire de littérature dans une de nos Facultés et il l'aurait remplit avec éclat. Après la mort de Renan, des étrangers venaient entendre Soury pour avoir une idée de l'éloquence et du geste du maître disparu.' *Annuaire, Ecole Pratique des Hautes Etudes*, 1915 (Paris, 1916) 72–3; Maurras, 'Jules Soury', 81–2 also associated Soury with 'la grande prose française' and someone 'qui donne la plus haute et la plus honnête idée du langage humain'.
81. Barrès, *Le Journal*, 11 May, 1894, 1.
82. Barrès, *Le Journal*, 24 November, 1899, 1. A eulogist remarked that Soury's teaching was 'la plus grande jouissance de sa vie. Après sa conférence il donnait à quelques auditeurs des renseignements

supplémentaires, et alors le maître debout comme les élèves, le temps passait si vite que l'heure de la fermeture (10 heures du soir) arrivait quelquefois avant que la conversation fût achevée. Le maître avait parlé pendant cinq heures et demie sans éprouver le besoin de diner ou de se reposer', *Annuaire, Ecole pratique*, 73.

83. Maurice Barrès, *Mes Cahiers* (Paris: Plon, 1930) t. 1, 66–74, 78–82, 83–6, t. 2, 117–21, 160–2, t. 3, 78, 87–9, 100–3. Barrès calls Soury 'le fou sublime', t. 1, 67 after attending his course on 1 May, 1896. See also Vettard, 'Maurice Barrès et Jules Soury', 685–95, and Sternell, *Maurice Barrès*, 254–67.

84. Fonds Barrès BN NAF contains nearly 100 items of correspondence from Soury to Barrès. For access to this uncatalogued collection in 1986 and permission to order microfilm, I wish to thank Florence Callu, Conservateur, Dept. des Manuscrits BN and Josué Seckel, Service des lecteurs, BN. The BN also possesses Barrès' library with numerous inscribed volumes from Soury and a scrapbook of published clippings by or about Soury. For the phrase, 'un des fils de mon esprit dont je suis le plus fier ... il veut bien m'appeler maître', see Fonds Barrès, letter 22 October, 1899. For Soury's denial that Barrès plagiarized him, see *ibid.*, 23 October, 1905.

85. On 13 October, 1899, (*ibid.*), Soury wrote to Barrès: 'grace à vous, je puis déjà prendre rang dans l'armée nationale', and he expressed his wish to distance himself from Dreyfusard professors at the Ecole de Chartes and the Ecole des Hautes Etudes. Later he credited Barrès with suggesting the title for his *Campagne Nationaliste* (*ibid.*, 23 August, 1905).

86. Anatole France, *Le Temps*, 8 November, 1891.

87. *Ibid.*

88. Soury letter to France, 17 October, 1891, NAF 15438. In a following letter of 25 October, Soury said that if the prospect of a bloody operation in his home, 'même sur le cadavre', bothered France, the autopsy could be performed 'chez moi, et pour vous seul'.

89. Anatole France, *Le Temps*, 17 July, 1887, 30 March, 1890, 23 April, 1893.

90. Soury letter to Edmond de Goncourt, 30 May, 1888, NAF 22476, 70–1. Soury's low opinion of Zola is stated in *l'Echo de Paris*, 15 January, 1895, 2.

91. See Paul Bourget, *Le Disciple* (Paris, 1889) 1–25, ch. 1 'Un philosophe moderne'. A few details were age, social origins, physical appearance and dress, celibacy, types of publications. For a scholarly assessment of *Le Disciple*, see Victor Brombert, *The Intellectual Hero, Studies in the French Novel 1880–1955* (London: Faber, 1960) 52–67. On Bourget as one of Soury's students, see Mousson-Lanauze, 'Jules Soury', 31.

92. *L'Echo de Paris*, 15 January, 1895, 2, published Soury's rebuttal to the 'bankruptcy of science' issue as part of an *enquête* of leading

academicians conducted by Bernard Lazare. *La Justice* 8 April, 1895, edited by Clemenceau, published Soury's 'La Science', a speech intended for the banquet honouring the chemist Berthellot, a major participant in the debate over science.

93. Fonds Barrès, 22 October, 1899, 24 August, 1901; Mousson-Lanauze, 'Jules Soury', 34.

94. Maurice de Fleury, 'Un Maître'.

95. Fleury, *Introduction à la Médecine de l'Esprit* (Paris, 1897), 169, viii, 209.

96. See AN Soury, 5 January, 1901 for Liard quotation in letter from Liard to Soury, 21 November, 1899, and Soury, 'Ma Vie', 64–5. A review of Barrès' review of Soury's work thought the best label for Soury to be 'critic' rather than 'magician' or 'poet', as Barrès preferred, but agreed that Soury held special status as one who bridged science and literature. *Mercure de France* 33 (1900) 240–2. An article in *La Presse*, 11 May, 1898, called Soury the 'chef incontesté de la philosophie naturelle'; on the comparisons with Renan and Taine, see above n. 79; Gabriel Hanotaux, *Mon Temps,* vol. 2, (Paris, 1938), 461 recalled Soury by name along with five others in his library of French philosophers of the 19th century; the others were Comte, Littré, Renan, Cournot and Fouillée; Fleury, *Introduction,* 437 grouped Soury with Renan, Taine, Ribot and Liard as the outstanding philosophers of the Third Republic.

97. Reinach, *Affaire Dreyfus,* t. 4, 445–6; Gustave Kahn, 'La vie et les variations de M. Jules Soury', (clipping in Barrès scrapbook, BN, from *Gil Blas,* July 1900); Arthur Ranc, 'Patriotard et bon chrétien', *Le Radical* (31 March, 1902); 'Universitaires 'bien pensants', *La Fronde,* 28 January, 1900.

98. After the publication of *Campagne Nationaliste,* the numbers of students at Soury's course declined drastically. He successfully resisted retirement in 1909, however, and continued to teach at the Ecole until shortly before his death. See *Annuaires Ecole,* AN Soury, and various eulogies cited in n. 76. Soury's discredit during the Dreyfus Affair may in part account for his obscurity today. He does, however, receive mention as 'étonnant, admirable et funeste' in Marcel Gauchet, *L'Inconscient Cérébral* (Paris: Seuil, 1992), 123–6.

99. See Jean Serc, 'M. Jules Soury. Un clerical athée' *Mercure de France* (1905), 215–30 and *l'Echo de Paris,* 16 October, 1915, obituary notice signed 'Junius'.

100. Fonds Barrès, Soury to Barrès, 20 September, 1899; Barrès, *Le Journal,* 21 October, 1899; *Campagne Nationaliste,* 75–80.

101. Fonds Barrès, Soury to Barrès 23 September, 1894 : '... des gens qui n'ont ni notre culture ni peut-être notre structure cérébrale....' But, at that time, Soury recommended tolerance of cultural difference to the militant Barrès, a position he would radically change during the Affair.

102. Barrès, 'Il y a une littérature nationaliste', *Le Gaulois*, 16 July, 1902,
    1. Barrès commented on a *Traité d'hygiène populaire* by doctor
    Plique: 'j'y voyais constater que certains malades ne peuvent être
    soignés avec succès que dans leurs pays originaires et que les sanatoria
    sont les plus efficaces en Lorraine pour les Lorrains, en Auvergne
    pour les Auvergnats....'

103. George Mosse, *Toward the final solution. A history of European racism*
    (Madison: U. of Wisconsin Press, 1985), 150, 168.

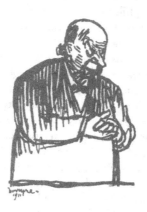

The sketch of Soury by André Rouvegre, first published in *Mercure de France*
(1911) is from Rouvegre, *Souvenirs de mon commerce* (Paris: Crèr 1921). No
photograph of Soury is known to exist.

8

Vicq d'Azyr,
Anatomy and a Vision of Medicine*

Caroline Hannaway

In the eighteenth century, scientific research was not seen as a political good in its own right. Nor did the profession of scientist, with its modern connotations of specialized knowledge and authority even exist. These are all inventions of the nineteenth century. Instead there were philosophers and men of letters (often indistinguishable from one another), and there were patrons and the king's ministers (likewise frequently the one and the same). It is important to bear these distinctions in mind when evaluating the way in which scientific careers were made in Ancien Régime France. In order to examine questions such as the extent of the support for scientific research, or the lack of it, the provision of requisite facilities for its conduct and the recognition given to its usefulness, one must begin by getting the categories right. Retrospective judgements made through the lenses of the nineteenth century are often misleading. In this essay, I wish to illustrate these points with reference to the way in which the great French comparative anatomist and physician Félix Vicq d'Azyr made his career and how he acquired the resources for doing so.

Félix Vicq d'Azyr was born in 1748 in the small provincial town of Valognes in Normandy.[1] He was the son of a physician who had a degree from Montpellier. Following his early education at a college in Valognes, he went to the University of Caen for his philosophical studies. He developed literary ambitions and considered an ecclesiastical career which would have allowed him time for *belles-lettres*. Although Vicq d'Azyr, reportedly at the urging of his father, decided on a career in medicine instead, his literary inclinations remained. He became a passionate collector of books and his contemporary and later reputation in the world of science and letters was founded to a certain extent on the eulogies he presented to the Royal Society of Medicine of Paris in his capacity as its permanent secretary.[2] The audience for the eulogies was not only his fellow physicians in the Society but also leading figures in political, social and literary circles. These public orations to listeners sensitive to the nuances of reference and style enhanced Vicq d'Azyr's status as a man of letters and demonstrated his erudition in matters of science and medicine. In 1788 he received recognition for his abilities in this genre with what he regarded as one of his greatest accomplishments – his admission to a seat among the 40 immortals of the Académie Française in replacement of Buffon.[3] The path he took to this high point of his career is revealing.

In 1765, like other provincial students seeking fame and fortune, Vicq d'Azyr left Normandy and travelled to Paris to study medicine. He undertook the required courses, exercises and theses to obtain the degree of doctor of medicine at the Faculty of Medicine of Paris but the formalized, some would say fossilized, nature of the instruction there was insufficient to satisfy his quest for knowledge. To further his education then, he availed himself of the opportunities in the capital beyond the university for studying the sciences and medicine. These were more numerous than has been generally recognized in accounts of medical education in Paris at this time.[4] Both the Jardin du Roi and the Collège Royal offered public courses in anatomy, botany, and pharmacy or chemistry which Vicq d'Azyr attended. He was tireless in his visits to amphitheatres, laboratories, hospitals, cabinets of natural history and libraries. He also followed the private courses offered by a number of teachers on subjects such as physics, chemistry, natural history, anatomy and surgery.[5]

These experiences had two effects. Vicq d'Azyr became convinced of the importance of the role of teaching in the advancement of knowledge and a shaping factor in his subsequent career was his desire to have suitable facilities in which to teach. As Sainte-Beuve, one of his later biographers, reports him saying, 'What a fine art that of teaching is! When, in effect, does a man offer another man the most flattering mark of his respect? It is without doubt when he falls silent in order to hear his fellow [speak], takes down his words, is imbued with his ideas (esprit).'[6] Vicq d'Azyr also developed a view of medicine which saw an important relationship between medicine and its ancillary sciences. Medicine for him was a science that comprehended the most useful parts of natural knowledge but it could not be studied in isolation. It was intimately linked to the natural sciences and the understanding of these was, he thought, essential to medicine's progress.[7]

Among the sciences, Vicq d'Azyr's chosen subject became anatomy for which he developed a passion. As his biographer Lalande described it, 'In winter he passed entire days in the midst of cadavers; he threw himself into dissection in an indefatigable way; he noted down everything unusual that he encountered and when he returned to his lodgings, he consulted the authors, ancient or modern, who had written on anatomy and made extracts of their ideas. [This] helped to develop the erudition that has been admired in his works. During the summer he repeated the physiological experiments of Haller, he studied natural history, and he went on botanical excursions.'[8] The anatomical theatre for demonstration through teaching and the dissecting room for research became the focus of Vicq d'Azyr's investigative life.

It was while following the lessons of Antoine Petit, who from 1769 to 1778 held the chair of anatomy at the Jardin du Roi, that Vicq d'Azyr developed his strong enthusiasm for anatomy and Petit became his model, his patron and his friend. Petit was a very successful teacher, reportedly drawing hundreds of students to his anatomical courses at the Jardin, and he also offered a range of private courses that were financially very rewarding for him.[9] As well as a way to establish one's reputation, economic considerations were of course part and parcel of private course teaching in eighteenth-century Paris.

Vicq d'Azyr's avid interest in anatomy was not confined to the study of man. Louis Daubenton introduced him to the importance of thinking about anatomy comparatively. As Vicq d'Azyr noted later 'It is to M. d'Aubenton, our master and our model, that the honour belongs of having created among us comparative anatomy properly so called. All that which relates to the general form and exterior of the skeleton and the large viscera of quadrupeds is set out in his writings. It was natural history that he proposed to illuminate by his investigations. From this point of view, he has succeeded, and to the merit of having begun the task, he has joined that of having fulfilled [i.e., his objective] it completely.'[10] The intellectual relationship between the two men acquired a personal dimension when Vicq d'Azyr married Monsieur Daubenton's niece.[11]

Vicq d'Azyr early in his career came to the conviction that the study of man had to be illuminated by the study of animals. As he explained, '[M]an must not be considered alone; he must be compared with the other animals: when thus brought together, they will form a tableau that is imposing in its extent and stimulating by its variety. Man alone does not seem as great; one does not see as well what he [really] is: the animals, without man, seem to be separated from their type and one does not know to what centre to relate them.'[12] Man's place in the order of nature was not understood if he was considered in isolation. He had to be perceived in relation to the rest of the animal kingdom. But Vicq d'Azyr planned to go beyond natural history and illuminate anatomy itself by his research. In his comparative anatomy, all the corresponding parts of humans and the entire range of animals would be analysed. To achieve this goal, human anatomy had to be pursued vigorously and in detail in all parts and organs: this included the articulations, ligaments, muscles, vessels, nerves and glands, as well as the internal structure of the viscera of the different classes of animals as yet unexamined.[13] Extensive research was needed to lay the foundations for this comparative anatomy project and it clearly could not be accomplished in private facilities. The resources of large institutions and the state were needed to get it underway and achieving access to these, as Vicq d'Azyr was to find, was not straightforward in the competitive world of scientific and ministerial patronage in France of the 1770s and 1780s.

On reaching the second phase of his medical training in 1772, that of the licentiate, Vicq d'Azyr was allowed to teach, and during the vacation from the regular courses at the Faculty of Medicine in 1773, he gave a very successful free public course in comparative anatomy in the Faculty's amphitheatre. His oratorical abilities were already apparent in his lectures and his insights enthralled his listeners. Not only students of medicine but also established physicians and surgeons of the capital flocked to hear the dynamic young teacher. The taste of success whetted Vicq d'Azyr's appetite for further teaching but the forum offered by the Faculty's amphitheatre did not long remain available. When the regular courses started again, Vicq d'Azyr could no longer use the amphitheatre.[14] He began, however, following Petit's example, to teach privately, offering an anatomy and physiology course in October 1773 in rooms on the Rue de la Pelleterie. This private course was offered again in October 1774 and November 1775 in an amphitheatre on the Rue de Glatigny. Besides the lecture demonstrations, opportunities were also offered for dissection. In 1776 the anatomy course was supplemented by an elementary course in surgery. These private courses, too, were well received and they enhanced Vicq d'Azyr's reputation as an anatomy teacher, but they were conducted in rented rooms that could hold only limited audiences.[15]

In seeking a public forum for continuing and expanding his teaching course in anatomy and pursuing research, Vicq d'Azyr sought to obtain a position at the Jardin du Roi. The Jardin was the premier institution in Paris for the teaching of botany, chemistry and anatomy. It had the amenities needed for instruction in these subjects and teaching exploited experimental demonstration. Its courses were free, open to the public, and much frequented by medical and surgical students. They were given in French, unlike the official courses for medical students at the Faculty of Medicine which were given in Latin. The professors received annual salaries. Moreover, under the intendancy of Buffon, teaching at the Jardin was conducted in the context of a broad natural history.[16] This prestigious institution seemed eminently suitable as a scientific home for a man of Vicq d'Azyr's views and he had good reasons to hope for a professorship. Not only were his patrons a part of the Jardin staff – Daubenton was the keeper and demonstrator of the cabinet of natural history and Petit the royal professor of anatomy – but in 1775 when Petit fell ill he designated Vicq d'Azyr to teach in his place. For three years, Vicq d'Azyr gave the Jardin's courses in anatomy and he had the expectation that, with Petit's patronage, he would assume Petit's position. If these hopes had been realized, Vicq d'Azyr's career might well have taken a different course; but in May 1777, to his dismay, the more established anatomist Antoine Portal was named as successor to Petit by Buffon and at the end of November 1778, when Petit retired to the countryside, Portal became the professor of anatomy. Vicq d'Azyr's quest to teach his subject in a public institution was thus blocked.[17]

Later Vicq d'Azyr's admirer Jean Verdier portrayed the consequences of this outcome in what are probably exaggerated terms in the *Encyclopédie Méthodique: Médecine*. According to Verdier the extended courses of Ferrein, an earlier Jardin anatomy teacher, and of Petit, which had been attended by eight hundred students were reduced to twenty lessons a year, ten on osteology and diseases of bones and ten on splanchnology (viscera), attended by a dozen students in a new amphitheatre built to hold twelve hundred. This Verdier portrayed as the sad consequence of Buffon's despotism.[18]

Another problem was that Portal had already secured the chair of anatomy in 1774 at the Collège Royal, the other public institution for teaching, and endeavours to find a chair there for Vicq d'Azyr bore no fruit.[19] The third available forum for anatomical teaching for a physician, the Faculty of Medicine of Paris, did not offer continuing professorships. The courses given by the Faculty were taught by regent doctors chosen by lot annually.[20] Vicq d'Azyr did have a turn at teaching the course in physiology and anatomy in 1780 and that in pathology in 1781 and was thus entitled to give a short public anatomy demonstration to medical students and others in the Faculty's amphitheatre but this was a one-time teaching opportunity.[21]

The other institution through which Vicq d'Azyr sought to develop his reputation as an anatomist was the Academy of Sciences. His early presentations were a series of memoirs on the anatomy of birds but the work that gained him membership in this august body was innovative studies of the structure of fish. At some time in 1773, he suffered an illness (the symptoms are suggestive of tuberculosis), and he was forced to give up his round of activities in the capital and convalesce at the seashore in his home province of Normandy. He used this period of retreat to investigate the anatomical and physiological structure of fish. His research led him to divide fish into three groups. He studied their bones, muscles and viscera, and their relationships with other living creatures such as reptiles, birds and quadrupeds. This new work was presented to the Academy of Sciences and earned him a place in the class of anatomists in 1774. Thereafter, he presented the results of much of his anatomical and physiological research to this body.[22]

Ironically, at the time when it seemed that his anatomical researches were proceeding down a philosophical path in comparative anatomy, it was an official request made of the Academy of Sciences that brought him back to medicine. In late 1774 the Comptroller General of Finances of France, Anne Robert Turgot, sought the Academy's help in controlling the widespread rinderpest epidemic that was devastating rural France. The Academy was asked to appoint a commission to investigate and Vicq d'Azyr was chosen to travel to the affected regions and determine personally what should be done. Vicq d'Azyr accepted this assignment although it meant his removal from Paris and the centre of things, as well as affecting his private course teaching.

His mission was to establish the nature of the disease and its means of communication, then to determine whether any proposed remedial measures were effective, and finally to find the best methods of bringing the disease under control.[23] Vicq d'Azyr threw himself into this arduous task, learning all he could of animal medicine from the publications available and touring extensively in the stricken provinces of Gascony, Guyenne and Picardy in the winter of 1774/5 and also in Normandy, Flanders and Artois in the winter of 1775/6. He investigated every aspect of the disease in a variety of areas, making frequent dissections of animals to determine the course of the disease and whether it was essentially similar in different regions. He drew up regulations governing movement of cattle and directed numerous measures on a large scale to prevent the spread of the disease, including disinfection practices and the use of troops as *cordons sanitaires* around infected areas.[24] In the course of these activities he became familiar with the bureaucratic network of royal intendants responsible for governing the provinces and the resources that could be called upon in disease outbreaks. As the nature of the epidemic made the slaughter of sick animals the only useful solution to the problem of the spread of disease, Vicq d'Azyr also used the opportunities this policy provided to try a number of physiological experiments on the sensibility and respiration of large domestic quadrupeds.[25] In the middle of his endeavours investigating the epizootic on behalf of the government, his anatomy research was not forgotten.

These provincial experiences affected Vicq d'Azyr in important ways and altered the course of his career. His travels had made him acutely aware of the economic and social problems of epidemics and epizootics. In a country as dependent on agriculture as was eighteenth-century France, rinderpest was a crippling blow to the economy affecting both human and animal populations. A lack of animals to work the fields caused want and deprivation for cultivators. Vicq d'Azyr realized that there was no organized corpus of information about epidemics and epizootics available, despite the endeavours of the veterinary schools to mitigate the effects of the latter, and he saw that responses to such disease problems in France were very much on an *ad hoc* basis. These perceptions led him to the idea that a more effective and timely response to epidemics and epizootics would be the establishment of a continuing source of advice with a network of experienced contacts in the provinces. Trained personnel would be available to travel to afflicted areas when needed and there would be a coordination of government and medical activities in response to disease outbreaks. This led him to propose a new medical venture – the founding of a Commission for Epidemics and Epizootics under royal patronage. The royal administration proved receptive to such a proposition at a time when ministers of physiocratic outlook were prominent in its ranks and Vicq d'Azyr's demonstrated willingness to assist in responding to perceived political needs gained him the patronage he needed to get his venture established.[26]

Vicq d'Azyr's provincial experiences also led to a broadening of his vision of medicine. The intimate linkages between the welfare of human and animal populations in rural areas led him to a perception of the unity of medicine that affected his thinking and writings throughout the rest of his life. From this point on, not only did he see comparative anatomy as the route to a true understanding of the nature and functions of all living beings; he also began to advocate the comparative study of human and animal diseases as well.[27]

In confronting the problem of epidemic disease both human and animal, Vicq d'Azyr reached back into classical tradition. Just as in his anatomical studies he evoked the ancient philosophical ideal of a comparative anatomy, so in confronting epidemics and working to develop a comparative medicine he drew upon the Hippocratic doctrine of an environmental and topographical understanding of health and disease – which was undergoing a notable revival in the eighteenth century. I have dealt elsewhere with the influence of airs, waters, and places and the role of the collection of meteorological data in the programme of the Commission for Epidemics and its successor, the Société Royale de Médecine, which were the products of Vicq d'Azyr's recommendations after his work in the provinces.[28] Two aspects of this programme deserve emphasis here. The first concerns the way in which Vicq d'Azyr exploited the knowledge of physical instrumentation that he acquired through his private study of the physical sciences to transform the simple noting of the elemental constitution of the atmosphere into the systematic recording of the weather and climate by means of such quantifying instruments as the thermometer, barometer and hygrometer.[29] In this way a classical conception of disease was linked up with the methods and instruments of the physical sciences. The second aspect was the insistence that the data should be collected in a systematic and co-ordinated way. Isolated observation, however accurate, was of no value unless it was brought into relationship with other observations of a similar nature. By these means, Vicq d'Azyr proposed to build up a complete environmental and topographical picture of the disease patterns affecting both humans and animals throughout the kingdom of France, in the way that his systematic comparative anatomy was intended to reveal with new precision the relationships between form and function of the different parts of the members of the animal kingdom seen as a whole.[30]

This programme in comparative medicine in the service of the state had a profound effect on the nature of the Société Royale de Médecine. This body was never conceived simply as an élite group of physicians domiciled in Paris who by their writings and example diffused the results of their learning to the provinces.[31] The model was different from that of the Academy of Sciences. Vicq d'Azyr's creation was a corresponding society which drew upon the political network governing the provinces and served to coordinate the contributions of a widely dispersed membership. In his journeys to confront the epizootics of 1774–6 Vicq d'Azyr had made every effort to seek out the knowledge and experience of local practitioners, physicians, surgeons, veterinarians and landowners, and he came to have a high appreciation of this provincial resource of knowledge.[32] Such local knowledge was built in to the overall plan of the Society. A comprehensive map of the condition of health and disease in France was predicated upon a continuing supply of local information. What was important was that the information be uniformly recorded, systematized and coordinated. While there were undoubtedly elements of a learned academy in Vicq d'Azyr's view of the Society, this body should not be seen only as a group of metropolitan savants advancing the science and ideals of the profession of medicine, but as the embodiment of a programme for understanding all disease in the natural world.

Vicq d'Azyr's experiences in the provinces were clearly formative in his view of medicine and the way in which it should be involved with the state. But he never lost sight of his ambitions to be a publicly recognized and supported teacher of comparative anatomy in Paris and to have facilities in which to do research. He reminded Turgot in 1775 of the sacrifices that his travels had entailed in the development of his career and he requested compensation. As a negotiated reward for his efforts there was built into the establishment of the Commission for Epidemics a professorship in human and comparative anatomy for Vicq d'Azyr. He was to teach a course in which he would be assisted in the dissections and other work by the six young physicians who were his close friends and who constituted the original core group of the Commission for Epidemics. The course was to be open to doctors and students of medicine and also surgeons and students of surgery.[33] The evidence shows that it was not only state-supported recognition of his teaching abilities that Vicq d'Azyr sought but also institutional facilities for carrying out his anatomical investigations. He negotiated for significant support for the establishment of an amphitheatre for teaching, a well-equipped dissection room and an office from which to direct the affairs of the Commission for Epidemics. Among the support personnel requested, there was a prosector and an aide to help manoeuvre the cadavers of the large quadrupeds it was proposed to dissect.[34] Vicq d'Azyr did receive funds to get the Commission underway and pay his expenses as chief correspondent with the provinces, but it is unclear to what extent the facilities relating to anatomy teaching were realized. Certainly there are references after

1778 to a course in the amphitheatre of the Société Royale de Médecine on the Rue du Sépulchre where Vicq d'Azyr had set up house after his return to Paris and he continued private teaching there as well, but this facility did not become a public teaching institution.[35]

Vicq d'Azyr's quest for an institutional home for his anatomical work was finally achieved in the 1780s at the veterinary school at Alfort. After the founder Claude Bourgelat's death in 1779, this institution became receptive to outside influences on the nature of its functions and programmes. Vicq d'Azyr's careful cultivation of political patronage aided him again in this situation. This time he succeeded in being installed in newly constructed facilities for the pursuit of anatomy at the veterinary school that matched his designated title of Professor of Comparative Anatomy. Moreover, he shared instruction and research at a reconstructed and reorganized veterinary school, with his friend Daubenton as professor of rural economy and with Antoine Fourcroy, his protégé, as professor of chemistry. The establishment of elaborate research facilities for this trio was part of an endeavour to transform the traditional nature and form of the instruction at the Paris veterinary school, which had previously focused on the care of horses, into a full-scale research and teaching institution devoted to the study of the health of the rural economy and to the teaching of a new type of veterinarian who would be at the forefront of animal medicine.[36]

It was at the veterinary school at Alfort that Vicq d'Azyr came closest to realizing his vision of developing a comparative medicine based upon a comparative anatomy. His anatomical teaching and research profited greatly from the resources that could be exploited at the school. Here at last was a place, in addition to the Jardin du Roi, where the various animals, not only domestic but also exotic, that were needed for his research programme became obtainable at government expense, and the preparations and specimens necessary to record results and use for teaching could be developed and maintained. Moreover, the results of research could be presented to acclaim at public sessions where science was put on display for the intellectual and political world, thus enhancing the reputation and prospects of the investigators.[37]

The first and only volume of the great treatise on anatomy and physiology that Vicq d'Azyr planned appeared in 1786. He began with the brain of man which he wanted to examine in relation to the brains of other animals, for in his view, 'The brain is, of all the organs, the one whose structure it is most necessary to study when wishing to develop general ideas on the nature of any genus or species whatsoever of animals, its principal dispositions are intimately linked to the general sensibility, the vigour or the feebleness of instinct, the strength of appetites, the force of affections, the extent of the intellectual faculties, and, in a word, all that can be termed the moral, the manners, in the physiological history of men and animals.'[38] Part of Vicq d'Azyr's quest was to contribute to the ongoing debate about the mind/body relationship through anatomical investigation. The beautifully illustrated first elephant folio volume of Vicq d'Azyr's *Traité* was dedicated to the king. It was hailed on its publication for its foundation in a wealth of research; but no second volume ever appeared.

It was Vicq d'Azyr's misfortune, at this very high point of his career, to see the economic policies and programmes of his patrons in the royal administration come under attack in the final years of the Ancien Régime. In 1788 the three professorships at Alfort came to an end after a change in ministerial patronage of such institutions. Although Vicq d'Azyr was allowed continued use of the facilities for research, other preoccupations distracted him from his anatomical pursuits. In the drawing up of the *New Plan for the Constitution of Medicine in France*, the Royal Society of Medicine's reform programme of 1790, there are elements of Vicq d'Azyr's belief in the value of developing a comparative anatomy and a comparative medicine. In the new pattern of medical education envisaged in the *Plan*, the dream was to have the Alfort veterinary school translated to Paris and placed next to the School of Medicine. The interrelationships of teachers and students and the sharing of resources, it was claimed, would illuminate both the anatomy and medicine of humans and animals.[39] And the medical section of the *Encyclopédie Méthodique*, begun under Vicq d'Azyr's aegis, demonstrates a broad-based conception of the medical art covering both human and animal welfare. It also contains Vicq d'Azyr's imposing plan for a course on human and animal anatomy and physiology.[40] But Vicq d'Azyr's promotion of his ideas was hindered by challenges brought by the Revolution to the scientific and medical institutions of the Ancien Régime. Attempts to adapt to the new order, the sad fate of his friends and the vulnerability of his own position undermined his career and health, and he died at the early age of 45 in 1794.[41]

In this paper I have attempted to integrate various aspects of Vicq d'Azyr's life and show how his pursuit of a career as an anatomist and anatomy teacher was significant in shaping his special vision of medicine. This work of integration is necessary, I believe, in order to recover a vision that does not play a prominent part in our understanding of the evolution of eighteenth-century medicine. Vicq d'Azyr was a noted physician in his lifetime, but in the history of medicine, his contributions seem peculiarly fragmented. His comparative anatomy seems to point not to developments in medicine itself, but to the advance of zoology in the hands of such later figures as Cuvier, Geoffroy St Hilaire and others. As a medical man he is depicted as the founder and moving spirit of an important medical society that was swept away in the Revolution only to be reconstituted as a fully fledged academy many years after his death. Yet, as I have suggested, there are important links between his accomplishments and activities that formed a distinctive vision of medicine that was constructed out of his efforts to fulfill his talents and ambitions in the particular circumstances of his times. His programme of a comparative medicine, with its underlying structure of a philosophical anatomy, was tailored to the political and institutional opportunities that were presented to him during his life. Thus was a philosophical and literary ambition transformed into a scientific and professional career in the only way that it could be in Ancien Régime France.

Notes

•Research for this paper was supported in part by a grant from the National Library of Medicine (1 RO1 LM02497), whose assistance is gratefully acknowledged.

1. Biographers of Vicq d'Azyr include Jacques Moreau de la Sarthe, 'Discours sur la vie et les ouvrages de Vicq d'Azyr', in Jacques Moreau de la Sarthe, (ed.), *Oeuvres de Vicq d'Azyr*, 6 vols (Paris, 1805), vol. 1, 1–88 (the *discours* is separately paginated from the rest of the volume); Pierre Edouard Lemontey, *Eloge Historique de Vicq d'Azyr, prononcé dans la séance publique de l'Académie Française du 25 août 1825* (Paris, 1825); C. A. Sainte-Beuve, 'Vicq d'Azyr', *Causeries du Lundi*, (Paris, 1854), vol. 10, 279–311; Jérôme Lalande, 'Eloge de Vicq d'Azir', *La Decade Philosophique, Littéraire et Politique*, An III, 3, no. 24: 513–21; 4, no. 25: 1–10. Vicq d'Azyr has not been the subject of a full-scale biography. Three medical theses have been devoted to his life and work: A.-J.-L.-M. Dufresne, *Notes sur la vie et les oeuvres de Vicq d'Azyr (1748–1794): Histoire de la fondation de l'Académie de Médecine* (Bordeaux, thèse de médecine, 1906); B. Leduc, *La vie et l'oeuvre anatomique de Vicq d'Azyr (1748–1794)* (Rennes, thèse de médecine, 1977); D. Delbos, *Un médecin normand à Paris: Félix Vicq d'Azyr (1748–1794)* (Caen, thèse de médecine,

1978). These theses are largely descriptive and draw upon the early nineteenth-century biographers.

2. Moreau de la Sarthe, 'Discours sur Vicq d'Azyr', 3–4, 82–4; Lalande, 'Eloge de Vicq d'Azir', 514. Vicq d'Azyr's eulogies are collected in the first three volumes of Moreau de la Sarthe, (ed.), *Oeuvres de Vicq d'Azyr*. For discussion of the eulogies, see Sainte-Beuve, 'Vicq d'Azyr', and Pierre Astruc, 'Les éloges prononcés par Vicq d'Azyr à la Société Royale de Médecine', *Le Progrès Médical*, 1951, 411–19. For an analysis of the eulogies as a tool for the social mobilization of talent and merit, see Daniel Roche, 'Talent, Reason, and Sacrifice: The Physician during the Enlightenment', in Robert Forster and Orest Ranum, (eds), *Medicine and Society in France: Selections from the Annales: Economies, Sociétés, Civilisations* (Baltimore: Johns Hopkins University Press, 1980), 66–88. This paper was originally published in *Annales E.S.C.*, 32 (1977), 866–86.

3. Moreau de la Sarthe characterizes the literary contribution of the eulogies as follows: 'Thus the historical eulogies of Vicq d'Azyr, which as a whole form one of the richest and most brilliant parts of the literary and philosophical history of the eighteenth century.' Moreau de la Sarthe, 'Discours sur Vicq d'Azyr', preface, iv. See also 70–1. For his opening address to the Académie Française, Vicq d'Azyr eulogized Buffon, his predecessor in the chair. See Vicq d'Azyr, 'Buffon: Discours sur sa vie et sur ses ouvrages. Prononcé à l'Académie française le 11 décembre 1788', in Moreau de la Sarthe, (ed.), *Oeuvres de Vicq d'Azyr*, vol. 1, 7–40. For an analysis of the background to Vicq d'Azyr's election to the Académie Française, see P. Thillaud, 'Vicq d'Azyr (1748–1794): Anatomie d'une élection', *Histoire des sciences médicales*, 20 (3) (1986), 229–36.

4. Laurence Brockliss has been investigating these resources. See, for example, his 'L'enseignement médical et la Révolution: essai de réévaluation', *Histoire de l'éducation*, May 1989, no. 42, 92–6. Pierre Huard, 'L'enseignement médico-chirurgical', in René Taton, (ed.), *Enseignement et diffusion des sciences en France au XVIIIe siècle* (Paris: Hermann, 1964), 223, lists a number of courses.

5. Moreau de la Sarthe, (ed.), 'Discours sur Vicq d'Azyr', 11. For information on teaching at the Jardin du Roi and the Collège Royal, see Yves Laissus, 'Le Jardin du Roi' and Jean Torlais, 'Le Collège Royal', in Taton, (ed.), *Enseignement et diffusion des sciences*, 285–319 and 261–75.

6. Sainte-Beuve, 'Vicq d'Azyr', 281.

7. Vicq d'Azyr, 'Notice historique sur les académies', in Moreau de la Sarthe, (ed.), *Oeuvres de Vicq d'Azyr*, vol. 2, 147; Vicq d'Azyr, 'Idée générale de la médecine et de ses différentes parties', *ibid.*, vol. 5, 45–6, 51.

8. Lalande, 'Eloge de Vicq d'Azir', 514–15. Moreau de la Sarthe also records how anatomy was at the centre of Vicq d'Azyr's thinking:

'But physiological anatomy occupied him in a special way. It became the science of choice for him, and inspired in him that keen interest which takes hold of thought, and makes a category of knowledge the one to which others are continually related by an active mind quick to seize upon all that can extend or enlighten the subject which captivates it.' Moreau de la Sarthe, 'Discours sur Vicq d'Azyr', 12.

9.   Laissus, 'Le Jardin du Roi', 330; Moreau de la Sarthe, 'Discours sur Vicq d'Azyr', 78; Sainte-Beuve, 'Vicq d'Azyr', 280. On Petit, see Dominique Latour, *Discours prononcé dans la salle des consultations gratuites de médecine et de jurisprudence d'Orléans. A l'occasion du buste de M. Petit* (Orleans, 1792).For a general description of anatomy at the Jardin, see Georges Barritault, *L'anatomie en France au XVIIIe siècle: les anatomistes du Jardin du Roi* (Angers: L'Imprimerie de l'Anjou, 1940).

10. Vicq d'Azyr, 'Deuxième Discours. De l'Anatomie comparée en général', in Moreau de la Sarthe, (ed.), *Oeuvres de Vicq d'Azyr*, vol. 4, 140. Also Moreau de la Sarthe, 'Discours sur Vicq d'Azyr', 8.

11. Moreau de la Sarthe, 'Discours sur Vicq d'Azyr', 77–8. Some sources, for example, Sainte-Beuve ('Vicq d'Azyr', 283) say that Vicq d'Azyr's wife was Madame Daubenton's niece.

12. Vicq d'Azyr, *Traité d'anatomie et de physiologie* (Paris, 1786), 7. Also 'There is as well a fruitful source from which the physiologist will draw useful knowledge and that is comparative anatomy. He who has only seen the brain, the heart, the stomach and the intestines of man, has only a limited idea of what the viscera are in the great chain of animals; he does not know their relationships and he is ignorant of the best part of that which he has to teach.' Vicq d'Azyr, 'Anatomie', in Félix Vicq d'Azyr *et al.*, (eds), *Encyclopédie Méthodique: Médecine*, 13 vols (Paris, 1787–1830), vol. 2, 576.

13. Vicq d'Azyr, 'Deuxième Discours. De l'Anatomie comparée en général', 141, 219–28; Vicq d'Azyr, 'Troisième Discours sur l'Anatomie. Exposition des caractères qui distinguent les corps vivans et idée générale de l'organisation des plantes et des animaux', in Moreau de la Sarthe, (ed.), *Oeuvres de Vicq d'Azyr*, vol. 4, 229–312. For an analysis of the theoretical structure of Vicq d'Azyr's comparative anatomy, see W. R. Albury, 'The Logic of Condillac and the Structure of French Chemical and Biological Theory', (Ph.D. Dissertation, Johns Hopkins University, 1972), 76–109.

14. Moreau de la Sarthe, 'Discours sur Vicq d'Azyr', 13; Lalande, 'Eloge de Vicq d'Azir', 515. Moreau de la Sarthe describes Vicq d'Azyr's appeal as a teacher as follows: 'A pure and frequently eloquent language, the contrast of youth and knowledge, a physiognomy full of expression; in fact, all the distinguishing marks that capture public esteem and quickly form a great reputation, were joined together in the new professor.'

15. Moreau de la Sarthe, 'Discours sur Vicq d'Azyr', 14–15. Information

on the dates of Vicq d'Azyr's private courses and their location has been obtained from course announcements in the *Journal de médecine, chirurgie et pharmacie*, 40 (1773), 383; 42 (1774), 476, 566; 44 (1775), 473–4.

16. The most recent work on Buffon is Jacques Roger, *Buffon: Un Philosophe au Jardin du Roi* (Paris: Fayard, 1989).

17. Moreau de la Sarthe, 'Discours sur Vicq d'Azyr', 14; Lalande, 'Eloge de Vicq d'Azir', 515; Sainte-Beuve, 'Vicq d'Azyr', 282–3; Laissus, 'Le Jardin du Roi', 330.

18. Jean Verdier, 'Anatomie (Jurisprudence de la médecine et de l'éducation physique)', in Vicq d'Azyr *et al.*, (eds), *Encyclopédie Méthodique: Médecine*, vol. 2, 630.

19. Torlais, 'Le Collège royal', 282, 284; Gustave Schelle, (ed.), *Oeuvres de Turgot*, 5 vols (Paris: Librairie Félix Alcan, 1913–1923), vol. 5, 39; Archives S.R.M., Carton 109, Letter of Joseph Lassone to Vicq d'Azyr.

20. Auguste Corlieu, *L'ancienne Faculté de Médecine de Paris* (Paris, 1877), 39, 124, 126–7.

21. Moreau de la Sarthe, 'Discours sur Vicq d'Azyr', 15; A. Pinard, H. Varnier, F. Widal, and G. Steinheil, (eds), *Commentaires de la Faculté de Médecine de Paris (1777–1786)* (Paris: Steinheil, 1903), 680, 703, 817, 819. For the course outline, see Vicq d'Azyr, 'Anatomie', in Vicq d'Azyr *et al.*, (eds), *Encyclopédie Méthodique: Médecine*, vol. 2, 236–544.

22. Moreau de la Sarthe, 'Discours sur Vicq d'Azyr', 16–17; Lalande, 'Eloge de Vicq d'Azir', 516–17; Lemontey, *Eloge de Vicq d'Azyr*, 4–5.

23. See Caroline Hannaway, 'Medicine, Public Welfare, and the State in Eighteenth-Century France: The Société Royale de Médecine of Paris (1776–1793)', (Ph.D. Dissertation, Johns Hopkins University, 1974), 82–95.

24. Vicq d'Azyr's collected recommendations and regulations are to be found in *Recueil d'observations sur les différentes méthodes proposées pour guérir la maladie épizootique qui attaque les bêtes à cornes, sur les moyens de la reçonnoitre partout ou elle manifester, et sur la manière de désinfecter les étables* (Paris, 1775). His account of his investigations and travels is Félix Vicq d'Azyr, *Exposé des moyens curatifs et préservatifs qui peuvent être employés contre les maladies pestilentielles des bêtes à cornes* (Paris, 1776). See also Léon Moulé, 'Vicq d'Azyr et la pathologie animale', *Bulletin de la Société française d' histoire de la médecine*, 17 (1923), 192–205.

25. Félix Vicq d'Azyr, 'Expériences relatives à la sensibilité et à la respiration', *Mémoires de la Société Royale de Médecine*, 1 (1776), 340–54; Lemontey, *Eloge de Vicq d'Azyr*, 7.

26. See Caroline Hannaway, 'The Société Royale de Médecine and Epidemics in the Ancien Regime', *Bulletin of the History of Medicine*, 46 (1972), 262–4.

27. Félix Vicq d'Azyr, *Mémoire instructif sur l'établissement fait par le Roi d'une Commission ou Société et Correspondance de médecine* (Paris, 1776), 30; Vicq d'Azyr, *Exposé*, 75. For a general history of comparative medicine, see Lise Wilkinson, *Animals and Disease: An Introduction to the History of Comparative Medicine* (Cambridge and New York: Cambridge University Press, 1992).

28. Hannaway, 'Medicine, Public Welfare, and the State', ch. 4.

29. *Ibid.;* Vicq d'Azyr, *Mémoire instructif,* 33–8; *Histoire de la Société Royale de Médecine,* 1 (1776), preface, xi.

30. Vicq d'Azyr, *Mémoire instructif,* 33–8.

31. Roche, 'Talent, Reason, and Sacrifice', has emphasized the role of Parisian academies and societies in diffusing knowledge and of Paris as the centre of élite medicine.

32. Vicq d'Azyr, *Exposé des moyens curatifs; Avis sur la correspondance de la Société Royale de Médecine, et sur les objets dont cette compagnie est chargée* (Paris, [1776]), 1–4.

33. *Arrest du Conseil d'Etat, qui établit une Commission de Médecine à Paris pour tenir une correspondance avec les médecins de province, pour tout ce qui peut être relatif aux maladies épidémiques et épizootiques,* 29 April, 1776, Articles IV, VII.

34. AN F17 1318.

35. For example, *Journal de médecine, chirurgie et pharmacie,* 46 (1776), 383.

36. For details on the transformation of Alfort, see Caroline Hannaway, 'Veterinary Medicine and Rural Health Care in Pre-Revolutionary France', *Bulletin of the History of Medicine,* 51 (1977), 439–40. See also Hannaway, 'Medicine, Public Welfare, and the State', 213–14.

37. Philibert Chabert, Pierre Flandrin, and Jean Huzard, (eds), *Instructions et observations sur les maladies des animaux domestiques,* 6 vols (Paris: 1782–1790), vol. 1, 82–5; *Journal de médecine, chirurgie et pharmacie,* 70 (1787), 556–8.

38. Vicq d'Azyr, *Traité d'anatomie et de physiologie,* Introduction.

39. *Nouveau Plan de constitution pour la médecine en France,* reprinted in *Histoire de la Société Royale de Médecine,* 1787 and 1788, 135–6.

40. See especially the preface to vol. 1 of the *Encyclopédie Méthodique: Médecine.* As well Vicq d'Azyr, Jean Huzard was the primary contributor of articles on animal husbandry and animal medicine. As indicated earlier, Vicq d'Azyr is the author of the article 'Anatomie', in vol. 2. For discussion of the *Encyclopédie Méthodique: Médecine* and Vicq d'Azyr's part in it, see Roselyn Rey, 'Les métamorphoses de l'Encyclopédie: le cas des sciences de la vie', *Recherches sur Diderot et l'Encyclopédie,* 12 (April, 1992), 41–58.

41. Sainte-Beuve, 'Vicq d'Azyr', 308–11; Lalande, 'Eloge de Vicq d'Azir', 8–9. Vicq d'Azyr had the misfortune to have attained the position of first physician to Queen Marie Antoinette in 1789. The Royal Society of Medicine was abolished along with the other academies and societies in 1793.

9

Medical Microscopy in Paris, 1830–1855

Ann La Berge

The story of the Paris Clinical School has been told many times in many ways, from those who first began to write its history – contemporary commentators and critics, including foreigners who studied in Paris and reported on their experiences – to recent secondary accounts ranging from Erwin Ackerknecht's 1967 survey – now the standard account – to Russell Maulitz's treatment of pathological anatomy and Jack Lesch's study of experimental physiology.[1]

While the Paris School is a well-known chapter in the history of medicine, some aspects of Paris medicine have been investigated hardly at all. Lack of personal papers has discouraged historians from attempting accounts of some of the leading figures such as Gabriel Andral, widely recognized as the 'father of haematology'. Other areas, such as medical microscopy and animal experimentation, have attracted little interest from historians.[2] The reasons are unclear. Whereas the use of the microscope in medicine figured prominently in contemporary accounts and debates, historians have generally either ignored the topic or made only passing reference to it. Perhaps justifiably so. Yet the nagging question remains: what, if any, was the role of microscopy in Paris medicine? Was the microscope a research tool which figured prominently in the French medical experience? Ackerknecht has tantalized us by suggesting that on the one hand 'France possessed a whole phalanx of outstanding microscopists', but on the other, by arguing that the French failure to embrace scientific, laboratory medicine – specifically, techniques such as microscopy – accounted in part for the decline of Paris medicine *vis-à-vis* German medicine after 1840.[3]

In this article I will show how shortly after the new compound achromatic microscope became available around 1830, Alfred

Donné pioneered medical microscopy in France, issuing a manifesto for the new approach in his 1831 MD thesis from the Paris Faculty and inaugurating the first public microscopy course in 1837. By the early 1840s, a microscopy community had developed in Paris, centred around the teachers of the new technology. At the same time the microscope was being used for teaching purposes in medical courses, such as physiology, and by utilizing the new instrument medical researchers began exploring new areas such as the microscopical study of body fluids and pathogenic plant and animal parasites. Some physicians embraced the improved instrument with great hopes of having a new diagnostic tool at their disposal, but in the pre-bacteriological era, the era of early medical microscopy, their successes were limited. Although the instrument was readily accepted for medical research, its applications to medical practice were few. Thus by the 1850s, the end of the early era of medical microscopy, the jury was still out on the utility of the microscope. Although Paul Broca, the leading spokesman of the second generation of medical microscopists could declare with confidence that the microscope was fully integrated into Paris medicine, in fact, few practitioners saw it as useful, and many remained sceptical of the microscope.[4] An active microscopy community embraced the instrument at first, taught microscopy skills, and recognized the value of the microscope in medical research, but by the mid-1850s, the instrument had failed to provide enough practical applications to assure its diffusion and acceptance by practitioners.

In France the medical applications of the microscope remained virtually unexplored until the 1830s, although scientists and amateurs had used the instrument since the seventeenth century.[5] There are many reasons why French physicians were reluctant to use the microscope. First, given the dominant theories of disease causation in the eighteenth century, the humoral and environmental theories, there was no medical reason to try to understand disease with the microscope. Second, in early nineteenth-century France a philosophy of radical empiricism which emphasized the use of the unaided senses in medical observation was dominant. This was the approach of Bichat, who said, 'Let us neglect all these idle questions where neither inspection nor experience can guide us. Let us begin to study anatomy there where the organs begin to fall into the range of our senses.'[6] Finally, and perhaps most critical, was the state of technology. Until the 1820s microscopes were hard to make, hard to use, and expensive. Images were often blurred and coloured fringes encircling the visual field distorted the image. Microscopy required considerable skill and training, which most physicians lacked, and a very delicate handling of specimens. Because the images were often unclear and the microscopes difficult to use, microscopy hardly seemed to be a promising method for preventing or diagnosing disease. Furthermore, before the 1820s (though actual details are lacking) most specimens were probably mounted dry. According to Brian Bracegirdle, author of a book on the history of micro-technique, with dry mounts not much detail is visible, and such specimens have little resemblance to life. Scientific research, he concluded, was almost impossible for all but the most extremely skilled investigators until the techniques of wet mounts, fixing, and staining were developed.[7]

By the early 1830s the situation had changed. The emergence of pathological anatomy as the central focus of Paris medicine and physicians' attempts to extend their investigations from the organ to the tissue, focused attention on a scientific approach to diagnosis. Pathological anatomy with its method of correlating symptoms in the living patient with lesions found *post mortem* had become one of the hallmarks of the Paris School.[8] The notion that one could dissect and analyse organs, tissues and body fluids to find disease provided an atmosphere in which the microscope might have something to offer. Equally as important, Joseph Jackson Lister and Charles Chevalier introduced compound achromatic microscopes in which the distortion factor was reduced from about nineteen to three per cent, and in which the fringes of colour around the object being observed were removed.[9] Some French scientists were already using microscopy in their work. Most notable was François Raspail, regarded as the father of histochemistry. Raspail, Chevalier and the naturalist A. C. M. Le Baillif greatly improved techniques of specimen preparation. By 1830 they were mounting most specimens in a fluid medium, and Chevalier introduced glass cover slips.[10] By the 1830s better and cheaper instruments made microscopes more attractive as research tools.

In the 1830s Parisian physicians began to use the microscope in their research. Scientifically-minded Parisian physicians embraced the new technology, which was rapidly diffused among the Parisian medical élite. By the late 1830s and 1840s a microscopy community had developed in Paris, clustered around four microscopy teachers, their students, and physicians and surgeons with whom they collaborated. Hermann Lebert, a Prussian by birth, began teaching microscopy informally in 1836; Alfred Donné, the only native microscopy teacher, offered the first public course in 1837; two Hungarian immigrants, David Gruby and Louis Mandl, began teaching in the 1840s, Gruby in 1842, Mandl in 1846. Lebert's disciples included the surgeons Aristide Verneuil and François Follin, microscopist and histologist Charles Robin, and pathologist (and later anthropologist) Paul Broca. Gruby's students included physiologists François Magendie, Claude Bernard and Pierre Flourens, and naturalist Henri Milne-Edwards. Donné's most famous student was Scottish pathologist John Hughes Bennett, and of Mandl we know he taught medical students, but we have no names.[11]

Donné, Gruby, Mandl and Lebert inaugurated the teaching of microscopy in formal and public as well as private settings in Paris and extended the microscope's applications from the natural sciences to medicine. They mapped out the field of early medical microscopy, their research suggesting in what areas of medicine the instrument could be useful, even indispensable, and where it was problematic owing to the state of scientific knowledge, the level of technological development, and techniques of specimen preparation. In some areas, such as the diagnosis of tuberculosis, early hopes were dashed, because microscopical observations did not improve diagnostic accuracy. For example, in the 1830s physicians held out the hope that a simple blood test might reveal the presence of cancer or tuberculosis. Such was not to be the case. In others, such as the diagnosis of a variety of common dermatoses, the microscope proved indispensable. The early medical microscopists – especially Lebert – put forward a full-blown theory of medical microscopy and its relationship to clinical medicine, proposing a model of how a new medical technology might occupy a position of centrality and importance in the research and practice of the clinician.

Alfred Donné, encouraged by Jean-Baptiste Bouillaud for whom he worked at the Charité hospital, introduced microscopy to the Parisian medical élite in 1831. He inaugurated medical microscopy in Paris and became the primary spokesman for the new approach to medical investigation. Donné received his MD from the Paris Faculty in 1831 with a thesis on the chemical and microscopical analysis of body fluids. He competed unsuccessfully for the *agrégation* in medicine at the Paris Faculty in 1835 and never held a faculty position. Setting himself up in private practice on the rue de Condé, he worked as *chef de clinique* under Bouillaud, embarked on a major research programme in microscopy, began to teach public microscopy courses, and became known for his expertise in treating infants and children. Donné was well-connected politically and socially. His father-in-law secured for him the position of assistant librarian at the Faculty of Medicine, and he was also appointed inspector-general of the University in charge of medicine.[12]

In his MD thesis, *Recherches physiologiques et chimico-microscopiques sur les globules du sang, du pus, du mucus, et de ceux des humeurs de l'oeil,* Donné forecast much of the work he would do in medical microscopy. He began by announcing the importance of microscopy for the study of pathological anatomy, noting that few had yet availed themselves of the instrument:

> The use of the microscope applied to the observation of tissues and liquids of the system is still rarely used by physicians; it would seem, however, that in an epoque in which anatomy has made such progress, that everything which we can directly observe with our senses in the various organs of the human body and that everything which can be attained by the thin blade of the scalpel is almost completely understood, observers ought rapidly to adopt an instrument which, doubling the power of their means [of observation] reveals to them an unknown world, and permits them to see and analyse that which up to now has escaped their detailed investigation.[13]

Donné addressed the reluctance of physicians to learn to use the microscope, suggesting two reasons why some resisted the new technology: general scepticism, based on a philosophy of radical empiricism, and the practical difficulties involved in using the instrument. On the first point he commented:

> Microscopical observations generally inspire little confidence from anatomists; this instrument appears to them more proper for procuring troublesome illusions than for precisely retracing the truth. They are sceptical of anything that they cannot see with their [naked] eyes and touch with their finger; they leave this type of research [microscope] to botanists, who have made good use of it for several years, to clarify plant physiology, and they do not believe they ought to include the microscope among the numerous useful apparatuses of their amphitheatres.[14]

The second reason why anatomists were reluctant to add the microscope to their research arsenal was the difficulty they had in using it. It required considerable practise and skill to use the instrument, and many were easily discouraged:

> Even though it seems, at first glance, that it suffices just to look [through the instrument] in order to see, it is certain that untrained people begin by seeing nothing when they are not well directed; their patience wears thin, runs out, and they reject the instrument which they do not at all know how to operate.[15]

The difficulty of using the microscope and resultant unfamiliarity with the instrument encouraged many to reject not only the instrument but also what had been discovered using it. Donné believed education was the key to acceptance. He saw the need for formal microscopy classes and believed that microscopy would provide an opportunity for him to establish a reputation in an area he regarded as the 'cutting edge' of medical research. Donné had learned to use the microscope from Le Baillif, a skilled amateur scientist, whose office was a meeting place in the late 1820s for many scientists, including microscopists Raspail, Mirbel and Turpin, and legal medicine specialist Matthew Orfila. Part of Donné's scientific programme was to teach the microscopic skills he had learned from Le Baillif to others. Donné inaugurated public microscopy classes in Paris in 1837.[16]

Microscopy, like other specialties and accessory sciences, was taught in private and public courses which were an integral part of medical study in early nineteenth-century Paris. The Faculty of Medicine made its facilities available for the public courses, which complemented the regular medical curriculum. Donné and Mandl used one of the Faculty's amphitheatres, while Gruby and Lebert taught microscopy in their private laboratories. The typical pattern was that a course in a new specialty would first be offered outside the Faculty, either in public or private courses, then eventually incorporated into the regular medical curriculum. For example, from the beginning of the century until 1835 pathological anatomy was taught in this manner. Only in 1835 was a chair in that specialty established at the Medical Faculty. Microscopy was, however, different from pathological anatomy and some of the nascent specialties like dermatology and paediatrics. Indeed neither Donné nor Lebert ever saw microscopy as a first-order specialty to be incorporated into the curriculum of the Faculty as a regular course. Rather both suggested that microscopy was a technique fundamental to many basic branches of medical science taught at the Faculty: anatomy, physiology, pathology, chemistry, natural history and legal medicine. Medical courses were also taught at the Collège de France – both Laennec and Magendie taught there, and later Claude Bernard – and clinics took place in the Paris hospitals. Erwin Ackerknecht has termed the whole conglomerate of Paris medicine with its great variety of institutions and teaching facilities 'the Paris hospital'.[17]

In order to offer a public course, a physician had to receive authorization from the Minister of Public Instruction. He would write to him explaining what he wanted to teach, attaching an outline or syllabus for the course. His letter was accompanied by a letter of recommendation from the Dean of the Paris Faculty of Medicine. Although courses were open to the public free of charge, most medical courses were intended primarily for medical students and *agrégés* at the Faculty of Medicine. The number of medical courses offered in any given year varied widely. For example, in 1857/8 there were 14 requests for courses, whereas in 1860/1 there were 36.[18]

Donné described his class, which was taught in the evenings. His description gives us a good insight into how microscopy was learned and taught in the early years of medical microscopy. He recounted that in 1837 he set up a private class at his own expense where he gave lectures and demonstrations in an amphitheatre equipped with 20 microscopes:

> Twenty microscopes lighted by lamps in order to have a fixed and constant light, and in order to be able to give lessons in the evening at an hour when the students are free from their principal occupations, are placed on tables in front of which they [the students] can circulate; each microscope carries a label indicating the nature of the object [being observed]; after the lesson, eight or ten students descend, from each side of the amphitheatre, into the enclosure where the instruments are, file by until they have viewed all the objects, and are replaced by others, in such a way that in a half hour or more, 100 to 140 auditors can examine the substances ... and acquire sufficient knowledge to state the exactitude of the facts.[19]

Donné then noted that while these demonstrations were a good introduction, they were not sufficient to teach students how to perform microscope analyses on their own. For this more in-depth study he offered special, smaller classes in which the students prepared the specimens and set up the demonstrations by themselves.[20]

Both in his teaching and research Donné was eager to make microscopy rigorously scientific, by which he meant precise, objective. Microscopical observation was particularly subject to observer error, was hard to objectify and hard to teach. It was difficult to fix the image so that more than a hundred students might observe the same thing. Illustrators tried to reproduce faithfully on paper what had been observed in the microscope, so that a fixed image would be available for study and serve as a permanent record. Nevertheless, students looking through the microscope often failed to see what was portrayed in a good illustration. In 1840 when Louis Daguerre announced his invention of photography to the Royal Academy of Sciences, Donné began exploring the possibility of applying the new technology to microscopy. Just a few months after Daguerre's announcement, Donné presented a photomicrograph, a photograph taken through a microscope, to the Royal Academy of Sciences. Donné had quickly realized the advantages photography would have for microscopy in providing a certain objectivity previously lacking. Now the image could be fixed, reproduced, published and studied.[21]

Like many of the leading Parisian physicians such as Gabriel Andral and Pierre Rayer, Donné was a neohumoralist who wanted to use chemical and microscopical analysis to study the structure of body fluids in order to diagnose disease. From 1831 until 1845 Donné published widely on the topic, with studies on saliva, pus, mucus, milk, blood and urine. The apogee of his teaching and research career was his 1844 comprehensive microscopy textbook accompanied by an atlas in which photomicrographs were presented along with illustrations. This work included and updated his earlier individual studies.[22]

Although our focus here is on Donné's teaching of microscopy, as for all the microscopy teachers, it is artificial to separate teaching from research. Early medical microscopists did both. Donné also excelled as a scientific researcher, making several discoveries with the microscope which have earned for him the dubious distinction of 'precursor'. He anticipated the cell theory with his discovery of the protozoon *Trichomonas vaginalis,* an event which signified the beginning of the understanding of the role of parasitic protozoa in pathology.[23] Donné also researched and described the abnormal blood condition characterized by an excess of white blood cells, or leukemia. In conjunction with his specialty of diseases of infants and children, he became the leading French authority on the microscopical analysis of human milk.[24]

Donné anchored the small and loosely-knit Parisian microscopy community in the early 1840s. Like the other microscopy teachers, he regularly sent his work to the Academy of Sciences and was, in addition, the Academy's reporter for the influential daily 'Establishment' newspaper, the *Journal des Débats.* Of his numerous students, we only know the name of John Hughes Bennett, the Scottish clinician and pathologist, who would himself become a microscopy teacher and leading promoter of medical microscopy.[25]

Among the four teachers David Gruby is probably the best known to historians of science and medicine, indeed the only one who has merited an article in the *Dictionary of Scientific Biography.* Gruby studied medicine at the University of Vienna under pathological anatomists Carl Rokitansky and Joseph Berres, who taught him microscopical pathology and encouraged his microscopy investigations. In 1839 Gruby received his MD, opened a private course in anatomy and physiology, and published his MD thesis, 'Microscopical Observations on Pathological Anatomy'. He also taught private microscopy courses, which were attended by visiting foreign physicians, such as Parisian surgeon Philippe-Joseph Roux, who was so impressed with Gruby's microscopy that he encouraged him to come to Paris to pursue it. Here was an opportunity for someone like Gruby to make his mark on Paris medicine, and also for Parisian physicians to benefit from his skills. The University of Vienna offered Gruby a position if he would convert from Judaism to Christianity, but he refused, left Austria, and taking Roux's suggestion, arrived in Paris towards the end of 1840. Gruby's most intense period of scientific activity was between 1840 and 1845, when he began offering private microscopy instruction and made important contributions in mycology.[26]

At the end of 1841 Gruby opened a private laboratory on rue Gît-le-Coeur, where from 1842 to 1854 he taught physiological and pathological anatomy and microscopy. Flourens, Magendie, Milne-Edwards and Bernard all studied with him, as well as students from England, Scotland, Norway, and Sweden. Onésime Delafond, professor at the Veterinary School at Alfort, with whom Gruby collaborated in his research, was also a student. Gruby spent much time at Alfort conducting animal experimentation with Delafond, teaching students microscopy in Delafond's laboratory, and thus inaugurating the study of microscopy at the veterinary school.

We have no details of Gruby's teaching methods or his microscopy classes. They were more informal and collegial than Donné's, since he taught only a few students, perhaps only one at a time, in his private laboratory. His students were colleagues in the scientific and medical community: Milne-Edwards was already an accomplished microscopist, having practised microscopy since the 1820s. Likewise, Magendie had been using microscopy since the late 1830s in both his teaching and research on blood circulation. Bernard probably learned to use the microscope from Gruby, but we have no information on this aspect of his medical education.[27]

Gruby's interest in dermatology, specifically the aetiology of common skin diseases, led to his accomplishments in mycology. Working at the Children's Hospital, Gruby noticed how widespread thrush and ringworm were and sought to discover their cause. In collaboration with Swedish proto-paediatrician F. F. Berg, he discovered the plant parasite that causes thrush, now known as *Candida albicans*. Using the microscope, he also identified the fungi that cause favus and ringworm. Working with Delafond at the veterinary school, he discovered several pathogenic animal parasites. He called the parasite he found in frog's blood *Trypanosoma*, the name used ever since for this genus. Gruby and Delafond also identified microfilaria, a parasitic hematozoon of dogs and discovered and described the parasites that caused several other kinds of skin disease. Most of Gruby's research was published between 1840 and 1845 as brief articles in the *Comptes-rendus de l'Académie des Sciences.*[28]

One of Gruby's colleagues and microscopy students was François Magendie, physiologist and pharmacologist, who held the chair of physiology at the Collège de France. From the 1830s Magendie regularly used the microscope in his teaching, where it added add a new dimension to physiological demonstrations. Magendie's use of microscopy in teaching and research is documented in his four-volume work, *The Physical Phenomena of Life*, a record of his teaching at the Collège de France in 1837–38. In these two years of courses, even before he began studying microscopy with Gruby, Magendie, in collaboration with Jean Poiseuille, used the microscope to show blood circulation to students. Magendie believed microscopical examination was central to an understanding of blood circulation in the capillaries, and he regularly used the instrument to demonstrate to students the circulation of blood in animals. Magendie and Poiseuille studied the movement of blood through the capillaries under the microscope, and Magendie wanted his students to be able to make the same observations. On 16 June, 1837, he discussed microscopical observations with his students and some of the problems related to using the microscope as a teaching tool:

> In order for you to judge for yourselves the questions we're going to address, it would be necessary for each of you to come one after the other to look through the eye-piece of the microscope, [an exercise] which is incompatible with our kind of teaching. However, I do not despair of giving all of you demonstrations of the movements of globules in the capillaries. I have at my disposal the dark room of the Collège de France, and if everything is ready on time, you will be able, by means of the solar microscope, to have a perfectly exact idea of all the principal phenomena.[29]

The solar microscope was especially good for observing circulation in animals, and was thus preferred by Magendie as a teaching tool. Although it did not provide the clarity of a compound microscope, the solar microscope offered advantages for teaching in that several students could view an object at the same time. To use the instrument, one inserted a tube in the hole of a shutter of a darkened room. In the tube were one or two lenses which concentrated the light from the sun on the object to be observed. The result was a brilliant image which shone on a large piece of white paper placed at a distance of 10, 15, or

20 feet. The greater the magnification, the weaker the image.[30]

On 23 June, the class was still examining the capillary action of blood and again had the opportunity to make microscope observations. Magendie spoke to the students:

> You will be able to examine the other specimens at the end of class.... They will give you a general idea of the tubular network and its anastomosis. To have a perfect description you must submit them to microscope inspection, follow with your eye the globules as they leave the arteries and not lose sight of them until they've arrived in the venous system.[31]

On 28 June, 1837, the class was devoted to an examination of circulation in animals, and microscope maker Charles Chevalier and Poiseuille arranged the microscopic demonstration for Magendie's students. Magendie reported:

> At the end of the class the professor [Magendie], followed by numerous students, went to the dark room at the Collège de France. Using the solar microscope, they examined the blood globules of several species of animal, capillary circulation in lizards, frogs, and tadpoles. M. Chevalier showed them the insect that causes scabies (*Acarus scabiei*) and several crystallized salts.[32]

After the next class on 30 June, Magendie addressed his students:

> You have been able to judge for yourselves the manner in which the blood moves in the infinitely small tubes. Those of you who have for the first time witnessed this spectacle must have been seized with admiration at the sight of these astonishing phenomena of which the solar microscope has displayed for us a living panorama.[33]

Magendie was discovering nothing new by using the microscope. Indeed in the seventeenth century Leeuwenhoek had identified blood cells, Malpighi had observed circulation in the capillaries, and Bonomo had identified the itch mite that caused scabies. What was important in the case of Magendie was his incorporation of microsopy as a form of classroom demonstration in his physiology classes.

Magendie believed microscopical examination was central to an understanding of blood circulation in the capillaries, one important area of physiology. But the problem, as he saw it, was that many physicians either did not have a microscope or did not know how to use one, leading to conflicting opinions on the structure and function of capillaries. There were many disagreements among investigators, Magendie maintained, 'because everybody does not have a microscope, and when they have one, often it is not good, and when they have an excellent one, everybody doesn't know how to use it.'[34]

Magendie also used the microscope for in-class pathological examinations, although far less often than for studying circulation. On several occasions, for example, he reported examining portions of diseased lungs from tubercular patients. Medical microscopists hoped to be able to diagnose tuberculosis either by an examination of sputum or blood. Based on his microscopical studies, Magendie had hypothesized that the disease was spread by the blood. During the 1830s and 1840s, with a resurgent interest in neohumoralism, physicians hoped that microscopical and chemical examination of the blood might reveal the presence of diseases such as tuberculosis and cancer, thus providing an easy method for early and accurate diagnosis. For these two diseases, their hopes were dashed. Examining the sputum from a tuberculosis patient, Magendie noted the presence of purulent globules. The problem he hoped, but failed, to solve with the aid of the microscope was the origin of the viscous liquid coughed up from the lungs.[35]

Magendie not only used the microscope for demonstration purposes, but also taught microscopy skills to his physiology students. On 28 March, 1838 he devoted the class to a discussion of the history and practice of microscopy. He also provided a detailed account of the techniques to be used in studying the blood under a microscope and of how to measure blood globules with a micrometer. Here was another opportunity for students to acquire microscopic skills. Magendie's students could learn the basics of microscopy while taking a physiology class. They did not have to study microscopy separately.[36]

Louis Mandl, like Donné, taught microscopy to large classes. Mandl, like Gruby, was in Paris by 1840, disseminating Johannes Müller's work on the microscopical study of cancer which had been done within the context of Schwann's cell theory. Indeed, Mandl's own studies on the histogenesis of tumours were simliar to Müller's. Beginning in 1846, Mandl offered a course, modelled on Donné's, on general and microscopical anatomy for medical students at the Ecole pratique at the Faculty of Medicine.[37]

In addition to group or private instruction, another method of teaching microscopy was by self-help books. Using such manuals, physicians and students might learn to use the microscope without formal training. Mandl was one of three microscopists who wrote microscopy manuals in the 1830s and 1840s, along with microscope maker Charles Chevalier and botanist Félix Dujardin, dean of the Faculty of Sciences at Rennes. Chevalier and Mandl's handbooks were published in 1839, Dujardin's small pocketbook in 1843.[38]

Mandl also produced between 1838 and 1846 a massive two-volume treatise entitled *Microscopical Anatomy,* a reference work in which he gave the history, bibliography and current research (including his own) on virtually every topic related to microscopy. In addition, he published a number of articles in the *Comptes-rendus de l'Académie des Sciences* and in the *Archives générales de médecine,* of which he was one of the editors.[39]

The fourth microscopy teacher was Hermann Lebert, who became by the late 1840s the recognized leader of French medical microscopy. Lebert studied medicine and natural science in Berlin until 1833, when he followed his teacher Schönlein (who was also Schwann's teacher) to Zurich. He received the MD from the University of Zurich in 1834, having studied with Schönlein and Oken. Lebert spent most of 1835 in Paris attending the clinics of some of the leading physicians and returned to Switzerland in 1836. By 1839 he was employed as a cantonal physician near Bex, and was attached to the water cure establishment at Lavey-les-Bains. Ackerknecht stated that Lebert started teaching microscopy in Paris in 1836, but Lebert did not mention it in his own account, and contemporaries gave Donné the honour of being the first to offer courses in medical microscopy in Paris. No doubt Lebert, already a skilled microscopist, may have taught microscopy informally to colleagues and students, however. In the early 1840s he began spending his winters in Paris (he mentions the winters of 1842/43, 1843/44, and 1844/45) and his summers practising medicine at Lavey-les-Bains. In 1845 his *Pathological Physiology,* one of the earliest treatises on tumours in which microscopy figured prominently, was published. It was here that Lebert put forward his theory of the specific cancer cell, according to which all tissue lesions contained cells having visible characteristics specific for the kind of lesion involved. Cancer cells, he maintained, appeared different from other cells when observed under the microscope. Lebert's theory of the specific cancer cell established his reputation within the Parisian medical community, even though almost all Parisian and foreign microscopists disagreed with him. Lebert finally settled in Paris in 1846. Like the other microscopy teachers, he never held an academic position in Paris. Nevertheless, by the late 1840s and early 1850s he was considered the leading microscopist in the city. In 1847 he opened a private medical practice and was awarded the Prix Portal by the Academy of Medicine for his work *Practical Treatise on Scrofulous and Tubercular Diseases,* in which microscopical observation held an important place.[40]

Lebert had more international connections than the other

microscopy teachers, collaborating with scientists and physicians in France and abroad. He practised medicine first in Switzerland, then in Paris, again in Switzerland, and finally in Germany, and he had professional colleagues and collaborators in each place. While still in Switzerland he did research and published a couple of articles on blood circulation and embryology with Genevan microscopist Jean-Louis Prévost. Lebert and Prévost became close friends, carried on a ten-year correspondence, and Lebert delivered Prévost's eulogy at the Société de biologie.[41]

Lebert worked with Rudolf Virchow at several points in his career, his friendship with him dating from 1845 when he went to Berlin to study surgery with Dieffenbach. Lebert, along with epidemiologist Ludwig Panum and microscopist Julius Vogel, published articles in Virchow's journal, *Archive for Pathological Anatomy, Physiology, and Clinical Medicine,* and later in his career he contributed to Virchow's six-volume *Handbook of Special Pathology and Therapy,* the first volume of which was published in 1854. Lebert's work, *Diseases of the Blood and Lymph Glands,* appeared in 1861 as part 2 of volume 5. By this time Lebert was teaching and practising medicine in Breslau.[42]

Ackerknecht claimed that Lebert had a strong influence on Virchow's thinking. Virchow, according to Ackerknecht, realized the limitations of gross pathological anatomy and wanted to make pathology into a science in its own right – based on clinical experience, animal experimentation, and pathological anatomy. This was the approach of Lebert (*Physiologie pathologique*) and earlier of Bichat (*Anatomie générale*). Virchow strongly urged the use of microscopy in pathology, acknowledging, however, that it had often been badly used, and therefore, in the minds of some physicians, had fallen into discredit.[43] Virchow had a close friendship with Lebert and picked up many microscopy skills from him, but he did not adopt Lebert's ideas of specific tubercles or cancer cells. Virchow showed in his work on tuberculosis that Lebert's 'tubercles' were not new, specific cells arising out of the blastema, but were in fact degenerating cells. And he always vigorously denied the existence of specific cancer cells.[44]

In Paris, Lebert collaborated with Donné, who, he said, gave him good research advice. Discussing the study of circulation, Lebert noted that microscopists usually used a frog's foot for demonstration and experimentation, while for studying inflammation they preferred a frog's tongue. Lebert credited Donné with showing him the benefits of using a frog's tongue to study circulation, noting that for a long time

Donné had used this method of demonstration in his microscopy course. 'When this skilful and ingenious observer showed me this experiment for the first time, I couldn't have been more pleasantly surprised to see that one could use such a great part of this organ for studies in pathological physiology.'[45] Lebert also collaborated with Donné on experiments on blood altered by pus: 'I did the first experiment on this subject in common with Donné, who very much wished to help us with his advice on this difficult study, and whose known skill for experimentation was a big help.'[46] In the first experiment Lebert got the experimental pus from the surgeon Velpeau at the Charité. Numerous similar experiments followed, with pus donated by physicians at the Parisian hospitals. The results of these experiments were inconclusive.[47]

Lebert's collaborators included many physicians and surgeons at the Parisian hospitals who provided him with morbid specimens. Such cooperation was critical to the success of early medical microscopy, since the microscopists themselves didn't hold hospital positions. Without such collaboration, microscopists interested in pathology couldn't do their work. But this kind of arrangement put the micros-copist in a subservient position – as a medical technician – and that is surely one of the reasons that Lebert and Broca stressed that microscopy could not be divorced from clinical medicine. Were microscopy to be a pursuit its own right, the micrographer would not have the social or professional status of the clinical physician or surgeon. Microscopists needed to acquire a professional reputation, to attain legitimacy in a new and controversial area of medical research and methodology. Mentioning his work with the famous Parisian clinicians lent authority to Lebert's work. And Lebert, as a foreigner, needed to show that he worked with the best of them. He specifically mentioned the help of Andral, Velpeau, Cruveilhier, Louis, Alphonse Bérard, Blandin and Guersant. Institutional affiliations also helped establish credibility. For example, Lebert acknowledged the assistance of the Anatomical Society, mentioning some members by name.[48]

Lebert's microscopy 'school', his disciples who were greatly influenced by his work, included Paul Broca, Charles Robin, François Follin and Aristide Verneuil. Even before he settled in Paris Lebert collaborated with Robin, whom Lebert met in August, 1844, when Robin gave his first paper at the Anatomical Society. In 1845 Matthew Orfila, dean of the Faculty of Medicine, sent Robin and Lebert to the coast of Normandy and Jersey to gather objects of natural history and comparative anatomy for a museum he was establishing. Robin and Lebert presented the results of their research on fish and molluscs to the Philomatic Society in 1845 and subsequently published a couple of articles on the topic.[49]

Lebert and his school made their own institutional contribution to the Paris scientific and medical world. They provided the nucleus of the Société de biologie, founded in 1848 by two surgeons, Follin and Houel, Charles Robin, Claude Bernard, and pathological anatomist Pierre Rayer, the first president of the organization. (Foreign correspondents included Kölliker and Virchow.) The goal of the organization was to promote biology and medical science and to provide a forum for discussion. Medical microscopists formed the nucleus of the society: Follin was one of the surgeons who regularly provided clinical observations (along with Eugène Bouchut, Charcot and Rayer) and Bernard, Broca, Follin, Lebert, Robin, Verneuil and Charcot regularly furnished pathological anatomical observations.[50]

Lebert went the furthest of the four microscopy teachers in providing a theoretical basis for medical microscopy and its integration into clinical medicine, providing us with the best French account of the theory and practice of early medical microscopy. Lebert's programme, like that of many of his contemporaries, was to make medicine scientific, using as his model the Baconian method of observation. During his student days in Berlin, he had been struck by the fact that medicine seemed to lag behind the natural sciences, and one of his lifelong goals was to make medicine a science in its own right. Using the microscope to investigate disease was one way to pursue this goal. Lebert recognized the contributions of pathological anatomy to this end, but also pointed out its limitations. What was now needed, he argued, was a neo-humoral approach: studies of vital secretions and morbid alterations of body fluids after death. He criticized the still-dominant gross anatomical method, advocating the application of chemistry and microscopy to pathology. Lebert emphasized the complementary nature of the scientific endeavour: clinical study, animal experimentation and microscopical observation had to be pursued together:

> For my part, I realized early that, if one wanted to arrive at more precise notions in pathological physiology, it was necessary, in addition to chemical research, to have the concurrence of three other methods of investigation, namely: clinical study, animal experimentation and microscope observation.[51]

Lebert did not exaggerate the role of microscopy which, he contended, always had to be used in conjunction with other methods. He emphasized the centrality of clinical observation:

The microscope can be a great help in pathology, but its role only begins after the use of other methods capable of unveiling the nature of disease. Thus clinical observation will always be the basis of pathology. It will remain the centre of activity and the goal of all the efforts of the true physician.[52]

For Lebert the clinician held the position of primacy in medical investigation:

The chemist who will analyse a product of secretion, the microscopist who will study the details of a morbid tissue, will be able to provide valuable information, but this information – by itself – would only have a secondary value. Both can provide materials for medical doctrines, but only the clinician is capable of coordinating them [the information] in a regular manner.[53]

In this selection Lebert asserted that the microscopist need not seek a separate and preeminent role apart from the clinician. Microscopists and chemists who merely assisted clinicians were laboratory technicians, but the clinician who was also a microscopist had the judgement and experience to put all the information together and interpret it. Lebert wanted to establish his credentials as a clinician who used the microscope, who availed himself of all the means of scientific investigation at his disposal. But he did not want to make his name as a micrographer. Microscopy must not be detached from clinical medicine and treated separately. Instead the two should be integrated.

Lebert's theory and practice of microscropy were most succinctly presented at the beginning of the *Atlas* which accompanied the two-volume *Pathological Physiology* (1845). This short document provides the clearest account of the techniques of early medical microscopy in the French literature of the period. Lebert began by stressing that microscopical examination must be grounded in pathological anatomy:

It is indispensable, before beginning the examination of a pathological specimen with the microscope to do a very careful dissection [with the naked eye] beforehand; next you continue with the magnifying glass or the simple microscope. Without a good preliminary dissection, microscope study only confuses and spreads errors, and all those who have closely followed the recent progress of comparative anatomy know very well that the naturalists who have cultivated this science almost exclusively by microscope examination without constraining themselves by a minutely exact dissection, have fallen into greater errors than those who cultivated comparative anatomy without using the microscope.[54]

The next step was the preparation of the specimen. The techniques of specimen preparation were not highly developed or widely known, and so Lebert's careful description assumes a greater importance than we might at first imagine. What is now common knowledge needed to be made explicit in the early years of this new medical technology. Lebert provided a detailed account of how the early nineteenth- century student of medical microscopy should proceed. He counseled that a very small quantity of liquid or a very thin section of tissue spread between two slips of glass allowed the microsopist to distinguish all the elements the most clearly. Sometimes a diluting liquid such as water would need to be added, but the observer should guard against rapid deterioration of the specimen: some liquids could not be diluted with water. In such cases the addition of a neutral salt, blood serum or liquid egg white might improve observation. Chemical reagents were most useful when one combined chemical analysis with microscope examination. Acetic acid was a good choice, because it made some cell walls transparent so that details of cell organization were more easily observed. For example, acetic acid allowed the observer to distinguish tuberculous matter from pus. But acetic acid had to be used with great caution, because when mixed with certain liquids, it promptly altered them. He advised letting the acid enter the specimen by capillarity between the two glass slips. Specimen preparation was always tricky, he warned, and only after much trial and error would the observer acquire the necessary skills.[55]

Another important procedural point concerned magnification. Lebert contended that one had to examine in succession the same object with varying magnifications ranging from weak to strong. Weak magnification of 30–50x sufficed for examining morbid tissue and all related to vascularity. Average magnification of 200–300x was better for studying the arrangement and disposition of molecular elements of which tissues were composed. While many microscopists were reluctant to use magnification stronger than 300x, Lebert asserted that to identify the characteristics of differing pathological elements, a stronger magnification of 500–800x was often required.

The instruments needed for specimen preparation included scissors, pointed tweezers and scalpels. Other instruments were not necessary, Lebert maintained, for the skill was in the microscopist's fingers, not in the instruments. The choice of time of observation was also an important procedural consideration. By the mid-1840s when Lebert was writing, optical instruments had been perfected so that observers could work at night with a lamp as well as in the day with natural light. Lebert recommended daylight for most research,

313

while contending that for strong magnifications and for seeing details that needed a bright, focused light, a lamp could be superior to daylight.

Final procedural recommendations included the use of micrometers for measuring the object observed and the importance of sketching the object while it was under the microscope so that it could be compared with other observations. Lebert also commented favourably on the new technique of photomicrography, pioneered by Donné. This use of the daguerrotype could render important services to microscopists, he said, by fixing the observation, which could then be studied by numerous observers.[56]

By the late 1840s medical microscopy was becoming entrenched in some areas of Paris medicine. Lebert was recognized as the leading microscopist, and a new generation of medical students was learning and practising medical microscopy. The early era, or first phase, of medical microscopy in France lasted until 1854. By that year the original medical microscopy community had been transformed and a major debate in the Academy of Medicine on the utility of the microscope marked a turning point in the history of French medical microscopy.

By 1854 three of the four original microscopy teachers had either left Paris or left microscopy. Donné departed in 1848. As adviser to the royal family, he was in political trouble during the Revolution. Shortly after Louis Napoleon came to power, Donné left Paris to become rector first at the Faculty of Medicine at Strasbourg and then at Montpellier, where he had a successful career for over 20 years in the French system of higher education.[57] Gruby did not continue to pursue his microscopical research after 1854, but instead acquired a second reputation as a practitioner known for his unorthodox but successful treatments and his famous clientele. In 1854 Gruby was authorized to practice medicine in France, and after that date he devoted himself exclusively to his patients, establishing a lucrative practice catering to many writers, artists and musicians, such as Alexandre Dumas (father and son), Frédéric Chopin, Franz Liszt and George Sand.[58]

Lebert became a well-known and highly respected clinician first in Zurich and then in Breslau. He left Paris in 1852 to assume a clinical post in Zurich. In his autobiography he claimed that combining research and the demands of a growing practice was too taxing, and so he decided to reduce his commitment to research and to focus on the practice and teaching of medicine. The position in Zurich allowed him to do this. In addition, Lebert felt that he was never fully accepted by the Parisian medical élite. He never held a clinical post while in Paris. Instead, he made his reputation on his research, microscopy teaching and, above all, on his theory of the specific cancer cell. But this was a minority theory, and Lebert was a German. Some colleagues accused him of systems building, that is, of constructing a whole medical system from a hypothetical cancer cell. He defended his position publicly in the debate on cancer that took place in the Surgical Society of Paris in 1852/3. In 1854 he was put up for election to the Academy of Medicine, but his candidacy was unsuccessful. Only in 1866, by which time he had moved to Breslau to practice medicine, was he elected a corresponding member.[59] None of the other three microscopy teachers was ever elected to the Academy of Medicine or the Academy of Sciences in any capacity.

Not surprisingly, with the departure of three of the four microscopy teachers, the number of microscopy courses declined. An American medical student who signed his name only 'B', wrote in 1854 about the great neglect of the microscope in Paris and claimed that there was only one microscopy teacher, Charles Robin, in the whole city. According to Henri Meding's 1853 survey of Parisian medical personnel and institutions, Robin taught microscopy in his private laboratory, which Meding singled out as the best scientifically equipped laboratory in the city. In fact, special courses were less needed by the 1850s, as microscopy became incorporated into other courses. Students could learn microscopy skills as part of other courses, such as pathology or physiology, or informally from colleagues and mentors.[60]

1854 marks the end of the early era of medical microscopy for another reason. That year the 13-session debate over the utility of the microscope for pathology began in the Academy of Medicine. Not one of the four microscopy teachers was present, since none of them were members of the Academy. Of the first generation of medical microscopists only Onésime Delafond was involved in the debate from inside the Academy. Mandl wrote a letter to the Academy clarifying his position on Lebert's cancer cell. The leaders of the second generation of microscopists, too young to be elected to the Academy, chronicled the debate from the outside: Broca, for the *Moniteur des hôpitaux*, Verneuil, for the *Gazette hebdomadaire*, Follin, for the *Archives générales de médecine*.

After 1854 microscopy was carried on by the 'Young Paris School', as Velpeau called them – to distinguish them from the original Paris School – the students of the first generation of medical microscopists, especially Lebert's students – Broca, Follin, Verneuil, Robin.[61] Broca, best known for his studies of the speech centres of the brain and as the founder of anthropology in France, was the leading disciple of Lebert and also taught microscopy informally. According to his biographer, Francis Schiller, Broca probably met Lebert in 1846 at the Charité hospital or in 1847 at the Hôtel-Dieu. Broca was a very enthusiastic student, and at one point in the late 1840s he was going to offer his own microscopy course to bring in some extra money, but nothing came of the plan. He did teach colleagues informally, however. Bouillaud, for example, recounted that Broca had given him a microscopy lesson.

Broca received his MD from the Paris Faculty in 1849. That same year the Academy of Medicine opened a competition for the best essay on cancer, and Broca submitted a 350–page manuscript which won the Prix Portal. Schiller describes the prize-winning essay as a well organized account of Lebert's principal teachings. The essay also contained Broca's own work in pathology, microscopy, and his discovery of how malignant neoplasms spread through the veins. Broca followed Lebert's basic philosophy, stressing the importance of a clinical approach combined with microscopy. For both Lebert and Broca there was no rivalry between clinical and laboratory medicine. Indeed they went hand in hand, each verifying and reinforcing the other. In the 1850s and 1860s, following Lebert's lead, Broca conducted tumour research. Before moving on to other areas of medical and scientific investigation, he wrote 46 papers on tumours and and published a two-volume *Treatise on Tumours*.[62]

Broca became a leading promoter of medical microscopy among the second generation of medical microscopists, chronicling the 1854–55 debate on cancer and the use of the microscope to diagnose cancer for the *Moniteur des hôpitaux*.[63] The Young Paris School preached the integrative approach of Lebert and Virchow, in which microscopy and clinical medicine went hand in hand. Broca expressed it like this: 'Let us bring together towards a common goal all the observational methods at our disposal, the clinic as well as pathological anatomy, the scalpel as well as the microscope, the study of tissues as well as the study of tumours.'[64] Former students like Robin, Broca, Follin and Verneuil were spokesmen for the utility of the microscope, and Robin and Broca taught microscopy. Some physicians and surgeons like Velpeau used it into their research and practice. Within a generation microscopy had been accepted by the Parisian medical élite. By the end of the debate in 1855, Broca, with great rhetorical flourish, proclaimed that a microscopical revolution had occurred and that microscopy had been integrated into Paris medicine.[65] Broca may have claimed too much. By the mid-1850s, microscopy had ceased to be a novelty and had become an accepted part of medical *research*. What was still at stake was the utility of the instrument for the *practice* of medicine and surgery, specifically its usefulness as a diagnostic tool to differentiate benign from malignant tumours.

A story from the 1860s illustrates the endurance of scepticism towards the instrument's utility for the practitioner. Victor Cornil, physician and microscopist, who was influenced in his microscopical work by Broca and Verneuil, recalled that when he defended his doctoral thesis in 1864 – a full ten years after the turning point in the history of medical microscopy – that his microscopical work was met with suspicion, even ridicule, by his examining committee:

> When I passed my doctoral thesis in 1864 on the histology of nephritis, one of my judges, very kindly in other respects, said to me, 'You have written an infinitely meritorious work, sir, but what the devil good does it serve? Have you found under your microscope the means of curing albuminuria?'[66]

Cornil's response shows that the intrument was primarily a diagnostic tool, but emphasizes the relationship of diagnosis to therapy and suggests the importance of a good understanding of anatomy and physiology for the practising physician who would treat patients with care.

> It was only too easy to respond that it was necessary to know the structure of the kidney in order to understand what happens when it is inflamed. That is the basis of our knowledge on this point. One certainly does not cure a victim of nephritis by examining urinary sediments under a microscope, but one makes a more correct diagnosis that helps in finding a medication.[67]

The introduction of the microscope into the Parisian medical community in the 1830s and 1840s provides an instructive case study of the acceptance and diffusion of a new technology and can be compared with the introduction and diffusion of the stethoscope and, later, Pasteurian science. For the microscope the pattern was one of introduction and rapid diffusion among a small group of research-oriented physicians and surgeons, but of slow diffusion, or even outright resistance, among Parisian practitioners and especially among the large army of average medical practitioners, most practising in the provinces. While leading Parisian physicians – the Paris School – readily accepted the utility of the instrument as a research tool, some of the Parisian medical élite questioned its role in medical practice. Indeed for most average practitioners there was a lag time of over 50 years from the introduction of the microscope within the Parisian medical community until widespread acceptance of its utility for the ordinary practising physician. It was not until the 1890s – 60 years after Donné introduced the microscope to Parisian physicians – with the introduction of diphtheria serotherapy that many practitioners began to see the advantages of using the microscope in medical practice.[68]

By contrast, the stethoscope, introduced in 1819, was more quickly accepted and diffused by researchers and practitioners alike. A comparison of the two instruments illustrates some key differences in their acceptance and diffusion. Until the era of bacteriology the microscope proved more problematic than the stethoscope. Within a few years after their introduction (the stethoscope in 1819, the microscope in the early 1830s), physicians acknowledged the diagnostic benefits of both instruments. But there was a major difference in skill required to use each instrument and how those skills could be acquired, in the kinds of disease each could diagnose, and in the applicability of each to medical practice and medical research. While the stethoscope was not easy for anyone to use, physicians could acquire necessary skills at the bedside of the numerous (20,000 or so at any given time) patients available in the Parisian hospitals for clinical research. By contrast, until laboratories were instituted in the hospital in the late nineteenth century, microscopy skills were learned by public classes and private lessons. Microscopy impressed contemporaries as more complicated and difficult to learn and not as easy to apply to the everyday practice of medicine as the stethoscope. Donné made this point in 1844:

> It is wrong to imagine that all its takes is to look into the microscope and [that] consequently everybody is capable of using this instrument as one uses opera glasses. Microscopical observation really constitutes a science which has its own principles and its rules, its difficulties and its methods, whose knowledge cannot be improvised any more than that of any other science.[69]

The diagnostic benefits of the stethoscope acquired a greater importance than those of the microscope, which is clearly one reason the latter met with greater resistance among Parisian physicians than did the stethoscope. The stethoscope enabled the physician to diagnose accurately the leading lethal disease of the nineteenth century – tuberculosis – as well as other lung and heart problems. But the immediate diagnostic benefits of the microscope were far less

318

obvious, being restricted in the early years after its introduction primarily to skin diseases caused by plant and animal parasites. It was not clear in this early period that the microscope had any great utility for medical practice, although some practitioners used it as a diagnostic aid. One good example was the surgeon Velpeau, who never relied exclusively on the microscope, and who in fact was sceptical of its practical diagnostic utility. He argued that for tumour detection the microscope was no better than naked-eye observation. Nevertheless, he routinely submitted tumour sections to Lebert and his students for microscopical examination. The microscope's utility in diagnosing certain skin diseases was recognized by leading dermatologists within a few years of Gruby's discoveries.[70] But, with the exception of skin diseases, most practitioners did not see that the microscope was of much help in their practices. If the microscope had enabled practitioners to diagnose tuberculosis or cancer by a microscopical analysis of blood or to distinguish benign from cancerous tumours, then the instrument might have assumed as central a place within the Paris School as did the stethoscope. But the microscope could do none of these things. Yet, the microscope was clearly seen as an aid to medical research. In this first phase of early medical microscopy, the instrument remained primarily a research tool, its use widespread among the Parisian medical élite, most of whom were actively engaged in both research and practice.

Notes

1. Erwin Ackerknecht, *Medicine at the Paris Hospital, 1794–1848* (Baltimore: Johns Hopkins University Press, 1967); Russell Maulitz, *Morbid Appearances: the Anatomy of Pathology in the Early Nineteenth Century* (New York: Cambridge University Press, 1987); John Lesch, *Science and Medicine in France: the Emergence of Experimental Physiology, 1790–1855* (Cambridge: Harvard University Press, 1984).
2. There is some discussion of animal experimentation in physiology in John Lesch, 'The Paris Academy of Medicine and Experimental Science, 1820–1848', in William Coleman and Frederic L. Holmes, (eds) *The Investigative Enterprise: Experimental Physiology in Nineteenth-Century Medicine* (Los Angeles: University of California Press, 1988), 100–38.
3. Ackerknecht, *Paris Hospital*, 125; Harry Paul, 'The issue of decline in nineteenth-century French science', *French Historical Studies 7* (1972), 416–50; Robert Fox and George Weisz, 'Introduction: The institutional basis of French science in the nineteenth century', in Robert Fox and George Weisz, (eds), *The Organization of Science and Technology in France, 1808–1914* (New York: Cambridge University Press, 1980), 1–28.

4. Paul Broca, 'Séance de l'Académie', *Moniteur des hôpitaux*, 23 January, 1855, 73.
5. Stanley Reiser, *Medicine and the Reign of Technology* (New York: Cambridge University Press, 1978), 72–5. The popularity of microscopes for amateurs continued unabated. For use of microscopes by amateurs in the United States, see John Harley Warner, 'Popular Microscopy in America', *J. Hist. Med.* 37 (1982), 7–33. An exception was physician Théophile Bordeu, who had used the microscope in the eighteenth century. See Elizabeth Haigh, *Xavier Bichat and the Medical Theory of the Eighteenth Century* (London: Wellcome Institute, 1984), 35, 124.
6. Ackerknecht, *Paris Hospital*, 8–9; Maulitz, *Morbid Appearances*, 13–14; Haigh, *Xavier Bichat*, 97–98. Quote in Haigh, 97. The quote is from Xavier Bichat, *Anatomie générale appliquée à la physiologie et la médecine*, 4 vols (Paris: Brosson and Gabon, 1801), vol. 2, 576. On the philosophy of ideology, see the classic article by George Rosen, 'The Philosophy of Ideology and the Emergence of Modern Medicine in France', *Bull. Hist. Med.* 20 (1946), 328–39.
7. Haigh, *Xavier Bichat*, 96–99; Reiser, *Reign of Technology*, 74–5; Brian Bracegirdle, *A History of Microtechnique* (Ithaca: Cornell University Press, 1978), 9.
8. Maulitz, *Morbid Appearances*.
9. Reiser, *Reign of Technology*, 76; Charles Chevalier, *Des microscopes et de leur usage* (Paris: Crochard, 1839), 79–105. John Quekett, *A Practical Treatise on the Use of the Microscope* 2nd edn (London: Baillière, 1852), 25–39.
10. Dora Weiner, *Raspail: Scientist and Reformer* (New York: Columbia University Press, 1964), 78–111; Bracegirdle, *History of Microtechnique*, 24–25; Chevalier, *Des microscopes*, 187–90.
11. Ackerknecht, *Paris Hospital*, 126. Ackerknecht says Lebert began teaching in 1836. Lebert does not mention it in his autobiographical account of his life and work, *Biographische Notizen* (Breslau: Korn, 1869).
12. Camille Dreyfus, 'Alfred Donné (1801–1878): Un précurseur en hématologie' *Nouvelle revue d'hématologie* 2 (1961), 241–55; A. Lennox Thorburn, 'Alfred François Donné, 1801–1878, discoverer of *Trichomonas vaginalis* and of leukemia', *British Journal of Venereal Diseases* 50 (1974), 377–80. *Agrégés* were assistant professors who could then compete for clinical positions when they became available. On Donné as proto-paediatrician, see Ann F. La Berge, 'Mothers and Infants; Nurses and Nursing: Alfred Donné and the Medicalization of Child Care in Nineteenth-Century France', *J. Hist. Med.* 46 (1991), 20–43. The head librarian at the Paris Faculty held professorial status. It is not clear exactly what the status of the assistant librarian was. See Ackerknecht, *Medicine at the Paris Hospital*, 35. The 'University' referred to the French system of higher

education. For an explanation of that system, see Terry Clark, *Prophets and Patrons: The French University and the Emergence of the Social Sciences* (Cambridge: Harvard University Press, 1973), 18.

13. Alfred Donné, *Recherches physiologiques et chimico-microscopiques sur les globules du sang, du pus, du mucus, et de ceux des humeurs de l'oeil* (Paris: Didot le jeune, 1831), 5.

14. *Ibid.*, 6.

15. *Ibid.*, 7.

16. *Ibid.*, 8. On Le Baillif and his students, see Chevalier, *Des microscopes*, 259–62.

17. On private courses, see George Weisz, 'Reform and Conflict in French Medical Science', in Robert Fox and George Weisz, (ed.), *The Organization of Science and Technology in France, 1808–1914* (New York: Cambridge University Press, 1980), 62–9; Pierre Huard and Marie-José Huart, 'L'enseignement libre de la médecine à Paris au XIXe siècle', *Revue d'histoire des sciences* 37 (1974), 45–62. On the teaching of pathological anatomy, see Maulitz, *Morbid Appearances*, 60; Ackerknecht, *Paris Hospital*, 167; and Pierre Huard and Marie-José Imbault-Huart, 'La vie et l'oeuvre de Jean Cruveilhier, anatomiste et clinicien', *Episteme* 8 (1974), 46–57; Donné, *Cours de microscopie complémentaire des études médicales* (Paris: Baillière, 1844), 8–9. On the development of medical specialties, see George Weisz's chapter in this volume.

18. Archives Nationales, Paris, F¹⁷ 6672, Dossiers, Cours de l'Ecole pratique, 1857–60, 1860–61.

19. Donné, *Cours de microscopie*, 8–9.

20. *Ibid.*

21. *Comptes-rendus de l'Académie des Sciences*, 9 (1839), 485–6. See also Alfred Donné, 'Procédés de gravure des images photogéniques sur plaques d'argent', *Comptes-rendus de l'Académie des Sciences*, 10 (1840), 933–4.

22. On microscopical analysis as a way of dissecting body fluids, see Reiser, *Reign of Technology*, 128–9; Alfred Donné, *Des propriétés chimiques des secrétions dans l'état sain et dans l'état morbide* (1834); *Recherches sur les caractères chimiques de la salive, considérés comme moyen de diagnostic dans quelques affections de l'estomac* (1835); *Mémoire sur les caractères distinctifs du pus, etc.* (1836); *Recherches microscopiques sur la nature du mucus* (1837); *Du lait, et en particulier celui des nourrices* (1837); *Nouvelles expériences sur les animalcules spermatiques* (1837); *Tableau des sédiments des urines* (1838); *Cours de microscopie* (1844); *Atlas de microscopie* (1845). I am not sure if Donné was the first to publish micrographs or not. Bracegirdle notes that the *Atlas* is of major interest because it exemplifies the use of very early photomicrography. See Bracegirdle, *History of Microtechnique*, 47.

23. Jean Théodoridès, 'Etat des connaissances sur la structure des

Protozoaires avant la formulation de la théorie cellulaire', *Revue d'histoire des sciences* 25 (1972), 27–44. See also the brief discussion in William Bulloch, *The History of Bacteriology* (New York: Dover, 1979; reprint of book originally published in 1938 by Oxford University Press), 162–3. For the report to the Royal Academy of Sciences, see 'Infusoires. Animalcules observés dans les matières purulentes et le produit des secrétions des organes génitaux de l'homme et de la femme', ext. d'une lettre de M. A. Donné in *Comptes-rendus de l'Académie des Sciences*, 3 (1836), 385–6. The main work in which Donné published his findings was *Recherches microscopiques sur la nature des mucus et la matière des divers écoulements des organes génito-urinaires chez l'homme et chez la femme* (Paris: l'auteur, 1837).

24. Camille Dreyfus, 'Alfred Donné'; Thorburn, 'Alfred François Donné'. Maxwell Wintrobe, *Hematology, the Blossoming of a Science* (Philadelphia: Lea and Febriger, 1985), 12–16. Wintrobe credits both John Hughes Bennett and Rudolf Virchow with the first description of the new disease, leukemia. On Virchow as the first person to discover leukemia as a pathological entity, see Walther Seufert and Wolf D. Seufert, 'The Recognition of Leukemia as a Systemic Disease', *J. Hist. Med.* 37 (1982), 34–50. On Bennett's claim and his disagreement with Virchow, see John Hughes Bennett, *Leucocythemia,* or *White Cell Blood* (Edinburgh: Sutherland and Knox, 1852). On John Hughes Bennett, see John Harley Warner, 'Therapeutic Explanation and the Edinburgh Bloodletting Controversy: Two Perspectives on the Medical Meaning of Science in the Mid Nineteenth Century', *Medical History* 24 (1980), 24–58. See Donné, 'Sur la constitution microscopique du sang', *Comptes-rendus de l'Académie des Sciences*, 6 (1838), 17–18 and *Cours de microscopie*, 135–6. For Donné's work on milk, see Alfred Donné, *Du lait, et en particulier celui des nourrices* (Paris: chez l'auteur, 1837).

25. John Hughes Bennett, *An Introduction to Clinical Medicine: Six Lectures on the Method of Examining Patients; Percussion; Auscultation; the Use of the Microscope; and the Diagnosis of Skin Diseases.* 2nd edn (Edinburgh: Sutherland and Knox, 1853).

26. V. Kruta, 'David Gruby', in *Dictionary of Scientific Biography*, vol. 5, 565–6. See also on Gruby, Raphael Blanchard, 'Notices biographiques. III. David Gruby, 1810–1898', *Archives de parasitologie* 2 (1899), 43–74; Jean Théodoridès, 'L'oeuvre scientifique du Dr Gruby', *Revue d'histoire de médecine hébraïque* 27 (1954), 27–38.

27. Blanchard, 'David Gruby', 61. Bernard is always mentioned by Gruby's biographers as one of his microscopy students, but Bernard himself doesn't mention it. Bernard never mentions it in his published works nor does Larry Holmes recall ever seeing any comments in Bernard's papers and laboratory notebooks. Frederic L.

Holmes, *Claude Bernard and Animal Chemistry: the Emergence of a Scientist* (Cambridge: Harvard University Press, 1974) and conversation with Larry Holmes.

28. Kruta, 'David Gruby', 565–6; Blanchard, 'David Gruby', 48–59.

29. François Magendie, *Les phénomènes physiques de la vie*, 4 vols (Paris: Baillière, 1842), vol. 3, 267–8. Jean Poiseuille studied blood pressure, inventing in 1828 an instrument called a hemodynamometer to measure blood pressure. The instrument was only used on aminals, however, since it depended on the dangerous procedure of opening an artery. On Poiseuille, see Reiser, *Reign of Technology*, 98–9 and Lesch, *Science and Medicine in France*, 186. For collaboration of Magendie and Poiseuille, see *Les phénomènes physiques*, vol. 3, 34–377, *passim*.

30. The information on the solar microscope is from Louis Mandl, *Traité pratique du microscope* (Paris: Baillière, 1839), 17–19.

31. Magendie, *Les phénomènes physiques*, vol. 3, 300.

32. *Ibid.*, 342.

33. *Ibid.*, 343.

34. *Ibid.*, vol. 2, 335.

35. *Ibid.*, 94, 152.

36. *Ibid.*, vol. 4, 340–52; vol. 3, 343, 354–6.

37. Louis Mandl, 'De la structure intime des tumeurs ou des productions pathologiques', *Archives générales de médecine* 8 (1840), 313–29; 'Histogenèse', in *Anatomie microscopique*, 2 vols (Paris: Baillière, 1838–47), vol. 2, 339–70. From Leland Rather, *The Genesis of Cancer* (Baltimore: Johns Hopkins University Press, 1978), 109; Blanchard, 'David Gruby', 61. For Mandl's microscopy course, there are two letters of interest in AN, F[17] 6695, Dossiers of *cours publics* offered by physicians. In a letter dated 23 March, 1846, Matthew Orfila, Dean of the Faculty of Medicine wrote to the Minister of Public Instruction, requesting a 1,000 franc encouragement to help Mandl teach his course in one of the Faculty buildings free to medical students. The course was to be similar in design to those Donné offered. The response, dated 9 May, 1846, was positive; an attempt would be made to find the money to help Mandl offer the course. In F[17] 6672, Dossier 1860/1, there is a letter from Mandl to the Minister of Public Instruction, dated 5 May, 1860 asking permission to teach a course on diseases of the chest, and tuberculosis in particular. There is also an undated letter of recommendation for Mandl from Paul Dubois, Dean of the Faculty of Medicine, to the Minister of Public Instruction, in which Dubois cites Mandl's histological and microscopical accomplishments.

38. Mandl, *Traité pratique du microscope* (Paris: Baillière, 1839); Chevalier, *Des microscopes et de leur usage* (1839); and Félix Dujardin, *Nouveau manuel complet de l'observateur au microscope* (Paris: Roret, 1843).

39. *Anatomie microscopique*. Beginning in 1837 Mandl regularly sent

papers to the Académie des Sciences. See, for example, 'Mémoire sur le pus, les mucus, et les épanchements différents', *Comptes-rendus de l'Académie des Sciences* 5 (1837), 478–9. Mandl was also one of the editors of the *Archives générales de médecine.*

40. All this introductory information on Lebert is from Francis Schiller, *Paul Broca: Founder of French Anthropology, Explorer of the Brain* (Berkeley: University of California Press, 1979), 59–76 and Lebert's own account, *Biographische Notizen,* 53 and *passim.* The quote is from Schiller, *Paul Broca,* 61. Correspondence to and from Lebert while he was physician at Lavey-les-Bains, 1839–46, before he moved to Paris permanently, is in Bibliothèque cantonale et universitaire de Lausanne, IS 4104, (1, 2, 3), Correspondance Lebert. Lebert, *Traité pratique* des *maladies scrofuleuses et tuberculeuses.* (Paris: Baillière, 1849).

41. 'Sur la formation des organes de la circulation et du sang chez les batraciens', *Annales des sciences naturelles (Zoologie),* 1 (1844), 193–229; 'Observations sur le développement du coeur chez le poulet', *Comptes-rendus de l'Académie des Sciences* 24 (1847), 291–2; Hermann Lebert, 'Eloge du Dr Prévost', *Mémoires de la Société de biologie* 2 (1850), 60–5.

42. Erwin Ackerknecht, *Rudolf Virchow: Doctor, Statesman, Anthropologist* (New York: Arno Press, 1981, reprint; originally published in 1953 by the University of Wisconsin Press), 6, 8, 12, 21, 53; *Handbuch der Speziellen Pathologie und Therapie,* 6 vols (Erlangen, 1854–76).

43. Ackerknecht, *Rudolf Virchow,* 53–4. Virchow, like his predecessors Donné, Lebert, Vogel, John Hughes Bennett and Müller, had at first subscribed to Schwann's cellular theory, according to which the amorphous blastema was the forerunner of the cell, or put another way, cells originated from blastema. Donné, Lebert, Vogel, Bennett and Müller had all studied the pathological changes in cells under the premises of blastema theory. Going against his predecessors, including Lebert, Virchow's great contribution was, according to Ackerknecht, not the reduction of pathology to cells, but the reversal of Schwann's blastema theory and the creation of a new cell theory. *Ibid.,* 56–7.

44. *Ibid.,* 77–8; Rather, *Genesis of Cancer,* 109–10. See the Academy of Medicine debate on cancer and the utility of the microscope in which Lebert's prominence was in great part due to his theory of the specific cancer cell: *Bulletin de l'Académie de Médecine* (1854–55), 7–447.

45. Hermann Lebert, *Physiologie pathologique* (Paris: Baillière, 1845), 5.

46. *Ibid.,* 312–14.

47. *Ibid.,* 313–14, 324–30.

48. *Ibid.,* 3–4.

49. Victor Genty, *Un grand biologiste: Charles Robin, 1821–1885* (Lyon: A. Rey, 1931), 18–19.

50. E. Gley, 'La Société de biologie et l'évolution des sciences biologiques

en France de 1849 à 1900', in E. Gley, *Essais de philosophie et l'histoire* (Paris: Masson, 1900), 168–9, 175, 272–4. Bernard and Robin were the first vice-presidents. Other members included Brown-Séquard and Davaine.

51. Lebert, *Physiologie pathologique*, viii, ix.
52. *Ibid.*
53. *Ibid.*
54. Herman Lebert, *Atlas. Physiologie pathologique*, 8.
55. *Ibid.*, 10–12.
56. *Ibid.*, 12–15.
57. Terry Clark explains the position of rector. Under the Ministry of Education there were 16 rectors, one for each Academy in France. The Academy was the basic administrative unit of the national educational system and included the Faculties and lycées. The rector was the administrative link between the Ministry of Education and the Faculties and lycées of each Academy. The dean of each Faculty reported to the rector. See Clark, *Prophets and Patrons*, 19.
58. J. H. Rille, 'David Gruby', *Dermatologische Wochenschrift* 12 (1926), 525; Blanchard, 'David Gruby', 62.
59. Lebert, *Biographische Notizen*, 32–3. *Bulletin de la Société de Chirurgie de Paris*, 3 (1852/3), 232–56.
60. Letter from 'B' in *The North-Western Medical and Surgical Journal* (Chicago), 3 (April, 1854), No. 4, 147. Thanks to John Harley Warner for bringing this source to my attention. In his survey of Parisian physicians and medical facilities, Henry Meding commented that Robin's laboratory was the first (the implication was, and the only) scientifically equipped laboratory in the city. Robin offered courses in general anatomy and pathological anatomy. Meding makes no mention of a separate microscopy course, but he noted that the laboratory was well equipped with microscopes. Robin incorporated microscopy into his anatomy and physiology classes. Henri Meding, *Paris médical* (Paris: Baillière, 1852–53), 349–51. Meding lists microscopists Follin, Broca and Verneuil all as teaching private pathology, anatomy and physiology courses. See 354, 357, 361–2.
61. Broca, 'Séance de l'Académie de Médecine', *Moniteur des hôpitaux*, 5 October, 1854, 945.
62. The following account is based on Schiller, *Paul Broca*, 59–76 and Paul Broca, *Traité des tumeurs* (Paris: Asselin, 1866), I–XVI; for Broca as Bouillaud's teacher, see *Bulletin de l'Académie de Médecine* (1854–55), 284. See also Broca's MD thesis, *De la propagation de l'inflammation. Quelques propositions sur les tumeurs dites cancéreuses* (Paris: Rignoux, 1849), 58. See also his prize-winning work for the Academy of Medicine: 'Anatomie pathologique du cancer', *Mémoires de l'Académie de Médecine*, 16 (1852), 453–824.
63. Broca, *Moniteur des hôpitaux*, 4 October, 1854–14 March, 1855. *Bulletin de l'Académie de Médecine*, (1854–55), 7–447.

64. Broca, *Traité des tumeurs*, 42.

65. For Broca's comment about a microscopical revolution, see *Moniteur des hôpitaux*, 23 January, 1855, 73.

66. Quoted in Jack Ellis, *The Physician-Legislators of France: Medicine and Politics in the Early Third Republic, 1870–1914* (New York: Cambridge University Press, 1990), 36. Originally cited in *Le Progrès médical*, 29 October, 1904.

67. *Ibid.*

68. Bruno Latour, *The Pasteurization of France*. Trans. Alan Sheridan and John Law (Cambridge, MA: Harvard University Press, 1988), 127–9. On these ordinary practitioners, see Hildreth's paper, this volume and also Martha Hildreth, *Doctors, Bureaucrats, and Public Health in France, 1888–1902* (New York: Garland, 1987).

69. Alfred Donné, *Cours de microscopie*, 32. On the stethoscope, see Reiser, *Reign of Technology*, 23–44.

70. Alfred-Armand Velpeau, *Traité des maladies du sein* (Paris: Masson, 1854) VI–XVI and 481–505. Bazin, Devergie and others were receptive, but Cazenave was still resisting in 1850. See Blanchard, 'David Gruby', 55–6.

10

Bacteriological Research and Medical Practice in and out of the Pastorian School

Anne Marie Moulin

From Salomon-Bayet to Latour and Leonard,[1] French historians have described a French society under Pasteur's influence at the end of the 19th century – a 'pasteurized society', to borrow the jocative title of Latour's book. The assumption that French society was indeed 'pasteurized' raises the issue of the role of the medical body. In this process were they the vectors or the actors? How did they adapt the main tenets of the pasteurian doctrine to their own professional goals and scientific interests? An alliance had been sealed between Pasteur and a part of the medical establishment the terms of which would be renegotiated in the following years between the 'Pastorian school' and the medical community. At stake was the emergence of a new style of medicine, laboratory-based:[2] 'Pasteur recreated medicine by introducing into it the spirit and the method of the exact sciences.'[3]

There is no doubt that in the last decade of the nineteenth century, sometimes after a period of scepticism, most physicians paid lip-service to what was represented as a sweeping medical revolution.[4] Since the romantic era of the 1830s, 'Revolution' had been celebrated as the fast track to progress and had been smoothly naturalized in medicine. The Pastorian revolution continues to be celebrated as the greatest revolution, the one that initiated the era of modern scientific medicine and the decline of mortality in the industrialized world.[5] The doctrines of contagionism and infectionism, once fierce enemies, now reconciled and formed the two buttresses of the new synthesis[6] that was at the foundation of the 'Pastorian revolution'.

Nevertheless one can legitimately wonder to what extent the Pastorian agenda actually did transform medical theory and practice.[7] In a satiric novel, the French writer (a former medical student) Léon Daudet describes a Gulliverian hell dominated by the

'Morticoles', a medical sect who has taken over the city and whose doctrines sound definitely pastorian. The main characters are obvious caricatures of Pasteur's supporters in the medical school, Bouchard and Brouardel. To these demonic figures, Daudet opposes his own masters, Tillaux and Potain,[8] who are still immune to the microbial obsession and provide human care to the sick. They maintain the humanitarian ethos of clinical (bedside) knowledge. Could doctors resist the 'emotional and epistemological transcendence of science'?[9]

Society was in many senses more easily 'pasteurized' than the medical corporation. Microbes were rapidly grasped by the popular audience as enemies to be fought. Politicians also seized upon the useful metaphor of 'microbes as a public plague'. The success of the 1886 campaign to create the Pasteur Institute reveals the extent to which society had accepted Pasteur's doctrines: donations came from all layers of the *petite* and *moyenne bourgeoisie*, as witness the nominal lists provided by the journals. Similar enthusiasm was displayed at the ceremonies commemorating each anniversary of the great man. France has been speckled with statues of the scientist-hero, that were erected by the Republican notabilities in each village. School textbooks have celebrated this pioneer of modern medicine[10] and Bruno Latour has not disdained to give the latest of this saga.

The medical response was far more complex than the popular one, since the doctors were confronted with a revision of their theories as well as their practices. In 1886, Emile Duclaux, a chemist and close collaborator of Pasteur, wrote: 'Medicine is a crumbling edifice. While tradition still maintains the general structure, it is more useful that everything crumbles. There is nothing that can be rescued except the building blocks. Were I a doctor, I would be the first to demolish it.'[11]

No doubt there were a few cases of absolute resistance among the physicians. The idea that a microscopical organism was the cause of disease was preposterous to many who followed Claude Bernard's and Charles Robin's sceptical stance about these new entities.[12] I will not deal here with the most vociferous opponents, such as the professor of internal medicine[13] Peter at the Charité Hospital, Pasteur's well-known challenger at the Academy of Medicine, or the surgeon Armand Desprès, called the 'dirty surgeon'[14] (because he put his surgical instruments into his pocket); nor with the obscure practitioners.[15] I will attend to those clinicians, professors, and *agrégés* in Paris who officially welcomed the new knowledge. They rallied behind the bacteriological revolution and sometimes became its spokesmen. Yet they still had to attune the recent discoveries to their own medical tradition and to their disciplinary framework.

In the first part of his scientific life, Pasteur had recruited his assistants primarily among the corps of the *agrégés-préparateurs*, the 'normaliens': Chamberland, Thuillier, Raulin, Gernez, Maillot and Duclaux.[16] Only later did he recruit physicians, who were legally required for the inoculation of human beings – among whom was Emile Roux. He collaborated then with the chairmen of medical departments and had Grancher and Vulpian make the rabies inoculations.

The pretext for the foundation of the Institute[17] was the success of the rabies curative inoculation. Although the initial project was launched upon these premises, it rapidly became evident to all that the project went far beyond these modest goals. Pasteur was creating an institute for research on all infectious diseases, encompassing plant and animal diseases – and he enlisted the whole society (doctors included) for the success of his enterprise.[18]

A *Comité de patronage* actively promoted the campaign for fund-raising and managed the funds from 1886 to 1888 (the actual erection of the building). In addition to representatives from the banks, the Paris City Council, the learned societies and the Press, it included many prominent physicians – such as the physiologists Vulpian,[19] Richet[20] and Béclard,[21] the neurologist Charcot,[22] the expert in legal medicine Brouardel, the internist Grancher[23] to name a few – the quintessence of the Academy of Medicine and a fine selection of professors from the medical school. The Committee also included spokesmen from both the Monarchist press and the Republican radicals. The political parties on both right and left were invited to contribute to the collective venture. In short, the Committee acted more as the protagonist of a broad social conspiracy than as an agency regulating public and private funds.

In 1886 only one of the four chairs of internal medicine was held by a fierce opponent of Pasteur; it was held by Peter. The others[24] were held by Germain Sée, Potain and Jaccoud. Among Pasteur's followers, Brouardel was the dean of the medical school, Cornil was professor of Anatomopathology,[25] Chantemesse professor of comparative medicine, Grancher was in charge of the chair of paediatrics.[26] Made cautious by the fierce debates at the Academy of Medicine, Pasteur claimed that he never infringed on the physicians' grounds, but instead only enlarged their previous territory. This shrewd statement protected him against any charge of illegal exercise of medicine and ingratiated the medical body to him. When in 1881 Pasteur successfully attenuated the anthrax strain, he claimed: 'We are now in possession of anthrax virus vaccines. These vaccines can protect against death, without being themselves mortal. They are living vaccines, cultivable, transferable anywhere without being altered: in short, prepared according to a particular method which nevertheless can be safely generalized, since it has been fully successful at least one time.'[27] In short, he offered guidelines for prevention of infectious diseases in the future – a programme of virus attenuation for vaccination and epidemiological investigation logically drawn from the germ theory of disease. It was this programme which was later credited with the dramatic changes in morbidity and mortality at the turn of the century.[28]

Yet by no means did Pasteur provide physicians with a complete set of medical postulates. He suggested that the role of bacteria was crucial in pathogenesis and even referred to the emergence of new epidemics in the future as the result of new host-parasite patterns. He did not seriously attempt to establish his own doctrine of immunity as the theoretical core of his vaccination programme. Instead he borrowed his main ideas on the topic from the bernardian tradition and adapted them from the new-fangled technology of bacterial cultures. For Pasteur, immunity resulted from the loss of an essential nutrient in the organism, just as a bacterium in a medium deprived of certain vitamins or minerals can no longer survive.

Pathologists had to complete Pasteur's nascent theory and to adapt his fermentation doctrine[29] to medicine. How did they react to the challenge of bacteriology ?

Pathologists as Allies

Charles Bouchard, professor of Internal Medicine, considered himself to be one of Pasteur's adepts, even if he did not directly collaborate with Pasteur. He came in the 1860s from Lyon to Paris where he had a brilliant career. With the neurologist Charcot, he published the authoritative textbook *General Pathology*, which was frequently re-edited through the Second World War. How did he integrate the new germ theory of disease into this text?

The germ theory of disease challenged current views of medical causation. For Bouchard,[30] the 'parasites' were but one of the four major causes of disease; the others were primitive dystrophies, nutritive disorders and nervous affections. Indeed he believed that most diseases were multifactorial. He interpreted infection in terms of a complex interaction between the host and the germ. Germ attenuation or 'immunity' was crucial because the evolution of the disease depended mainly on the host response which hinged upon 'recovery', 'acute' or 'chronic' disease. The germ exerted its deleterious effect only if the 'milieu' was receptive, but this was not an 'all-or-nothing' phenomenon.

While paying lip-service to the Pasteurian revolution and abundantly quoting from Pasteur's communications to the Academy of Sciences, Bouchard admonished his reader: 'Let us admit, at least provisionally, that each contagious disease is produced by a microbe. Let us await demonstration for those diseases whose germs have not yet been proved: we will greet without surprise the announcement of their discovery and without trouble the delays which might postpone their demonstration.'

Cornil was the first to teach microbiology in his laboratory of anatomopathology with his pupil Chantemesse; so also did Bouchard at the medical school of Paris in 1879.[31] Small facilities for research were provided for each chair from 1873, which allowed professors to develop a characteristic brand of scientific work.[32] Bouchard also created a bacteriological laboratory in the 1880s at Lariboisière Hospital. The lab was very primitive. Bouchard's assistants, Widal and Charrin, at first had no idea how to cultivate microbes. They hired private engineers to design their autoclaves. In the very beginning, an infuriated patient, perhaps suffering from delirium tremens, scared by the view of the glittering glassware, crushed it down to the ground – everything had to be started again. Cornil imparted to medical students the most recent data on bacteria from both the French and the German school; yet no kind of benchwork was available to them.

Microbiology did not emerge as an autonomous discipline in the medical school and remained ancillary to pathological anatomy or experimental pathology, hygiene or comparative pathology or even zoology. Although Bouchard actively advocated the introduction of microbiology into the medical curriculum,[33] he clarified the terms of the collaboration between microbiology and medicine: 'The doctor's role is not exclusively to hunt for microbes, although he has necessarily to cope with them. To say microbe for virus or contagion, does not mean to replace one word by another, it is to substitute a positive notion for ignorance or fantasy. The eminently practical question is subsequently raised: what are the conditions which make possible the growing of the microbe?'[34]

This statement was a claim that clinicians should retain control on a whole set of specifically medical questions, all related to the pathogenesis of disease, and microbiologists were only the depository of a partial answer. While urging the introduction of 'travaux pratiques',[35] Bouchard made it clear that doctors would not become scientists but that students needed the demonstration of the recent scientific output. The 'travaux pratiques' were laden with all kinds of positivist values, meant to strengthen students' belief in experimental 'facts'. Students would 'examine the sputum, identify the gonococcus, look for the presence of various bacteria, including Coli, typhoid fever bacillus, tuberculosis bacillus.'[36] The bacteriological diagnosis of diphtheria was mentioned in detail,[37] because it was understood that after 1894 diphtheria benefited from the complete sequence of modern medicine, from germ identification for diagnosis to treatment by curative serum.

Bouchard's student Widal illustrated his master's active syncretism as he attempted to reconcile clinical and laboratory knowledge. Unlike Bouchard, who emphasized the gap between human and animal experimentation, Widal claimed the experimental status of clinical knowledge and characterized the medical art as a clever use of the 'experiments of Nature', according to a strategy many times reassessed by physicians,[38] in order to legitimate what they call 'clinical research'. Widal[39] had also been the pupil of Brouardel and Cornil, already mentioned for their active interest in Pasteur's ideas. He became *préparateur* in Cornil's lab where he first worked with Chantemesse on the identification of typhoid fever bacillus and was a good friend of Emile Roux. From 1889 to 1895, he demonstrated slides and cultures to students. He became *agrégé* in 1895.

Not only did the germ theory of disease raise questions about pathogenesis, it also challenged current views of nosology. The doctors had to deal with a novel kind of anatomo-clinical parallelism.[40] They had to superimpose the new bacteriological order onto their former nosology. This was not an easy task. Fernand Widal for example, working at Lariboisière Hospital, identified streptococci in such different diseases as phlebitis, puerperal fever, erisipelas, not to mention the non-pathogen streptococci he found in the mouth. Widal failed to single out a cultural character for each pathogen. Another bacterial agent, the so-called Eberth bacillus, seemed first to fit with the clinical entity of typhoid, then numerous variants appeared which differed in cultures but produced the same affection. The heterogeneity of the group was illustrated by the failures of early antityphoid vaccination (which used only Eberth's bacillus). Although Fernand Widal has often been considered as the head of a Pastorian medical school, at the Faculté, he retained prudence in adopting the new nosology. He was far from Louis Martin's[41] confident statement in his clinical and bacteriological study on diphtheria in 1894: 'there is complete agreement between bacteriologist's and clinician's observations that are based on an undisputable diagnosis'[42] (a pleonasm for a bacteriological diagnosis).

Widal's most important contribution to 'Pasteurian sciences' is his description of 'serodiagnosis' (he coined the word), based on the blood properties of agglutinating microbes, in 1896.[43] Against Grüber who had described the agglutination reaction as a test for protective immunity, he claimed that he had invented a test for the diagnosis of a specific infection. Typhoid held a major rank among killing fevers in France and in the colonies. Widal communicated in 1894 to the Academy of Medicine the new technique, soon called in France the Widal test. The test contributed to the autonomy of typhoid among other fevers, if not for prognosis, at least for diagnosis. But with the important exception of Wassermann's reaction used after 1907 for screening syphilitic patients and based on Bordet's complement fixation phenomenon, serology remained mainly ornamental far into the twentieth century. For Widal himself, the bacteriological mode of thought was but one component of a complex approach that integrated the bacteria into the economy of the organism and unravelled the natural history of the disease.[44]

The 'Pastorians'

Only at the Pasteur Institute, did microbiology provide a *raison d'être* and the link between all research departments. Microbiology was the main axis of research; virology, microbial physiology and finally molecular biology were derived from it.[45]

Pasteur's most surprising achievement, at the end of his life, was to recruit an active cohort who would pursue his goals and perpetuate his views. After 1880, Pasteur's influence extended across disciplinary and institutional barriers to a small but active group of senior professors and younger assistants in the medical sciences. He allied himself with the influential veterinarians Bouley and Nocard, from Maisons-Alfort,[46] and with Vaillard from the military hospital Val de Grâce.[47] The first cohort was composed of Duclaux, Grancher, Chamberland, Roux, Metchnikoff, Nocard, Straus, Chantemesse, Vaillard, Calmette, Maurice Nicolle and Yersin. These early collaborators proclaimed themselves 'Pastorians'.[48] They were all very supportive of Pasteur's novel views, each one with different interests and strategies.

The foundation of the Pasteur Institute radically changed the landscape and gave opportunities for research teams, primarily composed of physicians, working on the premises. The institute scientists had to fulfill the expectations fostered by its foundation. They followed the empirical guidelines of Pasteur by trying all kinds of procedures to attenuate viruses. The antirabies vaccine had impressed the public and left a vivid memory in the collective imagination. Its impact was more limited on doctors, as the limited importance of rabies in mortality gave them a more balanced perspective. Tuberculosis was the major scourge for adults, and diphtheria had been recently shown to be one of the leading causes of child mortality. The antidiphtheria treatment came in time to rekindle declining enthusiasm[49] and strengthen expectations for laboratory-based therapeutic advances.[50]

The basic research came from Berlin and Paris. In Paris, Emile Roux and Alexandre Yersin demonstrated the toxicity of a substance liberated by the diphtheria bacillus into the medium broth. The substance was poisonous and explained the local symptoms and asphyxia determined by the formation of false membranes in the throat.[51] In 1881, Behring and Kitasato in Berlin attenuated this toxin by iodine and were able to raise sera from sheep and guinea pigs. They used this as a therapy in children, initially without much success.

Roux widened the scope of serum production by inoculating horses and experimenting on serum therapy at the Hôpital des Enfants Malades.[52] Jean-Joseph Grancher, his friend, had authorized him to experiment in his department at the hospital where he had already reduced the morbidity rate by simply isolating suspected patients. Roux started without objection a parallel series, leaving young patients untreated at the Trousseau Hospital. Louis Martin, then Grancher's resident, was the intermediary between the stables of the Institute and the paediatric wards.[53]

The results were published at the Budapest Conference of 1894 which marked a peak in Pastorians' popularity and prestige abroad. Mass production of curative serum was immediately launched in Germany and the United States in state-supported Institutes and increasingly in pharmaceutical companies competing between themselves.[54] Only in France did serum production remain attached to the Pasteur Institute, which was paradoxically a private institution devoted to public health.[55] The Institute enhanced its scientific prestige and identified a way of funding further research, even while retaining the logic of non profit advocated by the Pastorians (like Pasteur, Roux declined patenting his work).[56]

Grancher,[57] whose name has been associated with the serotherapy innovation, also illustrates the integration of Pasteur's train of ideas into the medical tradition. He became recognized when he chose the unitarian view of tuberculosis in 1873. He had met Pasteur himself in 1884 at the Copenhagen congress where Pasteur announced his rabies vaccination. It was Grancher who inoculated little Joseph Meister on 6 July, 1886. He collaborated with Pasteur from 1885 to 1887 in the small locale of the rue Vauquelin (as may be seen in Bayard's famous picture). Although not himself an academician, he defended Pasteur during the dramatic days of 1886 when Peter charged Pasteur with three patients' deaths. He helped create the pro-Pasteur *Bulletin Médical*, protagonist of the more reserved *Semaine Médicale*, and trusted it to his friend Dr Janicot.[58] His department at the Necker Hospital was a hotbed for pasteurianism. In an often celebrated attic, zealous assistants investigated microbial diseases: Veillon, later a member of the staff of the Pasteur Hospital, tackled the study of anaerobic germs.

While Grancher acknowledged the unitarian view proposed by the discovery of germs, he nevertheless remained attached to anatomo-pathological findings as the basis of nosology. He developed, for example, the method for the early detection of isolated cases of tuberculosis in families based on patient auscultation (typically a clinical skill) and applied to the tuberculous the method of isolation he had successfully applied for diphtheria in his own department.

Pathologists such as Grancher were interested in scientific investigations, but their main concern was with microbe attenuation *in vivo*, the mechanism of natural or artificial defence, in other words immunity. Pasteur had not given much credit to his own theory of immunity.[59] He had welcomed in his institute the Russian zoologist Elie Metchnikoff who had introduced the topic of phagocytosis into the study of immunity. Emile Roux confirmed 20 years later: 'You brought him nothing less than a fully elaborated doctrine.'[60]

When Metchnikoff antagonized the German school, comprised mostly of supporters of the 'humoral theory' (the predominant role of antibodies or chemical substances in the blood), by claiming that phagocytosis[61] was the body's main line of defence, most doctors followed Bouchard's rather conciliatory stance. Bouchard identified so-called 'natural immunity' with phagocytosis but made a distinction between natural immunity and the 'bactericid state' or artificial immunity elicited by vaccination and produced by the bactericid substances. Antibodies were secondarily produced in response to 'vaccinating substances' liberated by bacteria.

In other words, 'avant-garde' physicians such as Bouchard were concerned with the pathogenesis of disease and the necessity of invoking not only an external cause but also an internal determinism. They adhered to the idea that fermentation and putrefaction are normally operating inside the organism (Armand Gauthier's obnoxious 'ptomains', resulting from the splitting of proteins inside the organism). The idea of toxin was pivotal for that purpose. 'Microbes, ferments and toxins are inseparable terms and for this reason the discovery of the diphtheria toxin by Roux and Yersin in 1888 began a new era in bacteriology.'[62] Metchnikoff's favourite theory that the guts are a dangerous reservoir of germs can be seen as a reactivation of Broussais' central intuition that assimilated all diseases to gastro-intestinal disorders (Broussais' famous 'system'). For Bouchard, toxins liberated by the microbes and toxins elaborated by the cells during their normal lifetime were essentially the same.

Around 1900, a collaboration between the medical school and the Pasteur Institute was established along these lines. Experiments testing the notion that autointoxication was central to pathogenesis were conducted at the Pasteur Institute and at Necker, Cochin and Lariboisière hospitals. They suggested that, in the course of disease, the cells of the organism, when altered, liberate products which interact with the organism itself. The idea that the organism itself negotiated a compromise with the host and that its participation was required for the development of disease was a basic medical intuition experimentally put into sharp focus. Its adepts loosened the rigid bacteriological framework and shook some of its postulates, breaking the way to an alternative definition of immunity. Immunity had been primarily defined as an outwardbound function, it was tentatively reformulated as an internal process linked to each physiological event of the organism.

Noël Fiessinger, working at Cochin Hospital, repeatedly screened cirrhotic patients for antibodies directed at the liver. He selected these antibodies as good markers of clinical evolution. The antibody rate rose when the patient relapsed. Fiessinger concluded that 'the patient first protects his liver, then he protects himself against his liver'.[63]

Similar hypotheses were put forth for kidney diseases, anaemias and neurological syndromes. Even orchitis and sterility were discussed in relation to 'auto-antibodies' directed to the patients' own organs. By the time Castaing and Rathery described anti-kidney auto-antibodies in hospitalized patients,[64] Metchnikoff's assistants were raising anti-kidney cytotoxic sera in the guinea-pig.[65] The two groups converged upon a therapeutic strategy: they used a serum raised against auto-antibodies, an anti-antiserum which might tip the immunological balance. This idea was developed by Alexandre Besredka at the Institute and welcomed by Widal and his two assistants Chauffard and Brulé.

This exchange of acts and hypotheses best illustrates collaboration between Pastorian research and the medical avant-garde in hospitals. Interestingly, it was not a mere application of the germ theory of disease. It evolved instead from Metchnikoff's concern of the zoologist with the natural history of the disease, a track slightly deviating from the original Pasteurian guidelines. However, its influence was never broad in the medical landscape and waned around the First World War. Phagocytosis, once viewed as the organism's main line of defence againt pathogens fell into disrepute at the same time. Besredka called it 'a cursed doctrine'[66] and dedicated the rest of his life to rehabilitating the doctrine of cellular immunity.

Surgeons as Applicants

Unlike the physicians, the surgeons were not primarily concerned with the pathogenesis of disease — they held instead a very pragmatic view of bacteriology.[67] By the middle of the 19th century, they had considerably improved their techniques but remained plagued by an appalling rate of fatalities, especially when working in big hospitals.

Interestingly, the young intern who first started antisepsis in one surgical ward in France, Justin Lucas-Championnière,[68] did not take his lesson directly from Pasteur. He knew some English and went to Glasgow, then to Edinburgh, where Joseph Lister had been applying his method since 1867. In his *Principes de la chirurgie antiseptique*, published in 1876, he asserted that Lister's antisepsis was innovative: he stressed that it had nothing to do with the ancient 'topiques' used for wound dressing. He referred to Pasteur but only through the mediation of his fellow-surgeon Lister. The new method relied first on the importance given to the microbes of the air. The physicist Tyndall in London had viewed putrid wounds as the result of the exposure to 'microbian clouds', that depended on the local climate. In order to combat microbes from the air, Lucas-Championnière invented a spray which purified the atmosphere and remained in use for several generations.[69]

Then the antisepsis ritual shifted attention away from protection from atmospheric microbes to germs carried on the hands and instruments. Pasteur formulated the ironical vow that the surgeon himself be sterilized.[70] The operator was clearly designated as the main source of infection. A sense of guilt helped to promote the new order of antisepsis. Microbes were killed by the microbiologists' techniques used for lab cultures: the Pasteur oven (using dry heating), later the Chamberland autoclave which sterilized surgical material in metallic boxes. The new rituals were progressively adopted by the surgical wards.

In the late 1880s antisepsis was in turn displaced by a new doctrine, asepsis. Although asepsis also found its inspiration in the germ theory of disease, some surgeons, including Lucas-Championnière, never adopted asepsis: they had brought antisepsis to perfection through trial and error and did not see any strong empirical argument for abandoning their methods.

Interestingly, the practice of antisepsis in surgery suggested a treatment to the internist Bouchard. He irrigated his patients' guts with antiseptic solutions in the same way surgeons dipped their tools into the buckets of phenic acid. Bouchard assayed the antiseptic effect of all available drugs, mercury, quinine, salicylate and bismuth on typhic patients, without much success.

The ideal of sterility in the operating room brought together a generation of surgeons and was served by the generalized use of antiseptic solutions, among which the most famous was Dakin's[71] solution, still in use today. Only recently, surgeons have reintegrated a less radical view of their action, and considered the patient as the ultimate reservoir of germs, a potentially immunocompromised patient,[72] especially if manipulated and weakened by iterative surgery and long-term intensive care.

The Second Generation of Pastorians

We have seen how the medical body was receptive to the sweeping tide of Pasteurian new ideas. It was ready to discuss the new pathogenic agents and new treatments, and it integrated the main results into a broader view of the pathogenesis of disease. Now, how did this alliance between the laboratory and the clinic survive the passing of time? How did the personal link woven between the new species of researchers and clinicians evolve?

In the following years, the 'Pastorians'[73] increasingly appeared to be an autonomous community, with rules of their own and a pattern of recruitment and training strikingly different from the rest of the medical community.

Despite the efforts of professors such as Bouchard, microbiology did not become part of the medical curriculum before the First World War. In contrast, the Grand Cours organized in the Pasteur

Institute since 1889 by Roux himself, Metchnikoff and Duclaux, was first and foremost a practical school.[74] The students ('les élèves') each had a microscope and were trained to become skilled microscopists. Their teachers could boast of providing professional microbiologists to the world. The pastorians recruited themselves mainly from the military doctors and veterinarians sent by their schools to receive training at the Pasteur Institute which would make them fit for their future field practice. They usually did not follow the 'royal path' of the *internat*. Consequently, they did not embody the medical tradition but a new gospel, breaking from this tradition. They were 'des hommes sortant du rang'. The prototype was Emile Roux himself who had not followed the academic career and emphasized the preeminence of ideas over diplomas. 'In our house, we measure the importance of a man from the services he affords and the only title for promotion is scientific production. We welcome whoever brings forth interesting ideas.'[75]

The Pastorians wrapped themselves in Pasteur's cloak and benefited from the growing myth around his saga.[76] Another source of recruitment was the foreigners who came to Paris attracted by the prestige of cosmopolitan characters such as Metchnikoff and after 1918 tried thus to elude the professional barriers and the restrictions of practice imposed upon doctors from abroad.

In the years before the First World War, the formation of a community of experts dedicated to the germ theory of disease resulted in the estrangement of clinics from bacteriological research.

In 1894 pioneers had advocated a style for practical medicine which was common to clinicians and researchers: 'There is no safe diagnosis unless it is founded on bacteriology', Louis Martin said in his conference at the Pasteur Institute, in front of an audience composed of 'doctors completely alien to bacteriological work' and, he added, 'You can all make the diagnosis in a fast and easy way.'[77] In 1921 Noël Fiessinger retained an extreme position when he claimed that every physician had to set up a lab of his own. In a booklet many times re-edited, he gave the complete instructions for equipping a modest lab with a baker's oven ('four Pasteur') and a 'Roux étuve' for microbial cultures. But Fiessinger had worked in Morocco and his book was mainly for doctors working in the colonies. When Maurice Nicolle celebrated scientific improvisation in the field, he drew the lessons of his experience in the primitive conditions of his institute in Constantinople and first addressed isolated doctors working in similar conditions.[78]

In hospitals, independent microbiological work first flourished but was neglected as amateurish because it did not receive the pastorian stamp, such as Talamon's identification of pneumococcus[79] in 1882 or Enriquez's research on the diphtheria bacillus. Finally, the number of important bacteriological labs in hospitals remained limited until 1914.[80]

The Founding Fathers group spawned a second generation of researchers who tended to segregate from the clinicians. Because of the Medical school's inability to organize and promote laboratory-based research, the Pasteur Institute remained 'the only French centre for medical research'[81] until the Second World War. On the other side, the debate on medical reform which would transform doctors into fully fledged scientists retaining their clinical and teaching abilities was postponed. It was rekindled in the post-Liberation era of reorganization in 1945 but did not come to fruition until the Debré reform which founded academic medicine on a tripod: research, teaching and care of the sick, in1953.[82]

The pastorians defined themselves as a family, generated by the Grand Cours delivered by the Founding Fathers or by their heirs. As Pasteur had moved to the study of pathology, from plants to animals and finally to his crowning work, man, he had successively recruited specialists from all these fields. His last disciples were physicians who ultimately dominated the 'Pastorian' school, even while the original and successful character of the group remained interdisciplinarity. The school included veterinarians, botanists and agronomists – a clear illustration of the importance of 'hybrid' roles for the emergence of new disciplines.[83]

The pastorians always used the plural as they referred to 'pasteurian sciences' and 'pasteurian methods'. Pasteur himself had made available to his followers a broad spectrum of positions which ranged from soft recognition to adhesion to stringent guidelines. He had emphasized the impact of bacteriological techniques and discoveries on general welfare. Latour has demonstrated how Pasteur established himself at the crossroads of the universal traffic: after Pasteur, no way for giving birth, travelling, flirting or even simply walking down the street without meeting microbes and being wrapped by the epidemiological network which interwove all human lives. This grand definition, the most 'electoralist', gave rise to such solemn statements as Pasteur Vallery Radot 'All nations are tributary to Pasteur's discoveries.'[84] This definition was used by Pastorians in their official addresses to the political and the general audience.

But when they came to terms with medical fieldwork, the Pastorians' doctrine showed under other aspects: restricted pasteurism (a metaphor borrowed from the theory of relativity) consisted first of hygiene in a renovated sense. Pastorian hygiene can be characterized as scientific or bacterium-centred. Although it did not exclude social determinants it pushed them to the periphery: 'Whatever the life conditions are, they will be never able to create disease.'[85] Nevertheless, doctors still felt that special conditions fostered the emergence of disease; they continued to point to the negative effects of overwork, poor nutrition and inadequate housing as were evident from the toll of death in crowded cities and military barracks.

The second dimension of restricted pasteurism was that of an immunization programme, a tentative fulfilment of the year 1880's promise, partially achieved by anti-typhoid, anti-plague and anti-cholera vaccination.

The French legislation on public health during the Third Republic has often been quoted as an example of the pastorian influence. In fact, a close examination of the parliamentary debates shows that this legislation amounts to little,[86] especially when compared with the grand programme brought on the floor by the Pastorian deputy who was also the chairman of the Consultative Council for Public Health, Chamberland.[87] This programme suggested the creation of a medical administration that would supervise all aspects of public health. These delays revealed profound contradictions between the hygienic convictions and the liberal ideology of most physicians.[88] The programme was tabled repeatedly at the Parliament and the final law of 1902 was but an *ersatz* of the original project.[89] This law made the century-old jennerian vaccine compulsory, encouraged disinfection in case of epidemics and obligated physicians to report a limited number of infectious diseases to the sanitary administration. Equally significant in that respect was the 1906 legislation that bore on food surveillance. The law detailed the bacteriological screening of wine, meat, milk and spirits, for which it required a reliable laboratory.[90]

Another divergence from medical tradition emerged. The doctors coped with individual patients, while the pastorians relied on epidemiological investigation and immunization strategies and aimed at a social engineering of diseases. This legacy was incompatible with the Pastorians' liberal ideology[91] (also part of Pasteur's heritage) and their distrust of the state bureaucracy. The 1892 law which promoted the French system of welfare was a compromise with medical liberalism and finally endorsed the principle of free choice of physician by the patient.[92]

But these contradictions vanished on the colonial terrain:

Pastorian teaching blossomed in the overseas French territories. The first to apply pasteurian doctrines were not the professors of the medical school but the military physicians, surgeons and veterinarians, committed to the manipulation of the environment, including humans as a 'factor'.[93]

A Pasteur institute was initiated in Saigon in 1891, even before a similar institution appeared in Lille, inside the metropolis. The pattern of the overseas Pasteur institutes typically associated a department for rabies inoculation (clearly a symbolic asset), a unit for the production of smallpox vaccine and various labs related to public welfare and to local industry. Pasteur's versatile interests from silk, wine and beer production to vaccines were offered as scientific guidelines. Medicine was thus the central but not the exclusive concern in the comprehensive programme of the overseas Pasteur institutes.

Only in the colonies was the coordination between those who designed sewers, provided pure water, regulated frontiers and instigated the quarantines, supervised and wiped out epidemics, and the public authorities, usually harmonious. Ernest Conseil in Tunis and Emile Sergent in Algiers, claimed that they were responsible for the emergence of a hygienized and pasteurized city. There, Pasteurian lab-based hygienists displaced the early hygienists from their utopian stance and brought in medical engineers. In the colonies, the contradictions between mass and individual medicine and anxiety over ethical problems of human experimentation disappeared or were eclipsed by more stressing considerations.

In the metropolis itself, the pastorian doctrine was in quest of a place of its own, an independent hospital adapted to its views and methods. The Pasteur Hospital was originally planned to accommodate bitten patients, according to the donor's (Mrs Lebaudy), legacy.[94] The project evolved into a hospital for the application of diphtheria serotherapy and ultimately became a hospital for the study of infectious diseases.[95] The hospital was supposed to promote both clinically-inspired fundamental research in the neighbouring institute and applied experimental therapy in the clinic.[96]

This model was not completely effective and although some prestigious professors attended as consultants, the hospital remained insulated from the medical school and the residents were never recruited via the *concours* of the *Assistance publique*. It mainly housed patients sent by the colonial physicians. New drugs against malaria, syphilis and sleeping sickness, were tried within its walls. By the 1930s the hospital had become somewhat an 'hôpital de quartier' and was hardly a commonground between researchers' interests and clinicians' goals. While the Rockefeller Hospital builders had explicitly considered the Pasteur Hospital as one model in 1907, by 1933, the Rockefeller Hospital was proposed in turn as a model for the reform of the Pasteur Hospital, as it had successfully gathered scientists and clinicians in the study of carefully selected diseases and attracted clinicians by being a centre of excellence.[97]

Academic physicians thus took an ambivalent stance toward the pasteurian agenda. On the one hand, they did not want to miss the latest medical revolution and claimed their share of Pasteur's legacy. On the other, as they saluted pasteurian *mots d'ordre* as 'facts' in their most flamboyant positivist style, they considered these 'facts' as controversial. While they recognized the advent of modern medical science, they altogether emphasized physiology's contribution to the interpretation of disease and resisted its reduction to a dictate of the fundamental laws for the exegesis of symptoms. They did not become full-time scientists while clearly trying to benefit from the prestige attached to science. Maybe they were also suspicious of the Pastorian doctrine's systematic nature or, as Gerald Geison beautifully puts it, more tolerant of ambiguity.[98] While they were happy to elevate themselves into the grand hierarchy of Comtist science, they admitted *in petto* as the Dechambre dictionary comments, 'The art of curing the sick does not lie in systems.' The history of the theoretical debates and practices surrounding the Pastorian school exemplifies the persisting instability of the biomedical sciences. Bacteriology and medicine, which had functioned briefly on the fusional mode, tended to separate. If their hybrid status[99] was not easily maintained after the period of conquest which hailed the foundation of the Institute, it has remained at the basis of our modern inquiry into the status of clinical research in medicine and the epistemological foundations of medical knowledge.

Acknowledgements

I am very grateful to Kim Pelis, from Johns Hopkins Institute for the History of Medicine, for editorial assistance and useful criticisms, to Joy Harvey for witty comments and information, and to Annick Guenel for invaluable bibliographic help. I want also to express my gratitude to the director of the Pasteur Museum, Madame Annick Perrot and to the director of the Archives at the Pasteur Institute, Madame Denise Ogilvie for their scholarly help. This work was supported by a grant from the INSERM, Institut national de la santé et de la recherche médicale, Paris.

Notes

1. Claire Salomon-Bayet, *Pasteur et la médecine pastorienne*, (Paris: Fayard, 1985); Bruno Latour, *Les microbes* (Paris: A. M. Métailié, 1984); Jacques Léonard, *La médecine entre les savoirs et les pouvoirs* (Floch, Mayenne 1981). The forthcoming book of Gerald Geison, *The Private Science of Louis Pasteur*, should also be illuminating in that respect.

2. For a general view, see Stanley J. Reiser, *Medicine and the Reign of Technology*, (Cambridge: Cambridge University Press, 1978).

3. Etienne Burnet, *Microbes and Toxins* (New York: Putnam, 1912), 108. In 1897, Metchnikoff addressed the students of his microbiology course at the Pasteur Institute in these terms: 'Microbial theories have penetrated into the doctors' minds.' Course handwritten manuscript, Museum, Pasteur Institute, Paris.

4. 'La théorie des germes eut à son origine quelques contradicteurs, mais devant l'évidence des faits, les résistances qu'on lui avait d'abord opposées se sont évanouies et n'ont plus reparu.' P. Miquel et R. Cambier, *Traité de microbiologie pure et appliqué à la médecine et à l'hygiène*, (Paris: C Naud, 1902), VI.

5. Even if medical responsibility has been subject to controversy (See Ivan Ilich's *Medical Nemesis*, (Paris, Seuil, 1975) and Thomas McKeown's *Role of Medicine*, (Princeton: Princeton University Press, 1981). Hereafter any medical innovation has to be assessed against this general frame.

6. François Delaporte, *Disease and Civilization*, (Cambridge: MIT Press, 1986).

7. For a critical examination of 'medicalization' in French society during the 19th century, see Olivier Faure, 'La médicalisation de la société dans la région lyonnaise au 19e siècle (1800–1914)', unpublished Ph.D. Dissertation, Lyon 1989.

8. Léon Daudet, *Les Morticoles* (Paris: Fasquelle, 1894).

9. Charles E. Rosenberg, 'The Therapeutic Revolution: Medicine, Meaning, and Social Change in Nineteeenth-Century America', *The Therapeutic Revolution, Essays in the Social History of American Medicine*, Morris J. Vogel and Charles E. Rosenberg (eds), (Philadelphia: University of Pennsylvania Press, 1979).

10. See for example, the French biologist Jean Rostand's popular account *Hommes de vérité, C. Bernard, L. Pasteur, C-J. Davaine*, (Paris: Stock, 1968).

11. 'La Médecine est un édifice où plus rien ne tient debout. La tradition maintient encore le plan et l'ordonnance générale, mais il y a utilité que tout tombe parce qu'il n'y a rien de bon à tirer de ce qui existe que les matériaux. Si j'étais médecin, je donnerais, je crois, le coup de pioche qui ferait tout crouler!' Emile Duclaux, quoted by Mary Robinson (Mme Duclaux), *Vie de Emile Duclaux* (Laval: Barnéoud,

1906), 161.

12. In my native city, a well-known surgeon, at the turn of the century, used to spit with predilection in the wounds. He claimed that he stimulated the inflammatory process, so that the scar fabric would be substantially stronger.

13. Until 1893.

14. Jack D. Ellis, *The Physician-legislators of France* (Cambridge: Cambridge University Press, 1990), 178.

15. Russell C. Maulitz, '"Physician versus bacteriologist": the ideology of science in clinical medicine', *The Therapeutic Revolution*, C. Rosenberg (ed.), 91–107.

16. Postgraduate students in the physical sciences at the prestigious Ecole Normale Supérieure.

17. The only comprehensive work on the Pasteur Institute is Albert Delaunay, *L'institut Pasteur, des origines à aujourd'hui*, (Paris: Editions France-Empire, 1962) which is an account written by an insider. The novelist Pierre Gascar's *Du côté de chez Monsieur Pasteur* (Paris: Odile Jacob, 1986) is a book which captures some of the house atmosphere but cannot stand for a historical piece of work.

18. Delaunay, 'L'institut Pasteur'.

19. Alfred Vulpian, born in 1828, professor of pathological and comparative anatomy, member of the Academy of Medicine, honorary dean of the medical school.

20. Charles Richet, professor of physiology at the medical school of Paris.

21. Member of the City Council of the Seine Department, permanent secretary of the Academy of Medicine.

22. Born in 1825, member of the Academy of Medicine and of the Academy of Sciences, professor of neurology.

23. Born in 1843, professor of paediatrics at the Necker Hospital from 1892.

24. Antoine Prévot, *La Faculté de médecine de Paris, ses chaires, ses annexes et son personnel enseignant* (Paris: Maloine, 1900).

25. When he obtained the chair of anatomopathology, Cornil dedicated his first lecture to Pasteur: 'Ma première parole, au début de ce cours, sera pour glorifier le maître ... qui a révolutionné la partie de la science que j'ai l'honneur d'enseigner à la faculté....' Les découvertes de Pasteur et leurs applications à l'anatomie et à l'histologie pathologique, plaquette, Paris 1895.

26. Yves Auffray, 'L'enseignement de la médecine au 19ème siècle', Thèse de doctorat de médecine, Rennes 1963.

27. Louis Pasteur, 'Compte rendu sommaire des expériences faites à Pouilly-le-Fort, près Melun, sur la vaccination charbonneuse', *Comptes-rendus de l'Académie des Sciences* 92 (1881), 1383.

28. For a discussion of 'vital statistics' in the 19th century, see Philip Curtin, *Death by Migration*, (Cambridge: Cambridge University Press, 1989), 1–39.

29. Which referred a whole range of processes to the action of tiny beings, omnipotent in Nature.

30. Paul Le Gendre, *Un médecin philosophe, Charles Bouchard, son oeuvre et son temps (1837–1915)* (Paris: Masson, 1924).

31. See Emile Roux, 'Discourse for the 25th anniversary of the Pasteur Institute Foundation', 1913, 27.

32. Henri Roger, *Entre deux siècles. Souvenirs d'un vieux biologiste* (Paris: Expansion scientifique française, 1947).

33. Charles Bouchard, *Questions relatives à la réforme des études médicales*, (Paris: Steinheil, 1907).

34. Charles Bouchard, *Leçons sur les auto-intoxications dans les maladies (1885)*, (Paris: Savy, 1887), 5.

35. The chair of microbiology was not created before the 1920s, see Robert Fox and Georges Weisz, *The Organization of Science and Technology, 1808–1914* (Cambridge: Cambridge University Press, 1980).

36. Bouchard, *Questions*, 74

37. *Ibid.*

38. See A. Robert Good, 'Runestones in Immunology', *Journal of Immunology*, 117 (1976), 1417.

39. See Widal's biography by André Lemierre, *Un grand médecin français, Widal* (Paris: Expansion scientifique, 1955). On Widal as the pastorian head of a medical school, see his student Burnet's biography: Lydia Burnet, *Etienne Burnet, un humaniste de ce temps* (Tunis: Bascone, 1939), 80–3.

40. O. Amsterdamska, 'Medical and biological constraints: early research on variation in bacteriology', *Social Studies of Science*, 17 (1987), 657–87.

41. Later first director of the Pasteur Hospital.

42. Auguste Chaillou et Louis Martin, 'Etudes cliniques et bactériologiques sur la diphtérie', *Annales de l'institut Pasteur*, 7 (1894) 478.

43. Fernand Widal, 'Recherche sur les propriétés agglutinatives et bactéricides du sérum de convalescents de fièvre typhoïde', *Bulletins et Mémoires de la Société des médecins des hôpitaux de Paris*, 13 (1896), 681–2.

44. Fernand Widal, *Oeuvres scientifiques*, éditées par F. Bezançon, (Paris: Masson,1932).

45. Richard M. Burian, Jean Gayon, and Doris Zallen, 'Genetics in the history of French Biology', *Journal of the History of Biology*, 21 (1988) 357–402.

46. See Louis Nicol, *L'épopée pastorienne et la médecine vétérinaire*, (Paris: chez l'auteur, 1974). Maisons-Alfort is the premier veterinary school in France. Nocard was its director from 1887 to 1904.

47. Even if resistance persisted in the army. Leonard even talks of an anti-pastorian bolt ('verrou') in the middle of the army, Claire

Salomon-Bayet (ed.), *Pasteur.* The Val-de-Grâce was the main military hospital in Paris.

48. Maurice de Fleury is assumed to have coined the word 'pastorien', *Pasteur et les pastoriens* (Paris: Rueff, 1895).

49. Dr Paul Percy, *Ma première application du sérum antidiphtérique* (Le Mans/Monnoyer, 1895).

50. On the popular reception of serotherapy, see Evelyn Bernette Ackermann, *Health Care in the Parisian Countryside, 1800–1914,* (New Brunswick: Rutgers University Press, 1990), 94–108.

51. N. Bernard, *Yersin pionnier-savant-explorateur, 1863–1943* (Paris: La Colombe, 1955), 38–41.

52. Emile Roux, Louis Martin and A. Chaillou, 'Trois cent cas de diphtérie traités par le sérum antidiphtérique', *Annales de l'institut Pasteur,* 8 (1894), 640–61.

53. P. Weindling, 'From medical research to clinical practice: serum therapy for diphtheria in the 1890s' (forthcoming).

54. J. Liebenau, *Medical Science and Medical Industry* (Baltimore: Johns Hopkins University Press, 1987), 48–52.

55. During the financial crisis of the institute, in the 1970s, its director, Jacques Monod, when negotiating with the Minister of Health Simone Veil, argued that the State was morally indebted to the institute for one-century of services.

56. Roux declined any financial profit from anthrax vaccination, Letter to E. Chamberland, 28 May, 1885, Musée Pasteur, M G203. Pasteur officially transferred his royalties on veterinary vaccines to his institute, *Report to the comité de patronage, Pasteur Institute,* 25 March, 1887, Archives of the Pasteur Institute, Paris.

57. See Jacques Roussillat, *La vie et l'oeuvre du professeur Jacques-Joseph Grancher* (Guéret: Presses du Massif central, 1964).

58. Also later a member of the staff at the Pasteur Hospital.

59. See Anne Marie Moulin, *Le dernier langage de la médecine. Histoire de l'immunologie, de Pasteur au SIDA* (Paris: Presses universitaires de France, 1991), ch. 1.

60. Emile Roux, 'Jubilé Metchnikoff', *Annales de l'institut Pasteur,* 29 (1915), 357.

61. Phagocytes are scavenger cells in the blood able to take over pathogens or defective cells.

62. Burnet, *Microbes,* 129

63. Noël Fiessinger, 'Des anticorps hépatiques chez les sujets atteints de lésions hépatiques en évolution', *Journal de Physiologie et de Pathologie générale,* 10 (1908), 673–81.

64. Paul Castaigne and Francis Rathery, 'Lésions des reins produites par injection d'émulsion rénale', *Comptes-rendus de la société de biologie* (1902), 563–5.

65. Charles F. Bolduan, *Immune Sera* (New York: Wiley, 1911). For a general discussion of auto-immunity, see Arthur M Silverstein, *A*

History of Immunology (San Diego: Academic Press, 1990), ch. VII;
Moulin, *Le dernier langage de la médecine*, ch. VIII.

66. Alexandre Besredka, *Histoire d'une idée, L'oeuvre de Metchnikoff*
(Paris: Masson, 1921).

67. See the historical survey by Paul Lecène, *L'évolution de la chirurgie*
(Paris: Flammarion, 1923), especially the chapter: 'La révolution
chirurgicale au 19e siècle', 230–60.

68. See Félix Lejars, *Eloge de Just Lucas-Championnière (1843–1913)*
(Paris: Masson, 1916).

69. Just Lucas-Championnière, *Le passé et le présent de la méthode
antiseptique* (Paris, 1899).

70. Louis Pasteur, 'Maladies virulentes, virus, vaccins et prophylaxie de la
rage' *Oeuvres* (Paris: Masson, 1933) VI, 123.

71. From the name of an American chemist who worked during the First
World War in Alexis Carrel's War hospital.

72. An extreme example of the prevailing influence of immunology in
today's medical thinking, as I tried to demonstrate in *Le dernier
langage de la médecine.*

73. A few biographies of the main Pastorians are available, but none
meets the present standards of historical scholarship. A few scholars
(among whom myself) are now working on the Pastorian
community.

74. Marguerite Faure, 'Cent années d'enseignement à l'institut Pasteur',
lecture given for the centennial of the Pasteur Institute, Paris 1988.

75. Noël Bernard, *Yersin, pionnier-savant-explorateur (1863–1943)* (Paris:
La Colombe, 1955), 34.

76. See Geison's forthcoming book, *The private science of Louis Pasteur.*

77. Louis Martin, *Annales d'hygiène publique et de médecine légale,*
Décembre 1894,. 518.

78. Maurice Nicolle, *Traité de microbiologie,* (Paris: Doin, 1902).

79. Edouard Rist, *Vingt-cinq portraits de médecins français* (Paris: Masson,
1955), 113.

80. In England, Reiser cites Guy's Hospital in London and the Royal
Infirmary in Edinburgh, the Johns Hopkins Hospital, the Mass
General Hospital and Bellevue in the United States, Reiser, *Medicine.*
The army created a bacteriology lab in 1891 at Algiers and in 1895 at
Marseille.

81. Harry Plotz, *Report to the Rockefeller Foundation on the Pasteur
Institute,* Archives of the Rockefeller Foundation, see A. M. Moulin,
'Death and Resurrection of Immunology', in *Immunology : Pasteur's
inheritance,* P. A. Cazenave (ed.), (Delhi: East Wiley, 1992).

82. Haroun Jamous, *Sociologie de la décision. La réforme des études
médicales et des structures hospitalières* (Paris: Editions du CNRS,
1969); *Professions or self-perpetuating systems, Professions and
Professionalization,* J. A. Jackson, (ed.) (Cambridge: Cambridge
University Press, 1970), 109–52.

83. As emphasized by Ben David.

84. Pasteur Vallery Radot, quoted by Noël Bernard, *De l'Empire colonial à l'Union française* (Paris: Flammarion, 1951), 152.

85. Louis Pasteur, *Oeuvres*, tome 7, 125.

86. A. L. Shapiro, 'Private rights, public interest, and professional jurisdiction: the French Public Health law of 1902', *Bulletin of the History of Medicine*, 54 (1980), 4–22.

87. Anonymous, *C. Chamberland (1851–1905)* (Sceaux: Charaire, 1908).

88. See Ellis, *The physician-legislators of France.*

89. Claudine Marenko et S. Godevarica, 'La vaccination des sujets en France, 1880–1980' (unpublished work, 1982, communicated by courtesy of the authors).

90. The lab had been founded in 1902. Its directors published an authoritative *Traité de Bactériologie pure et appliquée à la médecine et à l'hygiène*, P. Miquel and R. Cambier, C. Naud, (Paris, 1902).

91. See Duclaux's attitude toward state-sponsored hygiene in Emile Duclaux, *L'hygiène sociale*, (Paris: Alcan, 1902).

92. Faure, *Médicalisation*, tome IV.

93. Anne Marie Moulin, 'Patriarchal Science, the network of the overseas Pasteur institutes', in *Science and Empires*, C. Jami, A. M. Moulin and P. Petitjean (eds), (Boston: Kluwer, 1991), 31.

94. François Lejeune, *Contribution à l'histoire de la médecine. L'hôpital Pasteur de sa création à nos jours*, Thèse médecine, Paris 1969.

95. Pasteur Vallery Radot's *Report to the Lacroix Commission for the reform of the institute*, 1933, Archives of the Pasteur Institute, Paris, 22.

96. Louis Martin, 'L'Hôpital Pasteur', *Revue d'hygiène et de police sanitaire*, 22 (1900) 633–46; 'Le fonctionnement de l'hôpital Pasteur', *Ibid*, 25 (1903), 256–81.

97. Rapport Pasteur-Vallery Radot, *op. cit.* 18.

98. Gerald L. Geison, 'Pasteur, Roux and rabies: scientific versus clinical mentalities', *Journal of the History of Medicine*, 45 (1990), 365.

99. See the recent Christiane Sinding, *Le clinicien et le chercheur* (Paris: Presses Universitaires de France, 1991).

11

La Visite: Mary Putnam Jacobi and the Paris Medical Clinics

Joy Harvey

The medical system of the past, like a remote tribe, is best presented through the words of a 'participant observer', to use an anthropological term, an eyewitness who functions as a member of that tribe, but who can explain it to outsiders. It is considered ideal if this observer herself comes from a different culture than the one observed so that seemingly obvious performances and beliefs are noted. This kind of 'participant observer' provides more objective information since she can view events both from within and without the system.

Hospital clinics were a central feature of French medicine and medical education. They were very active during this period as can be illustrated by the proliferation of hospital gazettes and journals in Paris. I have discussed these gazettes elsewhere, to argue that French clinical medicine was alive and well between the years 1850–1875.[1] These weekly hospital gazettes provide careful running reports of individual clinics, clinical lectures, debates in the Académie de Médecine, analyses of the foreign literature and even satires on important individuals. What they lack is the sense of direct personal experience which can be provided best through the correspondence of unusual individuals.

This paper examines the letters and clinical observations of Mary Corinna Putnam (later Mary Putnam Jacobi). Her descriptions cover the period from 1866 to 1871, as she detailed her experiences in the Paris Hospital clinics, both before and after she was admitted as the first woman student by the Faculté de Médecine. Her accounts of the Paris clinics come from her letters to her family and through regular reports on Paris medicine she made for the New York journal *Medical Record*.[2]

I have called my paper 'la visite' partly because that is the proper

French term for what we would call clinical rounds. It is also a term which Putnam used. The title indirectly refers to the manner in which Putnam gained acceptance in the Paris clinics and the Faculté through a sequence of social visits to influential people in order to obtain patronage and political support. This round of visits was a requirement of the French system, in academic science as well as medicine.

Her description of French clinical medicine in both her correspondence and in published review articles, present a sequence of six hospitals and the service of more than one physician within these hospitals. She described clinical lectures, anatomical and scientific laboratories, and both informal and competitive examinations. Her anonymous contributions of Paris medical news for the *Medical Record* were signed PCM, her initials backward. They covered clinical lectures and medical debates between 1867 and 1870. In most cases, she followed the style and content of the Paris hospital gazettes. Although at first sight she appears to have made rather eclectic choices of clinics and debates, these choices often reflected her personal experiences in those clinics.

Mary Putnam's life is very well known so let me give only the briefest of backgrounds.[3] She was born in 1842 in England to a New York family which became distinguished for its famous publishing house, (G. P. Putnam and Sons). George Putnam, her father, published both books and *Putnam's Magazine*. She obtained degrees in pharmacy in the United States from the New York College of Pharmacy in 1863 (when she was 21) and in medicine from the Women's Medical College of Pennsylvania the following year. Only limited hospital experience was available to her as a woman in Philadelphia. Her attempt to expand that experience at the New England Hospital for Women and Children proved to be limited and frustrating.

At the urging of Doctor Elizabeth Blackwell, who thought she should follow in her own footsteps, she went to Paris in 1866. Dr Blackwell had studied in a Paris hospital as *sage-femme* or midwife at La Maternité, not as a doctor, although she had a medical degree. In contrast Putnam reacted against the 'old-fashioned' style of medicine as practised in that hospital. She had become enamoured of the growing 'scientific medicine' of the mid-century.[4] With the help of French physicians who knew and respected Dr Blackwell, she was allowed to attend hospital clinics partly as one of the courtesies routinely granted to foreign physicians. Eventually, she was admitted as the first woman attending the Paris Faculty of Medicine. Soon after she received permission, at the end of 1867, three other women enrolled early in 1868, among them the English woman doctor Elizabeth Garrett (later Anderson) who also was a protegée of Elizabeth Blackwell.

The admission of women to the Paris School was not as simple as it has been portrayed by either the French or the Americans. The French have tended to describe it from the point of view of the Dean of the Medical School, Adolphe Wurtz, the Minister of Public Instruction, Victor Duruy, or the first French woman to enter the school, Madeleine Brès, while the Americans have emphasized Putnam's admission.

In re-reading Putnam's weekly account I have become convinced that she had proven herself in a series of visits – both social and clinical. She showed that she had the capacity and grace to give a good account of herself in both the hospital ward and the salon. Had she not been one of the best young physicians in the clinical hospitals, one wonders whether permission to let women enter the Paris Medical School would have been given at this time.

One of the on-going debates in the hospital gazettes was the admission of women to medical education. Harry Mark has used the hospital gazettes to good effect in his discussion of this debate, showing the various political aspects and orientation of different journals.[5] Given the acrimonious nature of this debate, it might seem surprising that a woman physician was allowed to attend the clinical rounds. Nevertheless, Putnam entered debates over diagnosis and therapeutics along with the *externes* and *internes* of the hospitals, although she was not allowed in the formal lectures or the laboratory courses. One explanation is that permission to follow the clinics was a privilege routinely extended to foreign physicians with the consent of the physician who was chief of service. No permission from the medical faculty was required.

Putnam began to summarize the medical scene from her own point of view for the *Medical Record.* Her reports were rather closely modelled on discussions in the French hospital gazettes. She detailed both surgical and medical controverises, including arguments about therapeutics. Her reports highlighted the real specialty of the Paris clinic – the diagnostic puzzle. Even her humour echoed that of the hospital gazettes.[6]

In one of her medical record reports, she emphasized the features of the French system which she preferred: the well organized clinical rounds *(la visite)*, which offered opportunities for students to present their own observations. She also enjoyed the public debates which ranged from specialized scientific societies to the Académie de

Médecine. She singled out the advantages of competitive hospital placements for medical students as *externes* and *internes*, contrasting this system with the American one, in which students had to rely on the goodwill of a sponsoring physician.[7]

Writing to her parents, she described some of the social factors that opened doors for her in the clinics. Elizabeth Blackwell, then briefly in Paris staying with her sister Anna, was instrumental in obtaining introductions for her to major medical figures with whom Blackwell had close ties. Dr Benjamin Ball and (later) Ulysse Trélat, whose wife held a socially important salon, opened the clinical doors for her. Trélat, head of the famous hospital for women's nervous diseases and geriatrics, the Salpêtrière, was a distinguished physician in the Faculté de Médecine and had been a Republican deputy during the short-lived Second Republic.[8]

By 16 November, 1866, soon after Mary Putnam arrived, Dr Ball obtained permission for her to follow the hospital clinics. She entered the service of the Lariboisière, a general hospital, and the Salpêtrière which specialized in chronically insane women and poor elderly women. She also expected to attend the lectures offered by the Muséum d'Histoire Naturelle (which gave no degrees) and the Collège de France.

The choice of those two hospitals was made in part because of their large size, but in part because they were sufficiently remote from the medical school so that few entering medical students visited them. At Lariboisière there were about 20 *internes*. The chief of service was Hérard, who was, as she put it, '*agréable*'. '(He) keeps me by his side so that I can see everything most distinctly and takes pains to explain matters to me as he goes along.'[9]

By the end of February Putnam was spending four or five hours a day in the hospital clinics, finding, as she put it, that 'for the first time since I began my studies, I find myself in a field sufficiently large to be actively stimulating'.[10] She had by then added Beaujon to her list of hospitals. She visited there from 5 until 6.30 p.m., then dined, paid a social call, wrote up her cases, and arose again at 5.30 a.m. to walk across Paris to Lariboisière.[11]

At Salpêtrière, Putnam was on the service of Dr Moreau who had about ten years earlier made a stir with his theories about hereditary insanity. (He was the first to associate genius with epilepsy and insanity.) She wrote to the *Medical Record* about Moreau's theories in connection with B. A. Morel's theories of degeneration.[12] Moreau also brought her back home a few times in his carriage. This must have been a great relief, since she had to get across Paris very early in the morning to the other hospital (Lariboisière) in order to be in time for the 'visite' which began at 8 a.m. Her intention was to spend six months at these two hospitals and then move to other clinics.

Her reports to the *Medical Record* gave first-hand accounts of the clinics at Lariboisière (and later Gosselin's clinic at the Charité), but not of Salpêtrière, although she confided to her mother that the insane patients at the latter hospital had begun to fascinate her. Echoing an anti-clerical attitude which Charcot and other French psychiatrists would later emphasize, she declared to her mother that any tendency to believe in spiritualism would be swept away by the study of insane delusions and hallucinations.[13]

She moved from Moreau's service to one for hysterical patients in the Salpêtrière after three months. She described the chief of service as a 'very talkative old gentlemen, [probably Ulysse Trélat] which is an advantage to listening students', and expressed hope soon to add another hospital to her list.[14]

Describing differences in attitude between the English and French concerning the admission of women as medical students, Putnam commented that the Englishman would say it was indelicate, but the Frenchman would say that it was dangerous. She observed that the French social system was constructed on the principle that it was necessary to keep young men and women apart as much as 'flame and gunpowder'. Her decision to study in Paris was partly influenced by her belief that she was not 'dangerous', that Frenchmen would instantly see she was not, and that once this first difficulty was overcome, she would be accepted. For the most part, this proved to be true. She found that she was well received in the clinics on a very 'agreeable footing'. As she put it, 'I receive a certain special treatment composed of the frankness with which a physician generally treats his students, the deference and politeness due to a woman and the consideration accorded to a rather small person in a very large place where she has to encounter many difficulties. I find this composite reception exceedingly charming.'[15]

Only a week later, however, she encountered some surprises. One old professor of anatomy declined to have her in his class on the grounds that her figure was too good and would distract her fellow students! Her next anatomy professor kept commenting on her appearance until she had to suggest he paid too much attention to her rather than to the other students.[16]

By 16 April, 1867, still some time before her admission to the school of medicine, she reported she was attending three different clinics (in three different hospitals), two sets of clinical lectures given in an amphitheatre, and one anatomical class. Dr Hérard at Lariboisière had offered to introduce her to a fourth clinic – for diseases of the larynx.[17]

One of these three clincs was a surgical clinic at Beaujon Hospital in which she had the opportunity to hear a formal surgical lecture in an amphitheatre containing a hundred students. For the first time, she heard a lecture by a professor of the Faculté de Médecine. She was equally impressed by the behaviour of the students and the brilliance of the lecture. She did not identify him, but M. Jarjarvay may have been the lecturer since she later described his surgical lecture, pleased that he would bow to her, although he had initially ignored her.[18]

Putnam explained to her mother that medical clinics in France were practical classes on diagnosis. In Lariboisière the examination of the patients took place during the rounds (or *visite*) by either a student or the chief of service. Each student was asked to express an opinion in turn. In Beaujon Hospital, under the direction of Montard, the students examined the patients before the *visite* and reported on the cases. She had the privilege of attending the patients in the afternoon before anyone else, thus having the leisure to examine them and prepare a report on all the patients (sometimes 10 or 12) while the other students prepared only the cases they expected to report upon. She was pleased to note that Montard always called on her once or twice.[19]

Although it seemed to her mother that she had taken on a punishing schedule, Putnam denied this and said she was enjoying herself. It was not like being chained to a desk or reading in a library, she added. She calculated she spent from three to five hours a day in the hospitals, two or three hours a day in lectures, with three or four hours left for reading and visiting. But all this, she explained, was punctuated by walking and talking so that she did not feel tired. In addition, she found the hospital clinics both stimulating and, she warned her mother not be shocked, amusing.[20]

Putnam was not content simply to follow the clinical rounds. She went to the post-mortem room to determine the results of an autopsy performed on a woman whose case she had been following. In order to find the *interne* involved, she had to approach the porter's lodge in front of the residents' (*internes*) quarters, the *salle de garde*. M Jarjarvay's *interne*, with whom she attended Hérard's service, hunted up his fellow *interne*. She recognized the need for a young woman to be discreet. She could not be seen entering the *salle de garde* with the young doctor.[21] On a previous occcasion at Beaujon, she also had to 'exercise discretion on behalf of this same individual'. Was this the man to whom she would later briefly become engaged? She remarked of this (un-named) *interne,* that he was 'by far the most interesting of all'. Her parents may have suspected that her interest was becoming too personal, since she subsequently had to assure them that she had no intention of marrying anyone, especially not a Frenchman. 'The French devote their gallantry in one direction, fall in love in another, and marry in still a third.'[22]

Mary Putnam began to rate herself in comparison with the *internes* and *externes* in the hospitals. Although she said she did not think herself 'especially brilliant' and had made mistakes 'over which I gnash my teeth in secret', she felt that she 'exhibit(ed) no less facility' than the *internes* 'and I am sure that I have more than many of the *externes*'. She did add parenthetically that they, presumably, had more formal knowledge since they had not only finished their medical education but had won their places through competition. 'I made a careful comparison of my mistakes with theirs (*internes* and *externes* together), and the strictest impartiality would decide, I think, that there is no difference either in their quality or quantity. From the manner in which the physicians talk to me I have reason to infer that they place me on a level with their good students.'[23] One of the doctors (Chereau) had even lent her his first-rate microscope, and stayed three hours showing her how to use it, adding that some day she would be a distinguished professor.[24]

In her auscultation class in a clinic at Lariboisière she announced in triumph she was right three times in her diagnosis and everyone else wrong, although she had since made a few minor errors. She told with some amusement of a running argument that she and an *interne* at Beaujon conducted about whether a certain condition was gastric or typhoid fever but the *interne* always opted for typhoid fever. 'I will confide to you the fact that so far I have been nearly invariably in the right. He diagnosed a case of mumps the other day as a commencing typhoid!'[25]

Dr Hérard, whose service she had been following at Lariboisière, had just begun a series of clinical lectures. A *médecin des hôpitaux* for a long time, he had just become a clinician, which gave him an opportunity to lecture. '[T]hough I am beginning to feel the limit of his intellect, [he] is a most charming man', she added with her customary frankness. He kindly bowed to her in a very genial manner and made certain she was able to see when, for example, there was a very interesting case of leprosy.[26]

Among the most interesting professors she had met were

'Ranvier and Cornil at the microscopic laboratory where I work a couple of hours a day. Ranvier is a man who appears about 45 though he is in fact much younger; is an intense enthusiast for his science (microscopy), at the same time is constantly bubbling over with a certain airy light-hearted gaiety peculiarly French.'[27] Ranvier obtained for her the privilege of using the great library of the Ecole de Médecine, where she read privately in the office of the Librarian-in-chief.

Putnam's opinion of the English she encountered was not so favourable: the young women were escorted in families, 'conventional as a pack of sheep'. The young Englishman in her anatomical class was 'intensely insipid'. Although he was a 'good innocent youth but so daisy-like, sandy, and English'. She fantasized that he would return home to his family, which would include four well-educated sisters. He would tell them as he sat around his father's substantial mahogany table: 'Oh by the way there was a woman in our class – yes there was 'pon my honour and by Jove she always answered just as well as us fellows.' She imagined the sisters responding that 'they were sure they could never do such a thing' and the mama observing sternly, 'I should think not my dears, highly improper, highly improper'. She had imagined this scene so often that she could even tell the difference in the colour of the English curtains and the difference between the noses of the sisters and their identical receding chins. She added, with a bit of wicked humour, that it would be hard not to know ten times as much anatomy as the youth in question.[28]

She also attended the clinics of the cardiologist and neurologist Bouillaud, who had done some excellent work on cardiac diseases. (He is still remembered for his study of heart complications in diabetes.) Putnam described him as a very distinguished man whose ideas were 'now entirely out of date'. Although he still tried to promote his ideas, 'his clinics are almost deserted'.[29] The reason for his loss of popularity may be that he was also a phrenologist. He had been Paul Broca's teacher and had urged the search for localization of function in the central nervous system among his students. He had defended Broca's analysis of the speech area before the Académie de Médecine in 1864–5 as a proof of phrenology. The emptiness of his clinics indicates how much phrenology had become a pseudo-science following the attack by the secretary of the Académie des Sciences, Pierre Flourens.

Bouillaud's political views may also have made him *persona non grata* during the Second Empire. He was called the 'red dean', having been dean of the medical school during the short-lived

Second Republic.[30] Putnam commented that Bouillaud was a 'heroic old fellow.... He has been *très gentil* to me and I have fancied has an odd sort of fellow feeling for me as if I too were fighting in an unpopular cause and deserved encouragement.'[31]

With Bouillaud's interest in brain localization, it is not surprising that Putnam while on this service, should report on additional clinical support for Broca's speech area to the New York *Medical Record*. She described a case of a cyst of the brain in Broca's speech area which produced temporary aphasia, with the reappearance of speech once the cyst broke.[32]

After Putnam had begun to feel that her attempt at admission had reached a dead end, the social route became significant again. Soon after meeting Madame and Dr Ulysse Trélat in 24 October, 1867, at a reception for Elizabeth Blackwell given by her sister Anna then living in Paris, she began to move closer to her goal of entering the Ecole de Médecine. She had even begun to write a thesis as a way of gaining admission. The second form of *'visite'* was invoked to obtain patronage for her. She was introduced to socially important women who could make calls with her upon the wives of influential men.

One of the most important women proved to be Mme Garnier, the widow of a member of the Institute, who had been a professor of metaphysics at the Sorbonne. She described her patroness as looking like 'the Marquise in Muller's painting, *Appeal in the Terror*, only 15 years younger'. Putnam began to 'dine out' in the Parisian manner, at Mme Garnier's urgency, in order to meet important members of the ministry and the faculty. One of those she met through Mme Garnier was M. Danton, secretary to the Minister of Public Instruction, Victor Duruy.

Clearly, her growing skill in the French language (and undoubtedly her charm and social skills) made the French bureaucrats and their wives very sympathetic. She placed a secondary request with M. Danton, asking the Minister to grant permission to her to attend the histology course given by Charles Robin at the École Pratique des Hautes Études. Since this was the only formal course she planned to take in the first year, even if she was not admitted to the Ecole, she would still have accomplished part of her educational goals.

Mme Garnier, well over 50, climbed five flights of stairs to Putnam's little room to urge her to come to a dinner she had arranged to introduce her to the Dean of the Faculty of Letters. More importantly, the Secretary of the Minister of Public Instruction was also at the dinner. He told her, (in this informal setting), that he had obtained permission for her to attend Charles Robin's course in histology. He also thought that nothing would be simpler than to admit her to the Ecole de Médecine since the move had the support of the Minister, Victor Duruy. Putnam did not know it, but both Dean Wurtz and Duruy were anxious to forestall a move by the Empress Eugénie to open a women's medical school for medical missionaries, linking training for women physicians with religious proselytizing.[33] He added that he had at first refused Putnam's request in 1866 but since then he had observed her in some of the courses and clinics. As she explained this sudden reversal, the Minister of Public Instruction (Victor Duruy) had been looking for an opportunity to express his opinion in favour of women physicians.

Putnam was told to enrol as a foreign physician with a certificate of citizenship from the American ambassador. Her American medical diploma would be converted to a Bachelor of Science. On payment of a fee, amounting to about 500 francs, preliminary examinations would be waived, while the later examinations would require an additional 300 dollars. She was flattered at the thought of being the first woman to be admitted to the Paris school for a medical degree or to any large metropolitan school in the world. (In England, Elizabeth Garrett's degree was not from a school but from Apothecaries' Hall.)

Putnam believed it was important for women that an American degree from the Women's Medical College of Pennsylvania should be recognized by a great medical school. She added, modestly, that her admission was not due to any special merit unless one counted 'attending hospital clinics faithfully at 8 or 8.30 for a year and not flirting with the students'. She also realized that she had to pass every public examination in a satisfactory manner. Her rejoicing over her admission was premature.

The decision to let her apply for entrance dragged on, while she began to attend the Ecole Pratique, which included laboratories of histology and anthropology. She was very nearly disappointed since in spite of her assurances from the Faculty Secretary when her admission was put to a vote, she was rejected. Later she dedicated her thesis: 'To the one member of the faculty whose name I do not know who voted in favour of my admission.' Since this had not been voted upon by the whole medical faculty some of her French teachers thought this dedication unfair and she took it off the later copies.[34]

Although not yet in the Medical School, she had been admitted to one of the great surgical clinics at the Charité, 'one of the official clinics held by a professor of the Faculty' headed by Gosselin. This clinic had a direct link to the Medical School. She found it very crowded, but since she knew the *interne*, the other students made way for her, giving her a place near the professor. She had been introduced to him by Bouillaud in whose service she had been for some time. She described Gosselin's clinic for the *Medical Record,* emphasizing the punctual manner in which he organized his clinics, his insistence on careful observation, as well as careful attendance on patients by his *externes*, and again extolled his clinic as far superior to the teaching in the New York hospitals. She emphasized the benefit of specific amounts of time set aside for the *externes* and *internes* in the clinic. Gosselin started his clinic at eight or nine in the morning, continuing it for three hours, which allowed him to drill his students on procedure or to criticize them if they had used an inappropriate wound dressing.[35]

Attending a reception held by an important (non-medical) Frenchman, Putnam groaned at how stupid and how limiting it was for all the women to sit together and the men to talk apart. The evening wore on, 'as heavy as butterflies made of cast iron'. In contrast she described the excitement of her interaction with medical men in the clinics and laboratories: 'The hours at Sappey's or Cornil's laboratory, the ten minutes conversation with this bright-eyed student in Gosselin's ward, impetuous with his hot Meridional blood or that *externe* of Bouillaud with large slow head and patient character of Normandy – although connected with disease, suffering and death and often frightful ugliness – are sparkling and brilliant; everyone is alert, bright, often witty, always keen.'[36]

By January 1868, Putnam was finally allowed to follow all the courses offered by the Faculty of Medicine, but she still had to be admitted officially to take the preliminary examinations. There was some fear, which did not materialize, that the examinations would have to be given by the Faculty in Montpellier. When she was finally ready to take the examinations in the March of 1868, she wrote, as she had been instructed, to the Secretary of the Minister that she wanted to apply for the examination. The examination could be arranged either through the agreement of the faculty, or, if it seemed necessary, solely on the minister's authority. Duruy's secretary, Danton, then sent word to the Dean of the Faculty, the chemist Adolphe Wurtz, who had expressed support for women's acceptance. He replied that she had only to send word to the Minister directly that she was prepared and then to send word back to him (Wurtz).

Putnam waited an additional six weeks preparing for the examination. Again she passed through a very complex procedure, going first to M. Danton, Secretary to the Minister, explaining she was ready to receive her authorization. She then paid a healthy fee for the process, since she was skipping the literary and the first four examinations required for the ordinary student without a foreign bachelor's degree. She returned the next Friday and was told by a sub-official that they were looking for a precedent to authorize the exams. (There had been one precedent, a Mme Boivin, who had taken the examinations privately but was never considered a pupil at the Ecole de Médecine).

She then went to the vice-rector as she had been instructed, and there met the Secretary of the Faculté de Médecine who said he had the authorization and wondered what had become of her. He walked publicly with her in the Luxembourg Gardens, to the astonishment of the bands of students, she noted. She took advantage of the Secretary's attention to set up her committee for her first examination. She chose Sappey, in whose anatomical lab she had dissected at the École Pratique; Vulpian, 'distinguished and charming', whose course she had followed and whose private pupil she hoped to become and M. Hovel who was reputed to be gentle on examinations and had a good natured face'. She then had the good sense to read Vulpian's writings before the exam and to work in Sappey's lab doing some additional anatomical dissections, although it was June and illegal to dissect in summer.[37]

She had the help of a fellow *externe* who was preparing for the same examination, who explained to her 'precisely the way of working here, (and) found that it was easy enough and easy enough to succeed if this method were followed'. The method required working up sets of organ systems and learning each week every anatomical, physical, physiological and microscopic aspect of that system.

In June she took her first examinations, passing with a *très satisfait.* She and two other young men were examined. They were first required to do anatomical preparations at the École Pratique, locked in a room in order to prepare them. One student was so frightened he ran away before the second part of the exam. She next had to be publicly examined, so that she had to return home in order to dress properly.

She described this examination at length, at which Vulpian presided and which she handled coolly and well. She added that one of her rather dull fellow applicants was passed even though he made horrendous blunders. She was not passing an entrance examination, I should emphasize, but the first examination for the medical degree. She expected to spend two years in study and then to write her thesis. Following a further examination, she would receive her degree as Doctor of Medicine.

She was made to feel afterwards that the Faculty as a whole felt quite provoked by the manner in which her entrance had been forced upon it. Vulpian, whose course she was following, ceased to speak to her, although he later was very supportive to women physicians. Her professor Gosselin, whose clinic she attended at the Charité, confided in her before her exam that he had voted against her in the Faculty because he was very opposed to women practising and was afraid she might settle in Paris. Another formerly friendly physician was the Librarian-in-chief of the École de Médecine, M. Raige-Délorme. He seemed uneasy with her, but she reported she had won him over to her cause after he read a biographical sketch of Elizabeth Blackwell (which had just appeared in French).[38] Putnam Jacobi admitted to him that she did not like entering the École on the insistence of the Minister of Instruction without the approval of the entire faculty, but she added that 'when one can't get in the *grande porte* one has to go up the back stairs.'

Her political visits to important people did not end with her acceptance into the École de Médecine. Mme Garnier, who had helped to engineer this, arranged a dinner on her behalf which would allow her to meet again and to thank M. Danton (Duruy's secretary) and two members of the Institute (Paul Janet and César Franck). Putnam Jacobi had immediately notified the English physician Elizabeth Garrett (later Anderson), who was seeking a prestigious medical degree outside England. Elizabeth Garrett, along with a Russian woman, Goncharev, sister of the writer, and a French woman, Madeleine Brès then entered the École de Médecine. Only the French woman did not have a prior medical degree. Madeleine Brès and Putnam participated fully in the medical school clinics and lectures, but the two other women simply used their admission to take the examinations and write a thesis for their degree.

The French woman, Madeleine Brès, had trained first as a midwife. She had been in correspondence with Dean Wurtz since 1866 about admission to the Ecole de Médecine, but had been told she first would have to obtain the equivalent of a bachelor's degree. Brès was described by Putnam as 'a right smart woman but common in grain, and her husband is a horse jockey.... But she will do very well I think.... I allowed my colleague's rather irrepressible French vanity to have full play so I guess she found me an agreeable personage.'[39]

Mary Putnam met young Paul Réclus, who was just beginning his medical training in one of the clinics. Becoming a close friend of the entire Réclus family, she took the opportunity to move to a vacant room in his brothers' large apartment. Here she got to know not only Elie and Noémie Réclus but the geographer and political activist Elisée Réclus. The Réclus family's gentle anarchism radicalized her. In their company she experienced the Paris siege during the Franco-Prussian War and the Commune which followed.[40]

Her medical studies continued. After her first examination in the medical school, she began to spend her day in a very regular but absorbed and 'secluded' manner (her term). She went to the Childrens Hospital (*Enfants malades*) from eight to eleven in the morning, then library until six in the evening, then dinner and lectures four evenings a week. She also began a very small class in operative surgery given by an (un-named) Polish émigré and which she took with two others, a Greek and a French youth. On 3 June, she took her second examination and received *bien satisfait*. No letters to her mother exist describing this event, since she took the chance to accompany a patient and returned to the US for two months to see her family.[41]

Again Putnam began preparation for a third examination, taking a private course (*cours particulier*). For the first time she attended clinics at Hôtel-Dieu, in a clinic 'whose chief is one of the most distinguished physicians of Paris, a charming man who treats me with the most distinguished politeness. I am almost overwhelmed by his grand air.'[42] She painted a verbal picture of the Hôtel-Dieu as a little city with subterranean passages. 'Little processions of different physicians meet and cross and clash in a romantic and picturesque environment.'[43] Certainly this was one of the great hospitals of the time.

On 27 December, 1869 Putnam passed her third examination with decided success, with a *très satisfait*. She described this examination at some length. Jules Gavarret (who headed one of the science laboratories and who had written on the physics of blood with Gabriel Andral) and Adolphe Wurtz (Dean of the Faculté and a famous chemist) were her examiners. This was an important examination for her because it included the sciences of medical chemistry, physics and natural history. She hoped to teach medical chemistry at the Blackwell sisters' school in New York. Gavarret rather spoiled the effect of her knowledge of heat and electricity by 'leading her on' in the development of her ideas. Wurtz was more than delighted with her extensive knowledge of organic chemistry, especially her knowledge of his writings on little known scientific experiments he had made in association with German physiologists. She was doubly pleased to hear that after she had left the examination room, Dean Wurtz addressed the students. He commended her thorough knowledge and urged the other students to study as thoroughly as she had done.[44]

An American observer writing about this examination for the New York Tribune described the scene. The young men who preceded Putnam in her examination were frightened and tongue-tied in contrast to the cool, collected and well-trained girl. 'One stuttered and stammered so that it was heartbreaking to see. Finally tears coursed down his innocent nose. He could not describe a potato, he could not describe anything. His professors boosted him, and his young friends behind but it was to no avail.' The reporter was delighted to see the pleasure of Putnam's fellow students on her behalf when Wurtz rubbed his hands with delight at her answers and said to a colleague '*Oh très bien, très bien*', awarding her the highest marks. 'And this is the way, oh boys of Philadelphia, that women are treated in the greatest University in the world.'[45]

The same day, Elizabeth Garrett took her fourth examination, with a mark just below Putnam's, '*bien satisfait*'. Elizabeth Garrett stayed for the brief period in Paris with Putnam at the home of the Réclus family, expecting to take her fifth examination the following week. Unlike Putnam Elizabeth Garrett Anderson cannot be considered a product of the Ecole, since she did not attend lectures or clinics in Paris, but did all her work in London hospitals. Putnam observed, 'She will graduate much before me but not being able to study as devotedly as I am, she will possibly not pass so well. I like her extremely: she has all the best traits of the English character – sterling and faithful – not exactly brilliant but highly intelligent.'[46] Garrett came to Paris only for the required examinations but still graduated only a year before her, in March 1870, the first woman to do so.

Just as Putnam was about to take her fourth examination, the medical school was closed because of reaction by the medical students against the decision to free a relative of Napoleon III from jail. The students were so incensed that they rioted in his classroom and the school was subsequently closed for a month. With the school closed, even the hospital lecture system stopped. Putnam experienced the first halt to her studies. She found it impossible to get a card to attend the obstetrical clinics, although she could still work in the hospitals and libraries. This frustration boiled over into uncharacteristic anger at the milieu of time-servers and unscientific people amongst whom she found herself. She wrote that few people 'even in a great centre like this, really work hard and love their work and how many merely use it as a make-shift for money or reputation or a lazy *passe-temps*'.[47] She began to see some of the faults of the French system, expressing her suspicion of rich physicians or, she added, with a touch of that anti-clerical atmosphere she had imbibed, rich priests.

She had to assure her mother that she was not becoming too acclimatized to Paris. Of course, she insisted, she would return to practice and teach in New York. Her open admiration for some of the young men who surrounded her had made her mother suspicious that she had met some attractive young French doctor. She was right. Putnam was soon to make and then break an engagement to an (un-named) French doctor, an *interne* in one of the services she attended.

Putnam had been offered a position in Edinburgh in the medical school which Sophia Jex-Blake had started, but realized that political events might prevent her finishing the degree in time to meet Jex-Blake's deadline. Emily Blackwell had written to assure her of a position in New York at the Women's Medical School of the New York Infirmary. She wrote to her mother at length that she hoped to instil a scientific spirit into women medical students when she returned.[48]

The events of the Franco-Prussian War and the Commune greatly slowed her work on her degree. She was able to finish it only when the school reopened in 21 July, 1871, enabling her to take her last examination, for which she again received high honours. She defended her thesis, written during this terrible time, on fats, fatty acids and fatty degeneracy of the kidney, for which she received a bronze medal. This was, she announced, only the beginning of research she hoped to do on this topic.[49] By May of 1871, she asked her brother, George Haven Putnam, to let Dr Emily Blackwell know that she was already preparing her lectures for the chair of *materia medica* she had been offered a year before.[50]

When Putnam returned to New York, she became a member of the Medical Society of New York by November 1871. She was supported in her application to join by Dr Abraham Jacobi, president of that society. The thrust of his remarks on her admission, German trained as he was, was not to praise the excellence of her clinical experience in Paris, but to praise the medical society which in its wisdom had properly recognized a woman physician.[51] Under his sponsorship she was admitted soon after to the New York Pathological Society, the New York Neurological Society, and eventually to the New York Academy of Medicine.

When she and Abraham Jacobi married, less than two years

later, one wonders to what degree Jacobi, trained, as he was, in the German system, and a promoter of German medicine, appreciated the extensive French clinical training Putnam Jacobi had received.[52] Certainly, some of his friends assumed that she had little hospital experience before her return to New York.

Her first months of teaching in the American medical school produced in her some degree of impatience for her women students so completely untrained in science. She was not willing to teach the routinized and abbreviated course which her predecessor had developed. Instead she had launched a whole new course, with the hope of instilling a scientific spirit in her students. Elizabeth Blackwell urged her to simplify, teaching in the form 'all are accustomed to'. Blackwell added that she must understand that she had become more French than American. 'You really must go to school and relearn your own country.'[53] Although Putnam Jacobi adapted herself to the new situation, she continued to be a very demanding teacher with high standards. This delighted some, and terrified other, women students.[54]

Few young women medical students of the period were willing to imbibe the truly 'scientific spirit' she had dreamed of instilling in them, especially if that included vivisection. In the 1880s Putnam Jacobi chided Elizabeth Blackwell for thinking it was necessary to sell American women physicians on anti-vivisection, since she was practically the only woman physician in America who practised animal experimentation.[55] She was also the only woman physician to publicly defend animal experimentation before the courts with Dr Welch and other male physicians.[56]

Extensive clinical teaching through the hospitals proved to be almost impossible for women students to obtain. Even male students rarely had this kind of opportunity. Opportunities to attend clinics of large public hospitals were shockingly lacking. Young women could obtain clinical experience only at their own women's hospital, often on an out-patient basis only. The lack of scientific and clinical opportunities for women medical students angered Putnam Jacobi who believed the great hospitals belonged 'to the communities which support them'. No one group should claim monopoly over these institutions.[57]

To counteract this lack, Putnam Jacobi tried to strengthen the system of clinical teaching in the New York Infirmary (attached to the New York Women's Medical School), when she returned from Paris. She sought as many visiting privileges as she could obtain. The dispensaries (outpatient clinics) rather than the hospital wards, provided her with a way to expand clinical observation for her students. Some time in the late 1870s she started an outpatient paediatric clinic, a 'dispensary' at Mount Sinai, where both Dr Jacobi and his close friend Dr Ernst Krackowizer were important staff members. This dispensary was incorporated the following year into the regular hospital services, and a woman remained on the staff for the following ten years.[58]

She was innovative in her clinical teaching to both men and women in the Post-Graduate Medical School to which she was appointed clinical lecturer on children's diseases in 1882. Since the school had neither dispensary nor hospital at that time, Putnam Jacobi had her patients 'sent from her large clinic at the Mount Sinai dispensary. These patients could not understand and frequently resented being sent to another clinic for this purpose. The most important cases were brought, (at times forcibly), by the clinical assistant.'[59] Patients were unwilling, one supposes, to pay this kind of *visite*. The clinical system, so well set up in Paris, was impossible for an American woman physician to reproduce with limited resources. Doubtless it was even less pleasant for the patient.

This image of an assistant wrestling a patient reluctantly into a cab to a distant clinic shows us the negative aspect of the clinical method in a situation not conducive to it. A more positive insight into the clinical method comes from Putnam Jacobi's observations in the *New York Medical Journal* in 1887. She began with a quotation from John Stuart Mill 'How much life is required to produce a little poetry.'[60] 'Similarly,' she continues 'I think no one can sift clinical records without feeling inclined to exclaim: what an enormous amount of data are required to justify a few positive conclusions.'[61]

Putnam Jacobi continued to reflect upon the degree to which she had been imbued with the methods and techniques of the Paris clinical school. In her addresses to young women physicians, she advised them to avoid narrow specialization early in their education. In 1883, she urged young women to continue to compete with men for hospital positions within the large public hospitals from which they were excluded in America. 'When at least half the hospital population are women and sometimes a third are children; when female nurses are trained in large and increasing numbers within the hospital wards, it is absurd to allege that for motives of either delicacy or convenience, female physicians must be excluded.'[62] Private practice could never provide the wide understanding of disease or therapeutics offered by hospital clinical experience. Seventeen years later, she reiterated the same theme: 'So long as the public hospitals are not open to women, women remain deprived of the indispensable basis of their entire work.'⁶³ *La visite* was still, in Mary Putnam Jacobi's eyes, the best method of medical training.

Notes

1. Joy Harvey, '"Faithful to its old traditions": Paris Clinical Medicine from the late 1840s to the Third Republic'. Paper presented at conference: Reinterpreting Paris Medicine, Francis Wood Institute for the History of Medicine, College of Physicians, Philadelphia PA 22 February, 1992.
2. Mary Putnam Jacobi, *Life and Letters of Mary Putnam Jacobi*, Ruth Putnam, (ed.), (New York and London: G. P. Putnam's Sons, 1925) (hereafter, *Life and Letters*). Women's Medical Association of New York, *Mary Putnam Jacobi: A Pathfinder in Medicine* (New York and London: G. P. Putnam's Soñs, 1925) (hereafter, *Pathfinder*)
3. For biographical material see: Rhoda Truax, *The Doctors Jacobi* (Boston: Little Brown, 1952); Eugene P. Link 'Abraham and Mary P. Jacobi, Humanitarian Physicians' *J. History Medicine* 4 (1949), 382–92; Roy Lubove 'Mary Corinna Putnam Jacobi' in *Notable American Women* (Cambridge, MA: Harvard University Press, 1971), 2: 263–5. For a reinterpretation of some of her French experiences see Joy Harvey 'Medicine and Politics: Mary Putnam Jacobi and the Paris Commune' in 'Women in Revolution' M. Josephine Diamond editor, *Dialectical Anthropology* 15 (Fall/Winter 1990), 107–17 and another on her marriage with Abraham Jacobi, 'Mary Putnam Jacobi and Abraham Jacobi: Mixing Medicine and Politics' in Helena Pycior and Nancy Slack, (ed.) *Creative Couples* (New Brunswick, NJ: Rutgers University Press, forthcoming).
4. See Regina Morantz' very interesting analysis of the contrasting viewpoints of Blackwell and Putnam Jacobi in Regina Markell Morantz-Sanchez, *Sympathy and Science: Women Physicians in American Science*, (New York: Oxford University Press, 1985).
5. Harry Marks, 'Attitudes of French Physicians towards Women (1840–1900)' M.A. thesis University of Wisconsin, 1972.
6. Mary Putnam Jacobi's reports, 'Letters from Paris to the *Medical Record*' are conveniently collected in *Pathfinder*, 1–170. She signed them PCM (her initials backwards).
7. She also discussed reports of the Académie de Médecine which also routinely appeared in the French hospital gazettes and cited interesting cases and debates from a number of French hospital gazettes.
8. Anna Blackwell living in Paris, wrote a charming biographical piece about her medical sisters for the *English Woman's Journal* 1 (1858): 80–100. On Dr Ball and Elizabeth Blackwell see *Life and Letters*, 3 December, 1866, 104. The Blackwell sisters had introduced Putnam to Mme Laboulaye who in turn introduced her to Mme Garnier, later her strongest patron. See M[ary] P[utnam] to V[ictorine]

H[aven] P[utnam] (her mother) (22 December, 1867) *Life and Letters*, 158–60.

9. Mary Putnam to V[ictorine] H[aven] P[utnam], 13 November, 1866, *Life and Letters*, 102.

10. Mary Putnam to E[dith] G. P[utnam] (sister) 21 February, 1867, *Life and Letters*, 113.

11. Mary Putnam to E[dith] G. P[utnam], 17 March, 1867, 117.

12. *Pathfinder*, 8–9.

13. Mary Putnam to V[ictorine H[aven] P[utnam] 22 December, 1866, *Life and Letters*, 107. Paul Broca also worked some 20 years before at some of the same hospitals that Putnam Jacobi attended, also describing them to his family in regular letters. See Paul Broca, *Correspondance*. 2 vols (Paris: Schmidt, 1886).

14. Mary Putnam to V[ictorine H[aven P[utnam], *Life and Letters*, 109. Ulysse Trélat was a conservative but well respected physician at the Salpêtrière, who later assisted Putnam Jacobi in her attempts to enter the school.

15. M[ary] P[utnam] to V[ictorine] H[aven] P[utnam], 16 April, 1867 *Life and Letters*, 121.

16. M. P./V. H. P. 22 April, 1867, *ibid.*, 127.

17. M. P./V. H. P. 16 April, 1867, *ibid.*, 121.

18. M.P. to E. G. P. (sister), 5 May, 1867, *ibid.*, 130.

19. M.P. to V.H.P. 16 April, 1867, *ibid.*, 121–2.

20. *Ibid.*, 122.

21. M.P. to E. G. P. 5 May, 1867, *Ibid.*, 131 The young physicians were often accused of taking prostitutes into the *salle de garde*. For the medical jokes, erotic drawings and high spirits of the *salle de garde* where the *internes* resided, see a recent history of the *internat* Jacques Fossard, *Histoire polymorphe de l'internat en médecine et chirurgie des hôpitaux et hospices civiles de Paris*. 2 vols 2e édition, Paris 1982.

22. M.P. to V. H. P., 29 May, 1867, *ibid.*, 141.

23. M.P. to V. H. P., 16 April, 1867, *ibid.*, 123.

24. This was Dr Chereau, but she added with her usual frankness that Chereau 'is not himself très distingué ... if Dr Ball ... ever calls me distinguée, I shall believe it.' M.P. to V. H. P., 16 April, 1867, *ibid.*, 123–4.

25. M.P. to V. H. P., 22 April, 1867, *ibid.*, 129

26. M.P. to E. G. P., 5 May, 1867, *ibid.*, 130.

27. M.P. to V. H. P., *ibid.*, 139.

28. M.P. to V. H. P., 29 May, 1867, *ibid.*, 140.

29. M.P. to V. H. P., 22 December, 1867, *ibid.*, 160.

30. Francis Schiller, *Paul Broca. Founder of French Anthropology, Explorer of the Brain* (Berkeley: University of California Press, 1979). Bouillaud figures significantly in Broca's letters to his family in the 1848 period. See Paul Broca, *Correspondance*.

31. M.P. to V. H. P., 22 December, 1867, *Life and Letters*, 159–60.

32. 'Aphasia' 'Letters to the Medical Record', reprinted in *Pathfinder* 2–3; 73–5.
33. Dr Blanche Edwards-Pilliet insisted on this point in a speech. She had obtained the right to compete for the *internat*, equivalent to an American hospital residency. She discussed her battle as well as that of the earlier women doctors, including Mary Putnam in a speech 'Les femmes dans l'art de guérir depuis cinquante ans' before the Paris conference on women's work (*2e Congrès international des Oeuvres et Institutions Féminins* (1900, *C.R. des Travaux...par Mme Pegaud*) (Paris: Imp. Charles Blot, 1902) Vol. 4, 108–10.
34. This dedication is in the copy in the Academy of Medicine in New York. See discussion quoted from *Archives de Médecine* (Paris, July 1871) *Life and Letters*, 290–1.
35. 'Letters to the Medical Record', Paris, 2 January, 1868, *Pathfinder*, 81–92. This discussion of Gosselin dated from just before her entrance into the full-fledged medical education of France which included clinical work, formal lectures at the École de Médecine, some laboratory work at the École Pratique, and lectures at Collège de France, as well as library research. M.P. to V. H. P., 22 December, 1867, *Life and Letters*, 159–60.
36. M.P. to V. H. P., January, 25, 1868, *Life and Letters*, 169.
37. M.P. to V. H. P., 24 June, 1868, *ibid.*, 178–84.
38. Possibly this was a translation of the biographical sketch of both Emily and Elizabeth Blackwell written by Anna Blackwell, see note 8 above.
39. (1 January, 1869) *Life and Letters*, 204.
40. Joy Harvey 'Medicine and Politics: Mary Putnam Jacobi and the Paris Commune'.
41. *Life and Letters*, 215.
42. Unfortunately she does not identify her chief, but it was probably Vulpian, whose private course she had taken.
43. *Ibid.*, 221. Francis Schiller has given a detailed description of the Hôtel-Dieu in his biography of Paul Broca. See Schiller, *Paul Broca*, The new Hôtel Dieu was built in the 1870s.
44. M.P. to V.H.P., 27 December, 1869. *Life and Letters*, 226–9.
45. Paris correspondent to the New York Tribune, as quoted by Ruth Putnam, *Life and Letters*, 230–2.
46. *Ibid.*, 229.
47. 15 April, 1870, *ibid.*, 246.
48. M.P to V.H.P., January, 13, 1870, *ibid.*, 235.
49. Once she was working full time as a medical student her reports on French medicine became far more specifically oriented to her research interest in fatty degeneration of liver and kidneys. She continued to do work on this topic, publishing on 'fatty degeneration of the new born', after she had returned to New York. A nearly complete list of her publications is given at the end of Mary Putnam

Jacobi, *Pathfinder.*

50. M.P. to George H [aven] P[utnam], 7 May, 1871, *Life and Letters.*, 279.

51. Abraham Jacobi, 'Presidential address' New York Medical Society, December 1871.

52. Abraham Jacobi can be considered as a member of that famous group who pushed American medical education in the direction of the research model of the German universities. I discuss the relationship between husband and wife in a forthcoming chapter 'Mary Putnam Jacobi and Abraham Jacobi: Mixing Medicine with Politics' in Pycior and Slack, (eds), *Creative Couples op. cit.*

53. Elizabeth Blackwell to Mary Putnam [Jacobi] 31 December, 1871. *Life and Letters*, 306–8; on 307.

54. 'Mary Putnam Jacobi, Physician, Teacher, Author' in *Pathfinder*, xiii–xxx. See especially recollections by her student Martha Wollstein, xx–xxi.

55. Mary Putnam Jacobi to Elizabeth Blackwell cited in Regina Morantz-Sanchez, *Sympathy and Science.*

56. 'Statement of Mary Putnam Jacobi, of New York', *Vivisection Hearing before the Senate Committee of the District of Columbia 21 February, 1900 on the Bill (S.34) for the further prevention of cruelty to animals in the District of Columbia.* (Washington: Government Printing Office, 1900), 58–61.

57. Mary Putnam Jacobi, 'Address delivered at the commencement of the Women's Medical College of the N.Y. Infirmary', (30 May, 1883) *Pathfinder*, 391–402, 396.

58. Mary Putnam Jacobi, 'Women in Medicine' in Annie Nathan Meyer, (ed.), *Woman's Work in America*, (New York: Holt, 1891). She credits Dr Annie Angell as having first participated in this clinic with her. See 190–1.

59. *Pathfinder*, xxii.

60. The quotation by John Stuart Mill was part of a review of the poems of Alfred de Musset.

61. Mary Putnam Jacobi, 'Indication for Quinine in Pneumonia', *New York Medical Journal* (1887) *Pathfinder*, 419–45.

62. 'Address delivered at the commencement of the Women's Medical College of the N.Y. Infirmary' (30 May, 1883) *Pathfinder*, 391–402, 397.

63. Mary Putnam Jacobi, Address before the Women's Medical Association about 1900' in *Pathfinder*, 494–500.

Index

Index

Printed in the United States
by Baker & Taylor Publisher Services